Essentials of
Nursing Research
Methods, Appraisal, and Utilization

Denise F. Polit, PhD
President
Humanalysis, Inc.
Saratoga Springs, NY

Bernadette P. Hungler, BSN, PhD
Associate Professor
School of Nursing
Boston College
Chestnut Hill, MA

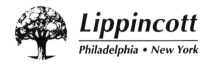

Lippincott
Philadelphia • New York

Fourth Edition

Essentials of Nursing Research

Methods, Appraisals, and Utilization

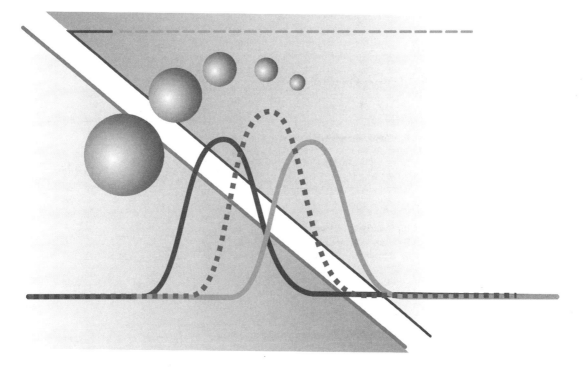

Acquisitions Editor: Margaret Zuccarini
Assistant Editor: Emily Cotlier
Project Editor: Susan Deitch
Production Manager: Helen Ewan
Production Coordinator: Kathryn Rule
Design Coordinator: Kathy Kelley-Luedtke

Fourth Edition

Library of Congress Cataloging-in-Publication Data
Polit-O'Hara, Denise
   Essentials of nursing research: methods, appraisal and utilization/Denise F. Polit, Bernadette P. Hungler.—4th ed.
      p.   cm.
   Includes bibliographical references and index.
   ISBN 0-397-55368-4 (alk. paper)
   1. Nursing—Research.   I. Hungler, Bernadette P.   II. Title.
RT81.5.P63   1996
610.73′072—dc20   96-28545
                                                                                                         CIP

Care has been taken to confirm the accuracy of the information presented and to describe generally accepted practices. However, the authors, editors, and publisher are not responsible for errors or omissions or for any consequences from application of the information in this book and make no warranty, express or implied, with respect to the contents of the publication.

The authors, editors and publisher have exerted every effort to ensure that drug selection and dosage set forth in this text are in accordance with current recommendations and practice at the time of publication. However, in view of ongoing research, changes in government regulations, and the constant flow of information relating to drug therapy and drug reactions, the reader is urged to check the package insert for each drug for any change in indications and dosage and for added warnings and precautions. This is particularly important when the recommended agent is a new or infrequently employed drug.

Some drugs and medical devices presented in this publication have Food and Drug Administration (FDA) clearance for limited use in restricted research settings. It is the responsibility of the health care provider to ascertain the FDA status of each drug or device planned for use in their clinical practice.

9   8   7   6   5   4   3   2   1

To Joanne—and to our past and future friendship

Preface

The nursing profession is increasingly involved in the development of a scientific body of knowledge relating to its practice. Not all nurses will engage in research projects of their own, but there is a growing expectation that **all** nurses will be able to read, understand, and critically appraise research reports. Additionally, the past decade or so has given rise to the expectation that nurses—especially those in clinical practice—will utilize the results of scientific studies as a basis for making decisions in their work. A major purpose of this fourth edition of *Essentials of Nursing Research: Methods, Appraisal, and Utilization* is to assist consumers of nursing research in evaluating the adequacy of research findings in terms of their scientific merit and potential for utilization.

This outstanding AJN Book of the Year Award-winning text has been widely hailed for its clear, concise, and "user-friendly" presentation. Written in a style designed to be nonintimidating, this textbook offers a clearly written, thorough, and accurate presentation of critical research concepts, without including any detailed information on the "how-to's" of conducting research.

New to This Edition

- **Balanced presentation of both qualitative and quantitative research.** For the first time, equal attention is given to both research approaches. Chapters consistently compare and contrast qualitative and quantitative studies with regard to each aspect of a study—from the posing of a question to the analysis and interpretation of research information. Given the growth of qualitative studies among nurse researchers, this treatment represents an important innovation that is unprecedented in nursing research textbooks.
- **A new chapter entitled "Qualitative Research Design and Approaches."** This chapter discusses major approaches to qualitative inquiry, the integration of qualitative and quantitative approaches, and examples of ethnographic, phenomenologic and grounded theory research.

• **Inclusion of two actual research studies.** Two complete research studies are presented for reading, analysis, and critiquing at the end of the textbook: one is qualitative and one is quantitative.

Organization of the Text

The content of this edition is organized into six main parts.

• **Part I—Overview of Nursing Research** serves as the overall introduction to fundamental concepts in nursing research. Chapter 1 introduces and summarizes the history and future of nursing research, discusses the philosophical underpinnings of qualitative research versus quantitative research, and describes the major purposes of nursing research. Chapter 2 presents an overview of the steps in the research process for both qualitative and quantitative studies and defines some key research terms. The chapter also describes research reports—what they are and how to read them.

• **Part II—Preliminary Steps in the Research Process** includes three chapters and focuses on the steps that are taken in getting started on a research project. Chapter 3 focuses on the development of research questions and the formulation of research hypotheses. Chapter 4 discusses two types of contexts for research studies—literature reviews and theoretical/conceptual frameworks. Chapter 5 is devoted to a discussion of ethics in research studies.

• **Part III—Designs for Nursing Research** presents material relating to the design of qualitative and quantitative nursing research studies. Chapter 6 describes some fundamental principles of research design and presents many specific aspects of quantitative research design. Chapter 7 discusses the various research traditions that have contributed to the growth of naturalistic inquiry and qualitative research. Chapter 8 presents various strategies for selecting samples of study participants.

• **Part IV—Collection of Research Data** deals with the collection of research data. Chapter 9 discusses the full range of data collection options available to researchers, including both qualitative and quantitative approaches. The chapter focuses primarily on self-reports, observational techniques, and biophysiologic measures, but other techniques are also mentioned. Chapter 10 discusses methods of assessing data quality.

• **Part V—Analysis of Research Data** is devoted to the organization and analysis of research data. Chapter 11 reviews methods of quantitative analysis. The chapter assumes no prior instruction in statistics and focuses primarily on helping readers to understand why statistics are needed, what tests might be appropriate in a given research situation, and what statistical information in a research report means. Chapter 12 presents a discussion of qualitative analysis, greatly expanded in this edition.

- **Part VI—Critical Appraisal and Utilization of Nursing Research** is intended to sharpen the critical awareness of consumers with respect to several key issues. Chapter 13 discusses the interpretation and appraisal of research reports. Chapter 14, the final chapter, is a guide to utilization for clinical practitioners.

Key Features

Many of the features successfully used in previous editions to assist consumers have been retained.

- **Assistance to Consumers of Nursing Research: What to Expect in the Research Literature:** Each chapter contains a section that includes numerous tips on what to expect in research reports vis-a-vis the topics that have been discussed in the chapter. In these sections, we have paid special attention to helping students *read* research reports, which are often daunting to those without specialized research training. These sections will enable students to translate the material presented in the textbook into meaningful concepts as they approach the research literature.
- **Guidelines for Critiquing Research Reports:** Each chapter has a section devoted to guidelines for conducting a critique. These sections provide a list of questions that walk the consumer through a study, drawing attention to aspects of the study that are amenable to appraisal by research consumers.
- **Research Examples:** Each chapter concludes with one or two actual research examples designed to sharpen the readers' critical skills. In most chapters, there is an example of both a quantitative and a qualitative study. Students are asked to evaluate features of these studies according to the chapter's critiquing guidelines. In addition, many real or fictitious research examples are used to illustrate key points in the text. The use of relevant examples is crucial to the development of both an understanding of and an interest in the research process. We also hope that the inclusion of many research ideas will stimulate an interest in further reading or pursuit of a utilization project of one's own.

Features for Student Learning

To enhance and reinforce learning, several features are used to help focus the student's attention on specific areas of text content:

- **Chapter Objectives:** Learning objectives are identified on the chapter opener to focus the reader's attention on critical content.
- **New Terms:** Each chapter begins with a list of new terms that are defined in context when used for the first time.

- **Tables:** Each chapter contains numerous tables that provide examples to support the text discussion or provide a comparison of selected research.
- **Chapter Summaries:** A detailed, yet succinct, summary that incorporates new terms and provides focus on salient chapter content is included in each chapter.
- **Suggested Readings:** Two lists of suggested readings, methodologic and substantive resources, are provided in each chapter to direct the student's further inquiry.

Teaching-Learning Package

Essentials of Nursing Research: Methods, Appraisal, and Utilization fourth edition, has an ancillary package designed with both the student and the instructor in mind.

- **The Study Guide** augments the text and provides the student with application exercises that correspond to each text chapter. This supports the learning of fundamental research terms that appear in research journals and provides the opportunity to practice the application of the concepts presented in the text and explore hundreds of research possibilities. This edition, for the first time, provides the answers to the application exercises at the end of the study guide.
- **The Instructor's Manual and Testbank** includes a chapter that corresponds to every chapter in the textbook. Each chapter of the instructor's manual contains the following: Statement of Intent, Comments on the Actual Research Examples in the Textbook, Answers to Selected Study Guide Exercises, and Test Questions and Answers.

It is our hope and expectation that the content, style, and organization of this fourth edition of *Essentials of Nursing Research* will be helpful to those students desiring to become intelligent and thoughtful readers of nursing research studies and to those wishing to improve their clinical performance based on research findings. We also hope that this textbook will help to develop an enthusiasm for the kinds of discoveries and knowledge that research can produce.

Denise F. Polit, PhD
Bernadette P. Hungler, BSN, PhD

Acknowledgments

This fourth edition, like the previous three, depended on the contribution of many individuals. We are deeply appreciative of those who made all four editions possible. In addition to all those who assisted us with the earlier editions, the following individuals deserve special mention.

Many faculty and students who used this text (and our graduate-level text) have made invaluable suggestions for its improvement, and to all of you we are very grateful. In particular, we would like to acknowledge the continuing feedback from the nursing students and nursing faculty at Boston College.

This edition of the book involved many revisions to more specifically address the needs of beginning students and to expand the discussion of qualitative research. We are indebted to the insightful comments of several anonymous reviewers, who contributed to the overall conceptualization of this edition.

We would also like to extend our warmest thanks to those who helped to turn the manuscript into a finished product, including Sara Coulter and Darci Clark. The staff at Lippincott-Raven Publishers has given us ongoing support and understanding. We would like to express our gratitude to many individuals, including Margaret Zuccarini, Emily Cotlier, Susan Deitch, and all the others behind the scenes for their contributions.

Finally, we thank our friends and family, who were patient and supportive throughout this enterprise.

Contents

Overview of Nursing Research

PART I

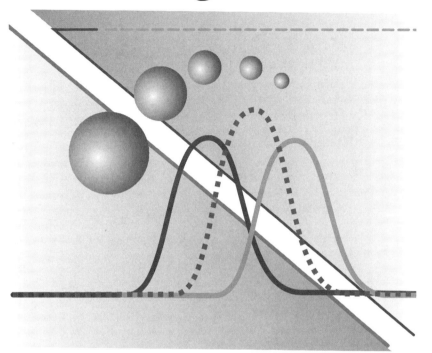

1

Introduction to Nursing Research

Student Objectives

On completion of this chapter, the student will be able to:

- describe ways in which research plays an important role in the nursing profession and discuss why learning about nursing research is important to practicing nurses
- describe general historical trends in the evolution of nursing research
- identify several areas of high priority for nurse researchers
- describe alternative paths to acquiring knowledge
- describe the major characteristics and assumptions of the two alternative paradigms used by nurse researchers
- identify similarities and differences between the traditional scientific method (quantitative research) and the naturalistic method (qualitative research)
- identify several purposes of qualitative and quantitative research
- distinguish basic and applied research
- define new terms in the chapter

New Terms

Applied research
Assumption
Basic research
Biomedical model
Constructivist paradigm
Consumer of nursing research
Control
Deductive reasoning
Determinism
Empirical evidence
Field
Generalizability
Inductive reasoning
Journal club
Logical positivism

National Institute of Nursing
    Research (NINR)
Naturalistic paradigm
Nursing research
Paradigm
Phenomenologic paradigm
Positivist paradigm
Producer of nursing research
Qualitative research
Quantitative research
Reductionist
Scientific approach
Scientific research
Systematic
Theories

Humans are curious and investigative by nature. Curiosity has prompted scientists to search for knowledge, which has, in turn, led to many discoveries that aid us in our daily lives. Nurses are curious about a variety of phenomena and are increasingly engaged in disciplined inquiries that benefit both the profession and its clients.

Nursing research involves a systematic search for knowledge about issues of importance to nurses. Nursing research has experienced remarkable growth in the past three decades, providing nurses with an increasingly sound base of knowledge from which to practice. Yet many health-care questions remain to be answered by nurse researchers—and many answers remain to be used by practicing nurses.

The purpose of this book is to provide you with the skills to read, understand, evaluate, and use nursing research reports. In this introductory chapter, we discuss the important role that research plays in establishing a knowledge base for the practice of nursing, and present an overview of nursing research approaches.

▧ NURSING RESEARCH IN PERSPECTIVE

A consensus has emerged among nursing leaders that nurses at all levels should develop research skills. In this section, we discuss the rationale for this view and present a brief summary of the historical development of nursing research.

The Importance of Research in Nursing

Practitioners in all professions need a base of knowledge from which to practice, and knowledge stemming from systematic research provides a particularly solid foundation. Many nurses are engaging in research to help develop, refine, and extend the base of knowledge fundamental to the practice of nursing. This expansion of knowledge is essential for continued improvement in patient care. Nurses who incorporate high-quality research evidence into their clinical decisions are being professionally accountable to their clients and are also helping nursing to achieve its own professional identity.

Nursing research also contributes to the profession by helping to define the parameters of nursing. Nursing is only one of several professions involved in the delivery of health care. Information from nursing investigations is beneficial in delineating the fairly distinct and unique role that nursing has in the delivery of health care.

The spiraling costs of health care and the cost-containment practices being instituted in health-care facilities represent another reason for nurses to engage in research. Nurses are being asked more than ever to document the social relevancy and the efficacy of their nursing practice to others, such as consumers of nursing care, administrators of health-care facilities, third-party payers, and government agencies. Nurses are increasingly focusing their research endeavors on the effectiveness of nursing interventions and activities for various groups of clients. Some research findings will help eliminate nursing actions that have no effect on the achievement of desired client outcomes. Other findings will help nurses identify the nursing care practices that make a difference in the health-care status of individuals and are cost-effective.

Nursing research is essential if nurses are to understand the varied dimensions of their profession. Research enables nurses to describe the characteristics of a particular nursing situation about which little is known; explain phenomena that must be considered in planning nursing care; predict the probable outcomes of certain nursing decisions made in relation to client care; control the occurrence of undesired client outcomes; and initiate activities designed to promote desired client behavior.

Roles of Nurses in Nursing Research

Nurses and nursing students have assumed a variety of roles in relation to research, forming a continuum that reflects their degree of active participation in the conduct of research. At one end of the continuum are those nurses whose involvement in research is indirect. **Consumers of nursing research** read reports of studies, typically to keep up to date on information that might be relevant to their practice or to develop new skills. Nurses are increasingly expected to maintain, at a minimum, this level of involvement with research.

At the other end of the continuum are the **producers of nursing research:** nurses who actively participate in the design and implementation of research studies. At one time, the majority of nurse researchers were academics who taught in schools of nursing, but research is increasingly being conducted by practicing nurses who want to find what works best for their patients.

Between these two extremes lie a variety of research-related activities in which nurses are engaging as a way of enriching their professional lives, including the following:

- Participation in a **journal club** in a practice setting, which involves regular meetings among nurses to discuss and critique research articles
- Attendance at research presentations at professional conferences
- Formal evaluation of completed research, for its possible utilization in the practice setting
- Discussions with clients about the implications and relevance of research findings
- Assistance in the collection of research information (*e.g.*, distributing questionnaires to patients or observing and recording patients' behaviors)
- Review of proposed methods for gathering research information with respect to their feasibility in a clinical setting
- Collaboration in the development of an idea for a research project
- Participation on an institutional committee whose mission is to review the ethical aspects of proposed research before it is undertaken
- Incorporation of research findings into nursing practice or nursing education

In all these roles, nurses who have some research skills are in a better position to make a contribution to the nursing profession and to the base of nursing knowledge. Because of this, almost all accredited baccalaureate nursing programs include research content as a requirement for nursing students.

At this point, you may have limited interest in learning about nursing research and may continue to wonder why a course in research methods is required. The following are some questions that students raise when beginning a course in nursing research, along with some responses:

I'm never going to do research, so why should I study research methods? First, many students become excited about research once they are exposed to it and go on to do some research of their own, even though they had not planned to do so. More important, however, a knowledge of nursing research can improve the depth and breadth of the professional practice of every nurse, not just those who perform the studies. Learning about research methods allows you to evaluate and synthesize new information (*i.e.,* become an intelligent research consumer) and to engage meaningfully in a number of other roles in relation to nursing research.

I'm studying nursing because I'm interested in people, not in dry facts and numbers, so why would I be interested in a research methods class? Almost all nursing research is about people and is intended to shed light on the mystery and complexity of some aspect of the human experience. Research reports tell us stories about that experience—generally not the stories of specific people, but rather of groups of people who share a common concern, problem, or characteristic. Learning about research methods gives us a key to unraveling the stories in research journals and also gives us skills to determine whether the stories are accurate and relevant.

Why are most research studies so difficult and intimidating to read? Most research studies are not as easy to read as anecdotal reports of patients' or nurses' experiences, in part because researchers have their own jargon—just like practitioners in any other field. This text will help you to learn research jargon and to become accustomed to researchers' styles of presenting research findings. This book will also help you to understand simple statistics. Statistics often seem formidable to students, but statistics simply represent a tool for evaluating the information that a researcher gathers—in much the same way as medical instrumentation provides tools for evaluating the physiologic functioning of patients.

Learning about nursing research methods can be a challenging task—and it can be a highly rewarding one. We hope this text helps you to acquire and appreciate the skills that will enable you to put current nursing information at your disposal for your own personal and professional development, for the improvement of patient care, and for the betterment of the nursing profession.

Historical Evolution and Future Directions of Nursing Research

Although nursing research has not always had the prominence and importance it enjoys today, it, nevertheless, has a long and interesting history. Most people would agree that nursing research began with Florence Nightingale during the Crimean War. For a number of years after Nightingale's work, however, little is found in the nursing literature concerning nursing research. Some have attributed the absence of nursing research during these years to the apprenticeship nature of nursing.

The pattern that nursing research followed subsequent to Nightingale was closely aligned to the problems confronting nurses. For example, most studies conducted between 1900 and 1940 concerned nursing education. As more nurses received university-based education, studies concerning students—their problems, differential characteristics, and satisfactions—became more numerous. And, when the staffing patterns of hospitals changed, fewer students were available to staff the hospitals throughout a 24-hour period. As a consequence, researchers focused their investigations not only on the supply and demand of nurses, but also on the amount of time required to perform certain nursing activities. During these years, nursing struggled with its professional identity, and nursing research took a twist toward studying nurses: who they were, what they did, how other groups perceived them, and what type of person entered the nursing profession.

It was not until the 1950s that a number of forces combined to put nursing research on the rapidly accelerating upswing it is still on today. An increase in the number of nurses with advanced academic preparation, the establishment of the *Nursing Research* journal, the availability of federal funding to support nursing research, and the upgrading of research skills in faculty are only some of the forces that provided impetus to nursing research.

By the 1970s, the growing number of nurses conducting research studies and the increase in discussions of theoretical and contextual issues surrounding nursing research created the need for additional sources of communication. Three additional journals that focus on nursing research—*Advances in Nursing Science, Research in Nursing and Health,* and the *Western Journal of Nursing Research*—were established in the 1970s. During that decade, there was also a change in emphasis in nursing research studies from areas such as teaching, administration, curriculum, recruitment, and nurses themselves to the improvement of client care. This shift, which may be attributed to the growing awareness by nurses of the need for knowledge to improve nursing practice, has persisted to the present time.

The 1980s brought nursing research to a new level of development. An increase in the number of qualified nurse researchers, widespread availability of computers for the collection and analysis of information, greater comfort in conducting research, and an ever-growing recognition that research is an integral part of professional nursing led nursing leaders to raise new issues and concerns. Greater attention was given to the types of questions being asked, the types of research methods that would maximize what could be learned, the protection of the rights of people who participate in studies, and the linking of research to theory. Several events in the 1980s provided impetus for nursing research. Of particular importance was the establishment in 1986 of the National Center for Nursing Research (NCNR) within the National Institutes of Health (NIH). The purpose of NCNR was to promote—and financially support—research training and clinical research focused on patient care. Additionally, the Center for Research for Nursing was created in 1983 by the American Nurses' Association (ANA). The Center's mission is to develop and coordinate a research program to serve as the source of national data for the profession. An important new journal was also established in the late 1980s: *Applied Nursing Research* includes research reports on studies of special relevance to practicing nurses.

After a long crusade by nursing organizations, nursing research was strengthened and given more national visibility in 1993 when NCNR was promoted to full institute status within NIH. The birth of the **National Institute of Nursing Research (NINR)** helps put nursing research more into the mainstream of research activities enjoyed by other health disciplines. Funding for nursing research is also growing. In 1986, the NCNR had a budget of $16.2 million, whereas in fiscal year 1996, the budget for NINR was about $55 million. In addition to the creation of NINR, two more research journals were inaugurated—*Qualitative Health Research* in 1990 and *Clinical Nursing Research* in 1991. Both journals emerged in response to the growth in clinically oriented and in-depth research among nurses.

During the 1990s, some of the research undertaken by nurses is being guided by priorities established by prominent nurse researchers, who were brought together by NCNR for two Conferences on Research Priorities (CORP). The priorities established by CORP #1, for research through 1994, were as follows: low birth weight, human immunodeficiency virus (HIV) infection, long-term care, symptom management, nursing informatics, health promotion, and technology dependence. In 1993, CORP #2 established the following as research emphases for a portion of NINR's funding from 1995 through 1999:

- Developing and testing community-based nursing models
- Assessing the effectiveness of nursing interventions in HIV/ acquired immunodeficiency syndrome (AIDS)
- Developing and testing approaches to remediating cognitive impairment
- Testing interventions for coping with chronic illness
- Identifying biobehavioral factors and testing interventions to promote immunocompetence

The future promises to be challenging and exciting for nurse researchers all over the world. Studies are increasingly likely to be directed toward the practice of nursing than they were in the past. In addition to pursuing new areas of research, there is a growing interest in building a firmer knowledge base by repeating studies, using the procedures used in previous research but with different clients, in different clinical settings, in different cultures, and at different times. There is also an increasing emphasis on developing mechanisms for utilizing the results of nursing research in actual practice, and this emphasis is likely to become stronger in the years ahead.

◩ SOURCES OF KNOWLEDGE

Think for a moment about any fact you have learned relating to the practice of nursing. What is the source of this information? Some of the facts you have learned are derived from research, but some are not. A brief discussion of alternative sources of knowledge for nurses serves as a backdrop for understanding how information from nursing research is different.

- *Tradition.* Within our culture and within the nursing profession, certain beliefs are accepted as truths simply based on custom. Many nursing problems are solved based on tradition and age-old practices. However, tradition may present some obstacles for maximally effective problem solving because traditions often are so entrenched that their validity or usefulness is not challenged or evaluated.
- *Authorities.* An authority is a person with specialized expertise and widespread recognition for that expertise. Reliance on authorities is, to some degree, inevitable because we cannot possibly become experts on every problem with which we are confronted. But, like tradition, authorities as a source of information have limitations. Authorities are not infallible, particularly if their expertise is based primarily on personal experience, yet their knowledge often goes unchallenged.
- *Personal Experience.* We all solve problems based on prior observations and experiences, and this is an important and functional approach. The ability to generalize, to recognize regularities, and to make predictions based on observations is a hallmark of the human mind. Nevertheless, personal experience has two primary limitations as a basis of understanding: first, each person's experience may be too restricted to be of general utility; and, second, personal experiences are often colored by biases.
- *Intuition.* Intuition is a type of knowledge that cannot be firmly explained on the basis of reasoning or prior instruction. Although intuition and hunches undoubtedly play a role in nursing practice—as they do in the conduct of research—it is difficult to develop policies and practices for nurses on the basis of intuition.
- *Trial and Error.* Sometimes we tackle problems by successively trying out alternative solutions. Although this approach may in some cases be practical, it is often fallible and inefficient. The method tends to be haphazard, and the solutions are, in many instances, idiosyncratic.
- *Logical Reasoning.* Reasoning is the mental processing of ideas to solve problems. Two intellectual mechanisms are used in reasoning. **Inductive reasoning** is the process of developing conclusions and generalizations

from specific observations. For example, a nurse may observe the anxious behavior of (specific) hospitalized children and conclude that (in general) children's separation from their parents is very stressful. **Deductive reasoning** is the process of developing specific predictions from general principles. For example, if we assume that separation anxiety does occur in hospitalized children (in general), then we might predict that the (specific) children in Memorial Hospital whose parents do not room-in would manifest symptoms of stress. Both systems of reasoning are useful as a means of understanding and organizing phenomena, and both play a role in research. However, reasoning in and of itself is limited because the validity of reasoning depends on the accuracy of the information (or premises) with which one starts, and reasoning may be an insufficient basis for evaluating accuracy.

- *Disciplined Research.* Research conducted within a disciplined format is the most sophisticated method of acquiring knowledge that humans have developed. Nursing research combines aspects of logical reasoning with other features to create systems of problem solving that, although fallible, tend to be more reliable than tradition, authority, personal experience, intuition, or inductive or deductive reasoning alone.

Nurses throughout the world have come to recognize the need to extend the base of nursing knowledge, and nursing research has become the most widely accepted way to achieve this objective. As we discuss next, disciplined research in nursing is richly diverse with regard to the questions asked and the methods used.

◩ PARADIGMS FOR NURSING RESEARCH

A **paradigm** is a world view, a general perspective on the complexities of the real world. Paradigms for human inquiry are often characterized in terms of the ways in which they respond to basic philosophical questions:

- *Ontologic.* What is the nature of reality?
- *Epistemologic.* What is the relationship between the inquirer and that being studied?
- *Axiologic.* What is the role of values in the inquiry?
- *Methodologic.* How should the inquirer obtain knowledge?

Disciplined inquiry in the field of nursing is being conducted mainly within two broad paradigms, both of which have legitimacy for nursing research.[1] This

---

[1] Other inquiry paradigms exist, such as several that collectively have been labeled *critical theory* or *critical inquiry* (*e.g.,* feminism, neo-Marxism). It is beyond the scope of this book to discuss these other paradigms.

section describes the two alternative paradigms and broadly outlines their associated methodologies.

The Positivist Paradigm

The traditional scientific approach to conducting research has its underpinnings in the philosophical paradigm known as the **positivist paradigm.** Positivism is rooted in 19th-century thought, guided by such philosophers as *Comte, Mill, Newton,* and *Locke.* Although strict positivist thinking (sometimes referred to as **logical positivism**) has been challenged and undermined, a modified positivist position remains a dominant force in scientific research.

The fundamental ontologic assumption of positivists is that there is a reality *out there* that can be studied and known (**assumptions** refer to basic principles that are believed to be true without proof or verification). Adherents of the scientific approach assume that nature is basically ordered and regular and that an objective reality exists independent of human observation. In other words, the world is assumed not to be merely a creation of the human mind. The related assumption of **determinism** refers to the belief that phenomena are not haphazard or random events, but rather have antecedent causes. If a person has a cerebrovascular accident, the scientist assumes that there must be one or more reasons that can be potentially identified and understood. Much of the activity in which a scientific researcher within a positivist paradigm is engaged is directed at understanding the underlying causes of natural phenomena.

Because of their fundamental belief in an objective reality, positivists seek to be as objective as possible in their pursuit of knowledge. Positivists attempt to hold their personal beliefs and biases in check, insofar as possible, during their research to avoid contaminating the phenomena under investigation. The positivists' scientific approach involves the use of orderly, disciplined procedures designed to test the researchers's ideas about the nature of the phenomena being studied and relationships among them. The methods associated with positivism and the scientific approach are discussed in a subsequent section.

The Naturalistic Paradigm

The **naturalistic paradigm** (which is sometimes referred to as the **phenomenologic** or **constructivist paradigm)** began as a countermovement to positivism with writers such as *Weber* and *Kant.* The naturalistic paradigm represents a major alternative system for conducting disciplined inquiry in the field of nursing. Table 1–1 compares the major assumptions of the positivist and naturalistic paradigms.

For the naturalistic inquirer, reality is not a fixed entity but rather is a construction of the individuals participating in the research; reality exists within a context, and many constructions are possible. Naturalists thus take the position of relativism: if there are always multiple interpretations of reality that exist in people's

Table 1–1. Major Assumptions of the Positivist
and Naturalistic Paradigms

Philosophical Question	Positivist Paradigm Assumptions	Naturalistic Paradigm Assumptions
Ontologic (What is the nature of reality?)	Reality exists; there is a real world driven by real natural causes.	Reality is multiple and subjective, mentally constructed by individuals.
Epistemologic (How is the inquirer related to those being researched?)	Inquirer is independent from those being researched; the findings are not influenced by the researcher.	The inquirer interacts with those being researched; findings are the creation of the interactive process.
Axiologic (What is the role of values in the inquiry?)	Values and biases are to be held in check; objectivity is sought.	Subjectivity and values are inevitable and desirable.
Methodologic (How is knowledge obtained?)	Deductive processes	Inductive processes
	Emphasis on discrete, specific concepts	Emphasis on entirety of some phenomenon, holistic
	Verification of researcher's hunches	Emerging interpretations grounded in participants' experiences
	Fixed design	Flexible design
	Tight controls over context	Context-bound
	Emphasis on measured, quantitative information; statistical analysis	Emphasis on narrative information; qualitative analysis
	Seeks generalizations	Seeks patterns

minds, then there is no process by which the ultimate truth or falsity of the constructions can be determined.

Epistemologically, the naturalistic paradigm assumes that knowledge is maximized when the distance between the inquirer and the participants in the study is minimized. The voices and interpretations of those under study are key to understanding the phenomenon of interest, and subjective interactions are the primary way to access them. The findings from a naturalistic inquiry are the product of the interaction between the inquirer and the participants. The methodologies associated with the two paradigms are discussed next.

Paradigms and Methods: Quantitative and Qualitative Research

The two alternative perspectives on the nature of reality have strong implications for the methods of knowledge acquisition. The methodologic distinction that is most often made focuses on differences between **quantitative research,** which is most closely allied with the positivist tradition, and **qualitative research,** which is most often associated with naturalistic inquiry—although positivists sometimes engage in qualitative studies and naturalistic researchers sometimes collect quantitative information. This section provides an overview of the methods associated with the two alternative paradigms. Note that this discussion accentuates the differences in methods as a heuristic device; in reality, there is often greater blurring—and richness—of methods than this introductory discussion implies.

The Scientific Method and Quantitative Research

The traditional **scientific approach** to inquiry refers to a general set of orderly, disciplined procedures used to acquire information. The traditional scientist uses deductive reasoning to generate hunches that are tested in the real world. In **scientific research**—the application of the scientific approach to the study of a question of interest—the researcher moves in an orderly and systematic fashion from the definition of a problem and the selection of concepts on which to focus, through the design of the study and collection of information, to the solution of the problem. By **systematic** we mean that the scientific investigator progresses logically through a series of steps, according to a prespecified plan of action. The researcher uses, to the extent possible, mechanisms designed to control the study. **Control** involves imposing conditions on the research situation so that biases are minimized and precision and validity are maximized.

In addressing research questions, the scientist gathers **empirical evidence**—evidence that is rooted in objective reality and gathered directly or indirectly through the human senses. The requirement to use empirical evidence as the basis for knowledge causes findings of a scientific investigation to be grounded in reality rather than in the personal beliefs or hunches of the researcher. Evidence for a scientific study is gathered according to a specified plan, using formal instruments to collect the needed information. Usually (but not always) the information gathered in a scientific study is quantitative (*i.e.,* numeric information that results from some type of formal measurement and that is analyzed with statistical procedures).

An important goal of a scientific study is to understand phenomena, not in isolated circumstances alone, but in a broad, general sense. The desire to go beyond the specifics of the situation is an important feature of the scientific approach. In fact, the degree to which research findings can be generalized (referred to as the **generalizability** of the research) is a widely used criterion for assessing the quality of a traditional research study.

The scientific approach—sometimes referred to as the **biomedical model**—has enjoyed considerable stature as a method of inquiry, and it has been used productively by nurse researchers studying a wide range of nursing problems. This is not to say, however, that scientific research can solve all nursing problems or that the scientific method has been without criticism. One important limitation is that the scientific method cannot be used to answer moral or ethical questions. Many of our most persistent and intriguing questions about the human experience fall into this area (*e.g.,* Should euthanasia be practiced? Should nurses be unionized?

Should abortion be legal?). Given the many moral issues that are linked to medicine and health care, it is inevitable that the nursing process will never rely exclusively on scientific information.

The scientific approach also must contend with problems of measurement. To study a phenomenon, the scientist attempts to measure it. For example, if the phenomenon of interest was patient morale, a researcher might want to assess if a patient's morale is high or low, or higher under certain conditions than under others. Although there are reasonably accurate measures of physiologic phenomena such as blood pressure, temperature, and cardiac activity, comparably accurate measures of such psychological phenomena as patient morale, pain, or self-image have not been developed.

A final issue is that nursing research tends to focus on human beings, who are inherently complex and diverse. The scientific method typically focuses on a relatively small portion of the human experience (*e.g.,* weight gain, depression, chemical dependency) in a single study. Complexities tend to be controlled and, insofar as possible, eliminated in scientific studies rather than studied directly, and this narrowness of focus can obscure insights.

Naturalistic Methods and Qualitative Research

Naturalistic methods of inquiry attempt to deal with the issue of human complexity by exploring it directly. Researchers in the naturalistic tradition emphasize the inherent complexity of humans, the ability of humans to shape and create their own experiences, and the idea that truth is a composite of realities. Consequently, naturalistic investigations place a heavy emphasis on understanding the human experience as it is lived, generally through the careful collection and analysis of narrative, subjective (*i.e.,* qualitative) materials.

Researchers who reject the traditional scientific approach believe that a major limitation of the classical model is that it is **reductionist** (*i.e.,* it reduces human experience to only the few concepts under investigation, and those concepts are defined in advance by the researcher rather than emerging from the experience of those under study). Naturalistic researchers tend to emphasize the dynamic, holistic, and individual aspects of the human experience and attempt to capture those aspects in their entirety, within the context of those who are experiencing them.

Flexible, evolving procedures are used to capitalize on findings that emerge in the course of the study. Naturalistic inquiry always takes place in the **field** (*i.e.,* in naturalistic settings), often over an extended period of time. The collection of information and its analysis typically progress concurrently in naturalistic research—as the researcher sifts through the existing information, insights are gained, new questions emerge, and further evidence is sought to amplify or confirm the insights. Through an inductive process, the researcher integrates the evidence to develop a theory or framework that helps explain the processes under observation.

Naturalistic studies result in rich, in-depth information that has the potential to elucidate the multiple dimensions of a complicated phenomenon. The findings from in-depth qualitative research are rarely superficial. However, there are several limitations of the approach. Human beings are used directly as the instrument through which information is gathered, and humans are an extremely intelligent and sensitive—but fallible—tool. The subjectivity that enriches the analytic insights in the hands of a skillful researcher can lead to petty and trivial "findings" among less competent inquirers.

A further potential limitation is that the subjective nature of the inquiry may give rise to questions about the idiosyncratic nature of the conclusions. Would two naturalistic researchers studying the same phenomenon in the same setting arrive at the same results? It is difficult to know, and the situation is further complicated by the fact that most naturalistic studies involve a relatively small group of participants. Questions about the generalizability of the findings from naturalistic inquiries can sometimes loom large.

Multiple Paradigms and Nursing Research

Paradigms should be viewed as lenses that help us to sharpen our focus on a phenomenon of interest—not as blinders that limit our intellectual curiosity. The emergence of alternative paradigms for the study of nursing problems is, in our view, a healthy and desirable trend in the pursuit of new knowledge. Although a researcher's world view may be paradigmatic, knowledge itself is not. The knowledge base in nursing would be slim, indeed, if there were not a rich array of approaches and methods available within the two paradigms—methods that are often complementary in their strengths and limitations. We believe that intellectual pluralism should be encouraged and fostered.

Thus far, we have emphasized the differences between the two paradigms and their associated methods so that their distinctions would be easy to understand. Subsequent chapters of this book will further elaborate on differences in jargon, methods, and research products. However, it is equally important to note that the alternative paradigms have many features in common, only some of which will be mentioned here:

- *Ultimate goals.* The ultimate aim of disciplined inquiry, regardless of the underlying paradigm, is to gain understanding about the world in which we live. Both quantitative and qualitative researchers seek to capture the true state of affairs with regard to an aspect of the world in which they are interested, and both groups can make significant—and mutually beneficial—contributions.
- *External evidence.* Although the word *empiricism* has come to be allied with the scientific approach, it is, nevertheless, the case that researchers in both traditions gather and analyze external evidence that is collected through their senses. That is, neither qualitative nor quantitative researchers are armchair analysts, relying exclusively on their own beliefs and views of the world for their conclusions. Information is gathered from others in a deliberate fashion.

- *Reliance on human cooperation.* Because evidence for nursing research comes primarily from human participants, the need for human cooperation is inevitable. To understand people's characteristics and experiences, researchers must persuade them to participate in the investigation *and* to act and speak candidly. In some areas of inquiry, the need for candor and cooperation is a challenging requirement—for researchers in either tradition.
- *Ethical constraints.* Research with human beings is guided by ethical principles that sometimes interfere with the researcher's ultimate goal. For example, if a researcher's aim is to test a potentially beneficial intervention, is it ethical to withhold the treatment from some people to see what happens? As discussed later in the book (Chapter 5), ethical dilemmas often confront researchers, regardless of their paradigmatic orientation.
- *Fallibility of disciplined research.* Although disciplined nursing research in both paradigms is often of high quality, a general caveat holds true: Virtually every research study contains some flaw. Every research question can be addressed in an almost infinite number of ways, and inevitably there are tradeoffs. In most situations, there are financial constraints that lead to less-than-ideal decisions. Even when tremendous resources are expended, there are bound to be some shortcomings. This does not mean that small, simple studies have no value. It means that no single study can ever definitively answer a research question. Each completed study adds to a body of accumulated knowledge. If the same question is posed by several researchers, each of whom obtains the same or similar results, increased confidence can be placed in the answer to the question. It is precisely because of the fallibility of any single study that it is important for you as a consumer of research to understand the tradeoffs and decisions that investigators make and to evaluate the adequacy of those decisions.

In summary, despite important philosophical and methodologic differences, researchers using the traditional scientific approach and more naturalistic methods share some overall goals and are faced with many similar constraints and challenges. In our view, the selection of an appropriate method depends to some degree on the researcher's personal taste and philosophy, but it also depends in large part on the nature of the research question, a topic we discuss at length in the next section. If a researcher asks what the effects of surgery are on circadian rhythms (biologic cycles), the researcher really needs to express the effects through the careful quantitative measurement of various bodily processes subject to rhythmic variation. On the other hand, if a researcher inquires about the process by which parents learn to cope with the death of a child, the researcher may be hard pressed to quantify such a process. Personal world views of the researchers help to shape the types of question they ask.

In reading about the alternative paradigms for nursing research, you likely were more attracted to one of the two paradigms—the paradigm that corresponds most closely to your view of the world and of reality. However, it is important to learn about and respect both approaches to disciplined inquiry, and to recognize their respective strengths and limitations. In this textbook, we attempt to provide a solid overview of the methods associated with both qualitative and quantitative research. We readily admit that more pages are devoted to the traditional scientific approach and quantitative research than to naturalistic methods and qualitative research. Our rationale for this imbalance is threefold:

- The methods associated with scientific research inherently are more deliberate and clearly defined. The fluidity that is the hallmark of naturalistic inquiry means that there are fewer "rules" that have to be understood in order to comprehend a study.
- The language of naturalistic inquiry is more conversational, and thus there is less technical terminology and jargon than in the case of the scientific approach. Qualitative analysis, for example, is inherently easier to understand than statistical analysis.
- The great majority of studies in nursing research continue to be quantitative.

Both qualitative and quantitative approaches have strengths and limitations, which are identified throughout this book. It is precisely because the strengths of one approach complement the limitations of the other that both are essential to the further development of nursing knowledge.

THE PURPOSES OF NURSING RESEARCH

The general purpose of nursing research is to answer questions or solve problems of relevance to the nursing profession. Research purposes in nursing can be further described in several ways.

Specific Aims of Quantitative and Qualitative Research

Various types of questions are addressed by nurse researchers, and certain types are more amenable to qualitative than to quantitative inquiry and vice versa. This section examines some of the specific aims of qualitative and quantitative research in nursing.

Identification

Qualitative researchers often conduct a study to examine phenomena about which little is known. In some cases, so little is known that the phenomenon has yet to be clearly identified or named—or has been inadequately defined or conceptualized. The in-depth, probing nature of qualitative research is well suited to the task of answering such questions as, "What is this phenomenon?" and "What is its name?" (Table 1–2) An example of a qualitative nursing study that involved questions of identification is Cohen's (1995) study of parental uncertainty with regard to chronic, life-threatening illnesses of their children. In her analysis, Cohen identified the concept of *triggers* that heighten parents' awareness of uncertainty and also identified seven types of triggers.

In quantitative research, by contrast, the researcher begins with a phenomenon that has been previously studied or defined—sometimes in a qualitative study. Thus, in quantitative research, identification typically precedes the inquiry.

Table 1–2. Research Purposes and Research Questions

Purpose	Types of Questions: Quantitative Research	Types of Questions: Qualitative Research
Identification		What is this phenomenon? What is its name?
Description	How prevalent is the phenomenon? How often does the phenomenon occur? What are the characteristics of the phenomenon?	What are the dimensions of the phenomenon? What variations exist? What is important about the phenomenon?
Exploration	What factors are related to the phenomenon? What are the antecedents of the phenomenon?	What is the full nature of the phenomenon? What is really going on here? What is the process by which the phenomenon evolves or is experienced?
Explanation	What are the measurable associations between phenomena? What factors caused the phenomenon? Does the theory explain the phenomenon?	How does the phenomenon work? Why does the phenomenon exist? What is the meaning of the phenomenon? How did the phenomenon occur?
Prediction and control	What will happen if we alter a phenomenon or introduce an intervention? If phenomenon X occurs, will phenomenon Y follow? How can we make the phenomenon happen, or alter its nature or prevalence? Can the occurrence of the phenomenon be controlled?	

Description

The main objective of many nursing research studies is the description and elucidation of phenomena relating to the nursing profession. The researcher who conducts a descriptive investigation observes, counts, describes, and classifies. Phenomena that nurse researchers have been interested in describing are varied. They include topics such as stress and coping in patients, pain management, adaptation processes, health beliefs, rehabilitation success, and time patterns of temperature readings.

Description can be a major purpose for both qualitative and quantitative researchers. Quantitative description involves the prevalence, incidence, size, and measurable attributes of a phenomenon. Table 1–2 summarizes some of the descriptive questions posed by quantitative researchers. As an example, Seifert, Frye, Belknap, and Anderson (1995) did a study to determine the characteristics of nurses' medication administration through enteral feeding catheters. These investigators wanted to describe such things as the *percentage* of patients receiving medications through feeding catheters and the *average* number of feeding catheter obstructions.

Qualitative researchers use in-depth methods to describe the dimensions, variations, and importance of phenomena. For example, Dellasega and Mastrian (1995) conducted a qualitative study designed to identify and describe specific stressors experienced by family members during and after making the decision to place an elder in a long-term skilled care facility. In-depth interviews with seven individuals led to a description of the decision-making process.

Exploration

Like descriptive research, exploratory research begins with some phenomenon of interest; but, rather than simply observing and describing the phenomenon, exploratory research is aimed at investigating the full nature of the phenomenon, the manner in which it is manifested, and the other factors with which it is related. For example, a descriptive quantitative study of patients' preoperative stress might seek to document the degree of stress patients experience before surgery and the percentage of patients who actually experience it. An exploratory study might ask the following: What factors are related to a patient's stress level? Is a patient's stress related to behaviors of the nursing staff? Does a patient's behavior change in relation to the level of stress experienced? For example, Picot (1995) conducted an exploratory quantitative study of African-American caregivers who provided care to an elderly demented or confused relative. Her study was designed to explore the relationship between the caregivers' coping and such factors as perceived caregiving demands, rewards, and costs.

Exploratory studies are undertaken when a new area or topic is being investigated, and qualitative methods are especially useful for exploring the full nature of a little-understood phenomenon. Exploratory qualitative research is designed to shed light on the various ways in which a phenomenon is manifested and on underlying processes. As an example, Jablonski (1994) explored the full dimensionality of the process and experience of being mechanically ventilated, based on in-depth interviews with 12 patients.

Explanation

The goals of explanatory research are to understand the underpinnings of specific natural phenomena, and to explain systematic relationships among phenomena. Explanatory research is often linked to **theories,** which represent a method of deriving, organizing, and integrating ideas about the manner in which phenomena are interrelated. Whereas descriptive research provides new information, and exploratory research provides promising insights, explanatory research attempts to offer understanding of the underlying causes or full nature of a phenomenon.

In quantitative research, theories are used deductively as the basis for generating explanations that are then tested empirically. That is, based on some previously developed theory or body of evidence, the researcher makes specific explanatory predictions that, if upheld by the data, add further credibility to the theory. For example, Bull, Maruyama, and Luo (1995) tested a complex theoretical model of factors influencing family caregivers' responses and health outcomes after an elder's discharge from the hospital for acute episodes of chronic illness.

In qualitative studies, the researcher often searches for explanations about how or why a phenomenon exists—or what a phenomenon means—as a basis for *developing* a theory that is grounded in rich, in-depth, experiential evidence. For example, Redfern-Vance and Hutchinson (1995) generated a theory designed to illuminate the social psychological processes of women who begin to change their behavior after repeatedly contracting sexually transmitted diseases.

Prediction and Control

With our current level of knowledge, technology, and theoretical progress, there are numerous problems that defy absolute comprehension and explanation. Yet it is frequently possible to make predictions and to control phenomena based on findings from research, even in the absence of complete understanding. For example, research has shown that the incidence of Down syndrome in infants increases with the age of the mother. We can predict that a woman aged 40 years is at higher risk of bearing a child with Down syndrome than a woman aged 25. We can partially control the outcome by educating women about the risks and offering amniocentesis to women over age 35. Note, however, that the ability to predict and control in this example does not depend on an explanation of *why* older women are at a higher risk of having an abnormal child.

There are many examples of nursing and health-related studies—typically, quantitative ones—in which prediction and control are key objectives. Studies designed to test the efficacy of a nursing intervention are ultimately concerned with controlling patient outcomes or with affecting the costs of care. For example, Smith-Hanrahan and Deblois (1995) investigated the impact of a postpartum early discharge program on maternal fatigue and functional ability. Many other nursing studies are designed to identify predictive factors in relation to patient outcomes.

For instance, the main purpose of a study by Hendrich, Nyhuis, Kippenbrock, and Soja (1995) was to identify factors that could be used to predict the risk of experiencing a hospital fall.

Basic and Applied Research

Sometimes the purpose of scientific inquiry is classified according to the direct practical utility of the information gained. **Basic research** is undertaken to accumulate information or to formulate or refine a theory. Basic research is not designed to solve immediate problems, but rather to extend the base of knowledge in a discipline for the sake of knowledge and understanding. For example, a researcher may perform an in-depth, qualitative study of the normal process of grieving.

Applied research is focused on finding a solution to an immediate problem. Applied research has as its final goal the systematic planning of induced change in a troublesome situation. For example, a study of the effectiveness of a nursing intervention to ease the grieving process would be considered applied research. We need basic research for the discovery of general principles of human behavior and biophysiologic processes, but applied research tells us how these principles can be put to use to solve problems in the practice of nursing. Qualitative and quantitative researchers engage in both basic and applied research, but in qualitative studies there is somewhat more emphasis on basic knowledge than on specific problem-solving information.

In nursing, as in medicine, the feedback process between basic and applied research seems to operate more freely than in the case of other disciplines. The findings from applied research almost immediately pose questions for basic research, whereas the results of basic research often suggest clinical applications to a practical problem.

◩ ASSISTANCE TO CONSUMERS OF NURSING RESEARCH

This book is designed primarily to help students develop skills that will allow them to read and evaluate nursing studies (*i.e.,* to become intelligent consumers of nursing research). In each chapter of this book, we present information relating to the methods used by nurse researchers, and then we provide specific guidance to consumers through two mechanisms: (1) tips on what they can expect to find, vis-à-vis the material discussed in the chapter, in actual research reports; and (2) guidelines for critiquing those aspects of a study covered in the chapter.

What to Expect in the Research Literature

During your nursing career, and probably while you are taking this course on research methods, you will read several reports prepared by nurse researchers that summarize disciplined studies. Here are a few tips to help you apply the materials in this chapter to these reports:

- Research studies can be found in dozens of nursing journals. Not only are there many nursing journals specifically devoted to research—and the number continues to grow—but most specialty journals (*e.g., Heart & Lung, Oncology Nursing Forum*) also publish numerous research reports.

- Although the emphasis in nursing studies has shifted to questions relating to nursing practice, the topics that have interested nurse researchers are extremely broad. Thus, there continue to be studies of nurses themselves as well as studies relating to the education of nurses, nursing administration, and public policy.

- Most nursing studies have multiple aims. Almost all studies have some descriptive intent. Some studies that are exploratory also have an underlying expectation that the results will serve a predictive or control function. Studies that are truly explanatory are the least common in the nursing literature.

- Most of the research conducted in nursing tends to be applied rather than basic in nature. However, researchers rarely specifically tell readers whether their intent is to address a pragmatic problem or to generate basic knowledge. The underlying purpose of a study generally has to be inferred, and, in many cases, it is ambiguous. This ambiguity stems from the fact that when knowledge is generated, it is often immediately useful (*i.e.,* it has an applied value), and when a practical problem is solved, knowledge is also gained (*i.e.,* it has a basic value).

- Most nursing research studies are quantitative, but the number of qualitative investigations is growing. In recent years, there has also been an increase in the number of studies that integrate qualitative and quantitative methods.

- When a study is qualitative or conducted within the naturalistic paradigm, there is often an explicit statement to this effect early in a research report, although this is less typical of quantitative studies. The researcher usually does not discuss his or her world view, but the paradigmatic approach is often defended in terms of the nature of the problem.

- Increasingly, nursing research journals are including both qualitative and quantitative studies. A few journals are either exclusively qualitative or devote considerable coverage to qualitative studies (*Qualitative Health Research, Western Journal of Nursing Research*), but most others include a greater preponderance of quantitative studies (*e.g., Nursing Research, Research in Nursing and Health, Applied Nursing Research, Clinical Nursing Research*).

Guidelines for a Preliminary Overview of a Research Report

Throughout this text, we offer guidelines for evaluating research reports. Generally, these guidelines focus on the methodologic aspects of a study (*i.e.,* on the methods that the researcher used to gather and analyze information). Because this chapter

Box 1–1

Questions for a Preliminary Overview
of a Research Report

1. How relevant is the research to the actual practice of nursing?
2. Does the study focus on a topic that is considered a priority area for clinical nursing research?
3. Is the research qualitative or quantitative? What is the underlying paradigm?
4. What is the underlying purpose (or purposes) of the study—identification, description, exploration, explanation, or prediction and control?
5. Is the study fundamentally basic or applied in nature?
6. What might the clinical applications of this research be? To what type of people and settings is the research most relevant?

did not present much information regarding research methods, we offer some questions in Box 1–1 that are designed to assist you in using information presented in this chapter in an overall assessment of a research report.

RESEARCH EXAMPLES

In each chapter of this book, we present brief descriptions of actual studies recently conducted by nurse researchers. (In the accompanying *Study Guide,* we offer descriptions of *fictitious* studies, followed by a critique.) The descriptions focus on aspects of the study emphasized in the chapter, and the critiquing guidelines can be used to assess many of the researcher's methodologic decisions. In most cases, a review of the actual report in the nursing journal would enhance the assessment process and would provide a useful supplementary assignment. In this chapter, you can use the guidelines in Box 1–1 to do a brief preliminary assessment of some of the features of the two studies that follow.

Research Example of a Quantitative Study

Okimi, Sportsman, Rickard and Fritsche (1991), who were interested in better understanding the roots of glaucoma, designed a study to examine the effects of caffeinated coffee on the intraocular pressure (IOP) of nonglaucomatous individuals. They noted that glaucoma is a condition due to optic nerve damage resulting from increased IOP, but that the factors contributing to elevated IOP levels are not well understood. Twelve individuals who volunteered to participate in the study received three different treatments: caffeinated coffee, hot water, and no fluid. Each person received one treatment per day on three successive mornings, in a totally random order. Each day, their IOP was measured (with an instrument known as a noncontact tonometer) at 1-hour intervals, for 3 hours after the treatment. The study revealed that, as a group, the study participants' IOP was higher after ingesting coffee than after receiving the other two treatments. Moreover, the increased IOP was maintained over a 3-hour period. The authors concluded that "there are enough indications of adverse effects of caffeine to advise caution in the use of caffeinated products" (p. 75).

Research Example of a Qualitative Study

Walcott-McQuigg, Sullivan, Dan, and Logan (1995) conducted a study to explore the factors influencing weight control behavior among college-educated African-American women. The researchers noted that African-American women have consistently been found to be more overweight than European-American women, and so they sought to identify potential cultural, social, and psychological factors influencing their weight control behavior. Face-to-face, in-depth interviews were conducted with 36 African-American women in their homes. The interviews explored personal weight control behavior among the study participants, factors such as emotions and beliefs that influenced the participants' behavior, and opinions about African-American women's weight control behavior in general. The interviews suggested six factors that influenced the women's individual weight control practices: emotions/feelings, beliefs, life events, self-control, discipline, and commitment. Factors related to the African-American culture were also identified by the women, such as eating and cooking patterns and cultural values relating to food, health, and body image. The authors concluded that "recognition of psychosocial determinants of weight control behavior may enable health professionals to design unique interventions relevant to African American women" (p. 502).

◎ SUMMARY

Nurses engage in research for a number of reasons. Research has an important role to play in helping nursing establish a scientific base of knowledge for its practice. Additionally, the systematic accrual of nursing information facilitates a better definition of the parameters of nursing and helps to document the unique contribution nursing makes to health care. There is a growing consensus that a knowledge of nursing research is needed to enhance the professional practice of all nurses—including both **consumers of research** (who read and evaluate studies) and **producers of research** (who design and undertake research studies). Nurses may assume a variety of additional research-related roles in the course of their practices.

Nursing research began with Florence Nightingale and gained slow acceptance until the 1950s, when it accelerated rapidly. Since the 1970s, the emphasis in nursing research has been on clinical practice. Nurses are increasingly studying problems such as health promotion, prevention of illness, the efficacy of nursing interventions, and the needs of special health-risk groups. The establishment of the **National Institute of Nursing Research** at the National Institutes of Health in 1993 attests to the growth and current importance of nursing research.

Nursing research begins with questions about nursing phenomena or with a problem to be solved. Disciplined research stands in contrast to several other sources of knowledge and understanding, such as tradition, voices of authority, personal experience, trial and error, and logical reasoning.

Disciplined inquiry in nursing is being conducted within two broad **paradigms**—world views with underlying **assumptions** about the complexities of reality. One paradigm is known as the **positivist paradigm.** Positivists assume that there is an objective reality that is not dependent on human observation for its existence and that natural phenomena are basically regular and orderly. The related assumption of **determinism** refers to the belief that events are not haphazard, but rather the result of prior causes. The **naturalistic paradigm**, by contrast, assumes that reality is not a fixed entity but is rather a construction of human minds— and thus "truth" is a composite of multiple constructions of reality. Each of these paradigms, with its associated assumptions, has implications for the methods of acquiring knowledge.

The positivist paradigm is associated with the traditional **scientific approach,** which is a systematic, disciplined, and controlled process often aimed at identifying underlying causes of phenomena. Scientists base their findings on **empirical evidence,** which is evidence rooted in objective reality and collected by way of the human senses or their extensions. The scientific approach strives for **generalizability** and for the development of explanations or **theories** about the relationships among phenomena. The scientific approach often involves the collection and analysis of numeric information (*i.e.,* it often involves **quantitative research**). Although the scientific approach offers a number of distinct advantages as a system of inquiry, it is not without its share of shortcomings, including its narrow focus on a small range of human experience and the difficulty of quantitatively measuring complex phenomena.

Researchers within the naturalistic paradigm place a heavy emphasis on understanding the human experience as it is lived, generally through the collection and analysis of subjective, narrative materials through flexible procedures that evolve in the **field;** consequently, this paradigm usually involves **qualitative research.** Research in both paradigms can contribute to the further development of nursing knowledge.

Research can be categorized in terms of its aims or objectives. Identification, description, exploration, explanation, prediction, and control of natural phenomena represent the most common goals of a research investigation. Within each broad aim, qualitative and quantitative researchers pose different types of questions. Research also can be described in terms of the direct, practical utility that it sets out to achieve. **Basic research** is designed to extend the base of information for the sake of knowledge. **Applied research** focuses on discovering solutions to immediate problems.

STUDY SUGGESTIONS

Chapter 1 of the accompanying *Study Guide to Accompany Essentials of Nursing Research,* 4th edition offers various exercises and study suggestions for reinforcing the concepts presented in this chapter.

Suggested Readings

Methodologic and Theoretical References

American Nurses' Association Cabinet on Nursing Research. (1985). *Directions for nursing research: Toward the twenty-first century.* Kansas City, MO: American Nurses' Association.

Guba, E. G. (Ed.). (1990). *The paradigm dialog.* Newbury Park, CA: Sage Publications.

Kuhn, T. S. (1970). *The structure of scientific revolutions* (2nd ed.). Chicago: University of Chicago Press.

Lincoln, Y. S., & Guba, E. G. (1985). *Naturalistic inquiry.* Beverly Hills: Sage Publications.

O'Sullivan, P. S., & Goodman, P. A. (1990). Involving practicing nurses in research. *Applied Nursing Research, 3,* 169–173.

Schlotfeldt, R. M. (1992). Why promote clinical nursing scholarship? *Clinical Nursing Research, 1,* 5–8.

Substantive References

Bull, M. J., Maruyama, G., & Luo, D. (1995). Testing a model for posthospital transition of family caregivers for elderly persons. *Nursing Research, 44,* 132–138.

Cohen, M. H. (1995). The triggers of heightened parental uncertainty in chronic, life-threatening childhood illness. *Qualitative Health Research, 5,* 63–77.

Dellasega, C., & Mastrian, K. (1995). The process and consequences of institutionalizing an elder. *Western Journal of Nursing Research, 17,* 123–140.

Hendrich, A., Nyhuis, A., Kippenbrock, T., & Soja, M. E. (1995). Hospital falls: Development of a predictive model for clinical practice. *Applied Nursing Research, 8,* 129–139.

Jablonski, R. S. (1994). The experience of being mechanically ventilated. *Qualitative Health Research, 4,* 186–207.

Okimi, P. H., Sportsman, S., Rickard, M. R., & Fritsche, M. B. (1991). Effects of caffeinated coffee on intraocular pressure. *Applied Nursing Research, 4,* 72–76.

Picot, S. J. (1995). Rewards, costs, and coping of African American caregivers. *Nursing Research, 44,* 147–152.

Redfern-Vance, N., & Hutchinson, S. A. (1995). The process of developing personal sovereignty in women who repeatedly acquire sexually transmitted diseases. *Qualitative Health Research, 5,* 222–236.

Seifert, C. F., Frye, J. L., Belknap, D. C., & Anderson, D. C. (1995). A nursing survey to determine the characteristics of medication administration through enteral feeding catheters. *Clinical Nursing Research, 4,* 290–305.

Smith-Hanrahan, C., & Deblois, D. (1995). Postpartum early discharge. *Clinical Nursing Research, 4,* 50–66.

Walcott-McQuigg, J. A., Sullivan, J., Dan, A., & Logan, B. (1995). Psychosocial factors influencing weight control behavior of African American women. *Western Journal of Nursing Research, 17,* 502–520.

Overview of the Research Process

Student Objectives

On completion of this chapter, the student will be able to:

- define new terms presented in the chapter
- distinguish terms associated with quantitative and qualitative research
- distinguish independent and dependent variables
- distinguish between a dictionary definition and an operational definition of a concept
- describe the flow and sequence of activities in quantitative and qualitative research
- identify and describe the major sections in a research journal article
- characterize the style used in quantitative and qualitative research reports

New Terms

Abstract
Attribute variable
"Blind" reviews
Categorical variable
Cause-and-effect (causal) relationship
Coding
Coinvestigator
Concept
Conceptual model
Conceptualization
Constant
Construct
Continuous variable
Criterion variable
Data
Dependent variable
Functional relationship
Gaining entrée
Heterogeneity
Homogeneity
Hypothesis
Independent variable
Informant
Interpretation
Investigation
Investigator
Journal article

Level of significance
Literature review
Operational definition
Outcome variable
Peer reviewers
Phenomena
Pilot study
Population
Poster session
Principal investigator
Project director
Qualitative data
Quantitative data
Raw data
Relationship
Representativeness
Research design
Research findings
Research project
Research proposal
Research report
Researcher
Respondent
Sample
Sampling plan
Saturation
Scientist

◧ BASIC RESEARCH TERMINOLOGY

Research, like nursing or any other discipline, has its own language and terminology—its own "jargon." Some terms are used by both qualitative and quantitative researchers (although in some cases the connotations differ), whereas others are used predominantly in connection with one or the other approach. New terms are introduced throughout this textbook. However, we devote a large part of this chapter to some basic terms and concepts whose meaning should be mastered so that more complex ideas can be grasped. The purpose of this chapter is to make the rest of this book more manageable by familiarizing readers with the basics of research terminology and with the progression of steps that are undertaken in a research project. The chapter concludes with a discussion of research reports, which are the bridges between producers and consumers of research.

The Study

Before turning to a discussion of the terms that are the building blocks of qualitative and quantitative research, let us consider a few basic terms that are used in research circles. Regardless of the methods used, when researchers address a problem or answer a question, it is usually said that they are doing a **study,** but the endeavor may also be referred to as an **investigation** or a **research project.**

Research studies with humans involve two sets of people: those who are doing the research and those who are providing information. In a quantitative study, the people who are being studied are sometimes referred to as the **subjects** or the **study participants,** as shown in Table 2–1. When the subjects provide information to the researchers by answering questions directly (*e.g.,* by filling out a questionnaire), they may be called **respondents.** The term *subjects* implies that people are *acted upon* by the researchers; however, in a qualitative study, the individuals cooperating in the study play an active rather than a passive role and are, therefore, referred to as **informants** or study participants.

The person who undertakes the research is called the **researcher** or **investigator** (or sometimes—more often in quantitative studies—**scientist**). A study may be undertaken by a group of people working together rather than by a single researcher. For example, a team of nurse researchers and clinical nurses might

Table 2–1. Key Terms Used in Quantitative and Qualitative Research

Concept	Quantitative Term	Qualitative Term
Person contributing information	Subject Study participant Respondent	— Study participant Informant
Person undertaking the study	Researcher Investigator Scientist	Researcher Investigator —
That which is being investigated	— Concepts Constructs Variables (independent, dependent)	Phenomena, topics Concepts —
System of organizing concepts	Theory, theoretical framework Conceptual framework, conceptual model	Theory —
Information gathered	Data (numerical values)	Data (narrative descriptions)
Connections between concepts	Relationships (cause-and-effect, functional)	Patterns of association

collaborate on addressing a problem of clinical relevance. When a study is undertaken by a research team, the main person directing the investigation is referred to as the **project director** or **principal investigator.** Two or three researchers collaborating equally are sometimes called **coinvestigators.**

Phenomena, Concepts, and Constructs

Conceptualization refers to the process of developing and refining abstract ideas. Research is almost always concerned with abstract rather than tangible phenomena. For example, the terms *good health, pain, emotional disturbance, patient care,* and *grieving* are all abstractions that are formulated by generalizing about particular manifestations of human behavior and characteristics. These abstractions are often referred to as **concepts.** (In qualitative studies, researchers often use the terms **phenomena** or **topics**).

The term **construct** is also encountered frequently in the research literature, especially with regard to quantitative studies. Like a concept, a construct refers to an abstraction or mental representation inferred from situations, events, or behaviors. Kerlinger (1986) distinguishes concepts from constructs by noting that constructs are abstractions that are deliberately and systematically invented (or constructed) by researchers for a specific purpose. For example, *self-care* in Orem's model of health maintenance may be considered a construct. In practice, the terms *construct* and *concept* are often used interchangeably, although, by convention, a construct often refers to a slightly more complex abstraction than a concept.

Theory

A **theory** is a systematic, abstract explanation of some aspect of reality. Concepts are the building blocks of theories. In a theory, concepts are knitted together into a coherent system in an effort to explain the way in which our world and the people in it function. Theories play a role in both qualitative and quantitative research.

In a quantitative study, the researcher often starts with a theory or a **conceptual model** (the distinction is discussed in Chapter 4). On the basis of a previously developed theory, the researcher develops predictions about how phenomena will behave in the real world *if the theory is true.* In other words, the researcher uses deductive reasoning to develop from the general theory some specific predictions that can be tested empirically. The results of the research are used to reject, modify, or lend credence to the theory.

In qualitative research, the investigators use the information gathered from the participants inductively as the basis for developing theory. The participants' input is the starting point from which the researcher begins to conceptualize, seeking to explain patterns and commonalities emerging from the researcher–participant interactions. The goal is to arrive at a theory that explains phenomena *as they occur,* not as they are preconceived. Inductively generated theory from a qualitative study are sometimes subjected to more controlled confirmation through quantitative research.

Variables

Within the context of a quantitative research investigation, concepts are usually referred to as **variables.** A variable, as the name implies, is something that varies. Weight, nursing diagnoses, blood pressure readings, preoperative anxiety levels, and body temperature are all variables (*i.e.*, each of these properties varies or differs from one person to another). To the quantitative researcher, nearly all aspects of human beings and their environment are considered variables. For example, if everyone had black hair and weighed 125 pounds, hair color and weight would not be variables. If it rained continuously and the temperature were a constant 70°F, weather would not be a variable; it would be a **constant.** But it is precisely because people and conditions *do* vary that most research is conducted. The bulk of all quantitative research activity is aimed at trying to understand how or why things vary and to learn how differences in one variable are related to differences in another. For example, lung cancer research is concerned with the variable of lung cancer. It is a variable because not everybody has the disease. Researchers have studied what variables might be linked to lung cancer and have discovered that cigarette smoking appears to be related to the disease. Again, smoking is a variable because not everyone smokes.

A variable, then, is any quality of a person, group, or situation that varies or takes on different values—typically, numeric values. Sometimes a variable can take on a range of different values (*e.g.,* height or weight); such variables are referred to as **continuous variables** because their values can be represented on a continuum. Other variables take on only a few discrete values (*e.g.,* pregnant/not pregnant, male/female, single/married/divorced/widowed). Variables of this type, which essentially place individuals into categories, are referred to as **categorical variables.**

Variables are often inherent characteristics, such as age, blood type, health beliefs, or grip strength. Variables such as these are sometimes called **attribute variables.** In some research situations, however, the investigator creates or introduces a variable. For example, if a researcher is interested in testing the effectiveness of drug A, as opposed to drug B, in lowering the blood pressure of patients with hypertension, some patients would be given drug A, and others would receive drug B. In the context of this study, drug type has become a variable because different patients are administered different drugs.

Two terms frequently used in connection with variables are **heterogeneity** and **homogeneity.** When an attribute is extremely varied in the group under study, the group is said to be heterogeneous with respect to that variable. If, on the other hand, the members of the group are highly similar to one another with respect to that variable, the group is described as homogeneous. For example, with respect to the variable of height, a group of 2-year-old children is likely to be more homogeneous than a group of 18-year-old adolescents.

Thus, quantitative research focuses on variables of interest and how they are interrelated. The **variability** of humans and their experiences is the basis for many questions of interest to nurse researchers.

Dependent Variables and Independent Variables

An important differentiation can be made between two types of variable in a quantitative research study, and it is a distinction that you should master before proceeding to later chapters. The distinction is between the dependent variable and the independent variable. Many quantitative studies are aimed at unraveling and understanding the causes underlying certain phenomena. Does a nursing intervention cause more rapid recovery? Does a certain procedure cause stress? The presumed cause is referred to as the **independent variable,** and the presumed effect is referred to as the **dependent variable.**

Variability in the dependent variable is presumed to depend on variability in the independent variable. For example, the researcher investigates the extent to which lung cancer (the dependent variable) depends on smoking behavior (the independent variable). In another study, a researcher might examine the effect of a special diet (the independent variable) on weight gain in premature infants (the dependent variable). Or an investigator might be concerned with the extent to which a patient's perception of pain (the dependent variable) depends on different nursing approaches (the independent variable). The dependent variable (sometimes referred to as the **criterion variable** or the **outcome variable**) is the variable the researcher is interested in understanding, explaining, or predicting. For example, in lung cancer and smoking research, it is the carcinoma that the research scientist is trying to explain and predict, not smoking behavior.

Frequently, the terms *independent variable* and *dependent variable* are used to designate the direction of influence between variables rather than cause and effect. For example, let us say that a researcher is studying nurses' attitudes toward abortion and observes that older nurses hold less favorable opinions about abortion than younger nurses. The researcher might be unwilling to take the position that the nurses' attitudes were *caused* by their age. Yet the direction of influence clearly runs from age to attitudes: it makes little sense to suggest that the attitudes influence the nurses' age. Although in this example the researcher does not infer a cause-and-effect connection between age and attitudes, it is appropriate to conceptualize attitudes toward abortion as the dependent variable and age as the independent variable.

Many of the dependent variables studied by researchers have multiple causes or antecedents. If we are interested in studying the factors that influence people's weight, for example, we might consider their age, height, physical activity, and eating habits as the independent variables. Note that some of these independent variables are inherently attribute variables (age and height), whereas others *could* be influenced by the investigator (activity and eating patterns). Just as a study may examine more than one independent variable, two or more dependent variables may be of interest to the researcher. For example, an investigator may be concerned with comparing the effectiveness of two methods of nursing care (primary versus functional) for children with cystic fibrosis. Several dependent variables could be designated as measures of treatment effectiveness, such as the length of stay in the hospital, the number of recurrent respiratory infections, the presence of cough, dyspnea on exertion, and so forth. In short, it is common to design studies with multiple independent and dependent variables.

It is important to understand that variables are not inherently dependent or independent. A variable that is the dependent in one study may be considered an independent variable in another study. For example, consider a study that examines the effect of contraceptive counseling (the independent variable) on unwanted pregnancies (the dependent variable). Yet another research project might study the effect of unwanted pregnancies (the independent variable) on the incidence of child abuse (the dependent variable). In short, the designation of a variable as independent or dependent is a function of the role that the variable plays in a particular investigation. Table 2–2 presents some additional examples of research questions from the nursing research literature and specifies the dependent and independent variables.

Operational Definitions of Variables

In a quantitative study, the researcher usually clarifies and defines the variables under investigation at the outset. To be useful, the definition must specify how the

Table 2–2. Examples of Independent and Dependent Variables
in Quantitative Nursing Studies

Research Question	Independent Variable	Dependent Variables
What is the effect of regular, active exercise during the last trimester of pregnancy on maternal weight gain and infant birth weight? (Horns, Ratcliffe, Leggett, & Swanson, 1996)	Amount of exercise	Maternal weight gain, infant birth weight
What is the effect of a high-calorie diet on energy intake and body weight in tumor-bearing rats? (Fridriksdottir & McCarthy, 1995)	Caloric density	Energy intake and body weight
What is the effect of pain on facial and cry behavior, heart rate, and palmar sweating in infants 0 to 12 months of age? (Fuller & Conner, 1995)	Pain level	Facial and cry behavior, heart rate, palmar sweating
Do nurses administer greater amounts of narcotic analgesics to men than to women? (McDonald, 1994)	Gender of patients	Amount of narcotic analgesics

variable will be observed and measured in the actual research situation. Such a definition has a special name. An **operational definition** of a concept is a specification of the operations that the researcher must perform to collect the required information.

Variables differ considerably in the facility with which they can be operationalized. The variable weight, for example, is easy to define and measure. We may use the following as our definition of weight: the amount that an object weighs in terms of pounds. Note that this definition designates that weight will be determined according to one measuring system (pounds) rather than another (grams). The operational definition might specify that the subjects' weight will be measured to the nearest pound using a spring scale with subjects fully undressed after 10 hours of fasting. This operational definition clearly indicates to both the investigator and to the consumer what is meant by the variable weight.

Unfortunately, many of the variables of interest in nursing research are not operationalized as easily and directly as weight. There are multiple methods of measuring most variables, and the researcher must choose the method that best captures the variables as he or she conceptualizes them. For example, patient well-being may be defined in terms of both physiologic and psychological functioning. If the researcher chooses to emphasize the physiologic aspects of patient well-being, the operational definition may involve a measure such as heart rate, white blood cell count, blood pressure, or vital capacity. If, on the other hand, well-being is conceptualized for the purposes of research as primarily a psychological phenomenon, the operational definition will need to identify the method by which emotional well-being will be assessed, such as the responses of the patient to certain questions or the behaviors of the patient as observed by the researcher.

Some readers of a research report may not agree with the way the investigator has conceptualized and operationalized the variables. Nevertheless, precision in defining the terms has the advantage of communicating exactly what the terms mean. Table 2–3 presents some operational definitions from several quantitative nursing research studies.

Qualitative researchers generally do not define the concepts in which they are interested in operational terms before gathering information. This is because of their desire to have the meaning of concepts defined by those being studied. Nevertheless, in summarizing the results of a study, all researchers should be careful in describing the conceptual and methodologic bases of key research concepts.

Data

The **data** (singular, datum) of a research study are the pieces of information obtained in the course of the investigation. In a quantitative study, the researcher identifies the variables of interest, develops operational definitions of those variables, and then collects the relevant data from the research subjects. The variables, because they vary, take on different values. The actual values of the study variables constitute the data for a research project.

In quantitative studies, the researcher collects primarily **quantitative data** (*i.e.,* information in numeric form). For example, suppose we were conducting a

Table 2–3. Examples of Operational Definitions from Quantitative Nursing Studies

Concept	Operational Definition
Postoperative pain in abdominal surgical patients	Sensory component of pain: patient's score on the Sensation of Pain Scale (a 10-point scale) and amount of narcotic intake 24 hours after ambulation (Good, 1995)
Parenting attitudes of fathers within 1 year of child's birth	Score on the Adult-Adolescent Parenting Inventory (AAPI), a 32-question inventory assessing agreement/disagreement with statements that indicate potential problems with parenting (Tiller, 1995)
Physiologic status in patients with chronic obstructive pulmonary disease	The ratio of forced expiratory volume in 1 second (FEV_1) to forced vital capacity (FVC), *i.e.,* FEV_1/FVC (Narsavage & Weaver, 1994)

quantitative study in which the variable of primary interest was *depression*. In such a study, we would try to measure how depressed different study participants were. For example, we might ask the question, "Thinking about the past week, how depressed would you say you have been on a scale from 0 to 10, where 0 means 'not at all' and 10 means 'the most possible'?" Box 2–1 presents some quantitative data from three fictitious respondents. The subjects have provided a number corresponding to their degree of depression—9 for Subject 1 (a high level of depression), 0 for Subject 2 (no depression), and 4 for Subject 3 (very mild depression). The numeric values for all subjects in the study, collectively, would comprise the data on the variable depression.

In qualitative studies, the researcher collects primarily **qualitative data,** which usually are narrative descriptions. Narrative information can be obtained by having conversations with the subjects, by making detailed notes about how subjects behave in naturalistic settings, or by obtaining narrative records from subjects, such as diaries. As an example, suppose we were studying depression qualitatively. Box 2–2 presents some qualitative data from three subjects responding conversationally to the question, "Tell me about how you've been feeling lately—have you felt sad or depressed at all, or have you generally been in good spirits?" Here, the data consist of fairly rich and detailed narrative descriptions of the participants' emotional state.

In both qualitative and quantitative research, the collection and analysis of the research data are typically the most time-consuming aspects of a study. The analysis of qualitative data is a particularly labor-intensive process.

Relationships

Researchers are rarely interested in a single isolated concept or phenomenon. Rather, researchers usually study phenomena in relation to other phenomena (*i.e.,* they explore or test **relationships**). Generally speaking, a relationship is a bond or a connection between phenomena; for example, researchers repeatedly have

Box 2–1

Example of Quantitative Data

Question:	Thinking about the past week, how depressed would you say you have been on a scale from 0 to 10, where 0 means "not at all" and 10 means "the most possible"?
Data:	9 (Subject 1)
	0 (Subject 2)
	4 (Subject 3)

Example of Qualitative Data

Question: Tell me about how you've been feeling lately—have you felt sad or depressed at all, or have you generally been in good spirits?

Data: Well, actually, I've been pretty depressed lately, to tell you the truth. I wake up each morning and I can't seem to think of anything to look forward to. I mope around the house all day, kind of in despair. I just can't seem to shake the blues, and I've begun to think I need to go see a shrink. (Participant 1)

I can't remember ever feeling better in my life. I just got promoted to a new job that makes me feel like I can really get ahead in my company. And I've just gotten engaged to a really great guy who is very special. (Participant 2)

I've had a few ups and downs the past week, but basically things are on a pretty even keel. I don't have too many complaints. (Participant 3)

found that there is a relationship between cigarette smoking and lung cancer. Both qualitative and quantitative studies examine relationships among phenomena.

In a quantitative study, the researcher is primarily interested in the relationship between the independent variables and dependent variables. Variation in the dependent variable is presumed to be systematically related to variation in the independent variable. Relationships are usually expressed in quantitative terms, such as *more than, less than,* and so on. For example, let us consider as a possible dependent variable a person's body weight. What variables are related to (associated with) a person's weight? Some possibilities include height, metabolism, caloric intake, and exercise. For each of these four independent variables, we can make a tentative relational statement:

Height: Taller people will weigh more than shorter people.

Metabolism: The lower a person's metabolic rate, the more he or she will weigh.

Caloric intake: People with higher caloric intake will be heavier than those with lower caloric intake.

Exercise: The greater the amount of exercise, the lower the person's weight.

Each of these statements expresses a presumed relationship between weight (the dependent variable) and a measurable independent variable. Most quantitative research is conducted to determine whether relationships do or do not exist among variables, and often to *quantify* how strong the relationship is.

Quantitative variables can be related to one another in different ways. One type of relationship is referred to as **cause-and-effect** (or **causal**) **relationship.** Within the positivist paradigm, natural phenomena are assumed not to be random or haphazard; if phenomena have antecedent factors or causes, they are presumably discoverable. For instance, in our example about a person's weight, we might speculate that there is a causal relationship between caloric intake and weight: eating more calories causes weight gain. As an example of a quantitative study that was concerned with causal relationships, Anderson, Lane, and Chang (1995) studied the effect of deep-water tub baths on heat loss in healthy newborns 2 to 3 hours postbirth.

Not all relationships between variables can be interpreted as cause-and-effect relationships. There is a relationship, for example, between a person's pulmonary artery and tympanic temperatures: people with high readings on one tend to have high readings on the other. We cannot say, however, that pulmonary artery temperature *caused* tympanic temperature, nor that tympanic temperature *caused* pulmonary artery temperature, despite the relationship that exists between the two variables. This type of relationship is sometimes referred to as a **functional relationship** rather than a causal relationship. As an example, Evans, Dick, and Clark (1995) studied the relationship between maternal sleep during the week before labor and labor outcomes (*e.g.,* length of time in labor, type of delivery, and so forth).

Qualitative researchers are not concerned with quantifying relationships, nor in testing and confirming causal relationships. Rather, qualitative researchers seek patterns of association as a way of illuminating the underlying meaning and dimensionality of phenomena of interest. Patterns of interconnected themes and processes are identified as a means of understanding the whole. For example, King, Collins, and Liken (1995) studied the values of caregivers of persons with dementing disease in relation to their patterns of using community services.

What to Expect in the Research Literature

Many terms that are part of the fundamental vocabulary of researchers were presented in this section, but these terms do not necessarily appear in reports in the nursing research literature. Here are some tips on what to expect regarding the concepts discussed in this chapter:

- Every study focuses on one or more phenomenon, concept, or variable, but these terms per se are not necessarily used. For example, a research report might say: "The purpose of this study is to examine the effect of primary nursing on patient satisfaction." Although the researcher has not explicitly called anything a concept, the concepts (variables) under study are type of nursing and patient satisfaction.
- In quantitative studies, researchers usually are interested in understanding the relationship between one or more independent variables and one or more dependent variables. Almost no research report, however, explicitly

labels variables as dependent and independent. In the example just used, type of nursing care is the independent variable whose effect on the dependent variable (patient satisfaction) is under investigation, but the research report for this study would probably not identify the variables in these terms. Nevertheless, the distinction between independent variables and dependent variables is important to master; our job of helping readers of this book understand critical methodologic decisions will be more straightforward if we can assume that the reader has grasped the distinction.

• In research reports, variables (especially independent variables) are sometimes implied rather than fully explicated. In the example we have been using, the problem statement indicated the researcher's interest in understanding the effect of primary nursing on patient satisfaction. Patient satisfaction, as we have indicated, is the dependent variable. It is a variable because not all patients are equally satisfied. Primary nursing, however, is not in itself a variable. Rather, *type* of nursing (primary nursing versus something else) is the variable; the "something else" is often implied rather than stated in the researcher's statement of the problem. Note that, if primary nursing were not compared to some other form of nursing care, then type of nursing care would not be a variable in this study.

• Some research reports have an explicit statement regarding the operational definitions of the key concepts, but most never use the term. Quantitative research reports do, however, provide information on how key variables were measured (*i.e.,* they specify the operational definitions even if they do not use this label). This information is generally included in a section of the report called "Research Measures" or "Instruments."

▧ MAJOR STEPS IN A QUANTITATIVE STUDY

One of the first decisions a researcher makes before embarking on a study involves the selection of a paradigm to guide the inquiry. As discussed in the previous chapter, the researcher generally works within a paradigm that is consistent with his or her world view, and that gives rise to the type of questions that excite the researcher's curiosity. The maturity of the concept of interest also may lead to one or the other paradigm: when little is known about a topic, a qualitative approach is often more fruitful than a quantitative one. After the appropriate paradigm is identified, the progression of activities differs for the qualitative and quantitative researcher.

In a quantitative study, a researcher moves from the beginning point of a study (the posing of a question) to the end point (the obtaining of an answer) in a logical sequence of predetermined steps that is similar across studies. In some studies the steps overlap, whereas in others certain steps are unnecessary. Still, there is a general flow of activities that is typical of a quantitative study. This section describes that flow; the next section describes how qualitative studies differ.

Phase 1: The Conceptual Phase

The early steps in a quantitative research project typically involve activities with a strong conceptual or intellectual element. These activities include thinking, reading, rethinking, theorizing, and reviewing ideas with colleagues or advisors. During this phase, the researcher calls on such skills as creativity, deductive reasoning, insight, and a firm grounding in previous research on the topic of interest.

Step 1: Formulating and Delimiting the Problem

The first step is to develop a research problem. Good research depends to a great degree on good questions. Without a significant, interesting topic, the most carefully and skillfully designed research project is of little value. Quantitative researchers generally proceed from the selection of broad topic areas of interest to the development of specific questions that are amenable to empirical inquiry. In developing a research problem to be studied, nurse researchers ideally consider its substantive dimensions (Is this research question of theoretical or clinical significance?); its methodologic dimensions (How can this question best be studied?); its practical dimensions (Are adequate resources available to conduct a study?); and its ethical dimensions (Can this question be studied in a manner consistent with guidelines for the protection of subjects?).

Step 2: Reviewing the Related Literature

Quantitative research is typically conducted within the context of previous knowledge. To build on existing theory or research, the quantitative researcher strives to understand what is already known about a topic. A thorough **literature review** provides a foundation on which to base new knowledge and generally is conducted well before any data are collected in a quantitative study.

Step 3: Defining the Theoretical Framework

Theory is the ultimate aim of science in that it transcends the specifics of a particular time, place, and group of people and aims to identify regularities in the relationships among variables. When quantitative research is performed within the context of a theoretical framework (*i.e.*, when previous theory is used as a basis for generating predictions that can be tested), it is more likely that its findings will have broad significance and utility.

Step 4: Formulating Hypotheses

A **hypothesis** is a statement of the researcher's expectations about relationships between the variables under investigation. A hypothesis, in other words, is a prediction of expected outcomes; it states the relationships the researcher expects to find as a result of the study. The research question identifies the concepts under investigation; a hypothesis predicts how those concepts will be related. For example, the initial research question might be phrased as follows: Is preeclamptic toxemia in pregnant women associated with stress factors present during pregnancy? This might be translated into the following hypothesis or prediction: Pregnant women with preeclamptic toxemia will report a higher incidence of emotionally disturbing or stressful events during pregnancy than asymptomatic pregnant women. Most quantitative studies are designed to test a priori hypotheses through statistical analysis.

Phase 2: The Design and Planning Phase

In the second major phase of a quantitative research project, the investigator makes a number of decisions about the methods to be used to address the research question and carefully plans for the actual collection of data. As a consumer, you should be aware that each methodologic decision the researcher makes during this phase has implications for the integrity and interpretability of the results. Thus, you must be able to evaluate the decisions to determine how much faith can be put in the findings. A major objective of this book is to help you evaluate methodologic decisions.

Step 5: Selecting a Research Design

The **research design** is the overall plan for obtaining answers to the questions being studied and for handling some of the difficulties encountered during the research process. The design normally specifies which of the various types of research approach will be adopted and how the researcher plans to implement scientific controls to enhance the interpretability of the results. In quantitative studies, research designs tend to be highly structured and to include tight controls designed to eliminate the effects of contaminating influences.

Step 6: Identifying the Population to Be Studied

The term **population** refers to the aggregate or totality of all the objects, subjects, or members that conform to a set of specifications. In quantitative studies, the researcher identifies the population to be studied during the planning phase. For example, a researcher might specify nurses (RNs) and residence in the United States as the attributes of interest; the study population would then consist of all licensed RNs who reside in the United States. The requirement of defining a population for a research project arises from the need to specify the group to which the results of a study can be applied. It is seldom possible to study an entire population, unless it is particularly small. Before selecting actual subjects, the quantitative researcher needs to know what characteristics the sample should possess.

Step 7: Specifying Methods to Measure the Research Variables

To address a quantitative research problem, some method must be developed to observe or measure the research variables as accurately as possible. In most situations, the quantitative researcher begins by carefully defining the research variables to clarify exactly what each one means. Then the researcher needs to select or design an appropriate method of operationalizing the variables (*i.e.,* of collecting the data). A variety of quantitative data collection approaches exists (*i.e.,* biophysiologic measurements, interviews, formal observations, and so on). The task of measuring variables is a complex and challenging process that permits a great deal of creativity and choice.

Step 8: Designing the Sampling Plan

Research studies, as a rule, use as subjects only a small fraction of the population, referred to as a **sample.** The advantage of using a sample is that it is more practical and less costly than collecting data from the population. The risk is that the selected sample might not adequately reflect the behaviors, traits, symptoms, or beliefs of the population. Various methods of obtaining a sample are available to the quantitative researcher. These methods vary in cost, effort, and level of skills required, but their adequacy is assessed by the same criterion: the **representativeness** of the selected sample (*i.e.,* the quality of the sample for quantitative studies is a function of how typical, or representative, the sample is of the population with respect to the variables of concern in the study). Sophisticated sampling procedures can produce samples that have a high likelihood of being representative. In a quantitative study, the researcher's **sampling plan** specifies in advance *how* the sample will be selected and *how many* subjects there will be.

Step 9: Finalizing and Reviewing the Research Plan

Normally, researchers have their research plan reviewed by several people or groups before proceeding to the actual implementation of the plan. When a researcher needs financial support for the conduct of a study, the research plan is usually presented as a formal **research proposal** to a potential funder. Students conducting a study as part of a course or degree requirement have their plans reviewed by faculty advisors. Also, before proceeding with a study, researchers may need to have their plan approved by a human rights committee to ensure that the plan does not violate ethical principles.

Step 10: Conducting a Pilot Study
and Making Revisions

Unforeseen problems frequently arise in the course of a project. The effects of these problems may be negligible but, in some cases, may be so severe that the study has to be stopped so modifications can be introduced; in a quantitative study, changes in the research design, the sampling plan, or the data collection instruments once the study is underway usually mean that data collected before the change must be discarded. Whenever possible, therefore, it is advisable to carry out a **pilot study,** which is a small-scale version, or trial run, of the major study. The function of the pilot study is to obtain information for improving the project or for assessing its feasibility.

Phase 3: The Empirical Phase

The empirical portion of a quantitative study involves the collection of research data and the preparation of those data for analysis. In many studies, the empirical phase is the most time-consuming part of the investigation, although the amount of time spent collecting data varies considerably from one study to the next.

Step 11: Collecting the Data

The actual collection of data in a quantitative study normally proceeds according to a preestablished plan. The researcher's plan typically specifies procedures for collecting data (*e.g.*, where and when the data will be gathered); for describing the study to the subjects; for obtaining the necessary informed consents; and, if necessary, for training those who will be involved in the collection of the data.

Step 12: Preparing the Data for Analysis

The data collected in a quantitative study are rarely amenable to direct analysis. Some preliminary steps are usually necessary before the analysis can proceed. One such step is known as **coding,** which refers to the process of translating verbal data into categories or numeric form. For example, patients' responses to a question about the quality of nursing care they received during hospitalization might be coded into positive reactions, negative reactions, neutral reactions, and mixed reactions. Another preliminary step that is now almost universal is transferring the data from written documents to computer files so they can be analyzed by computer.

Phase 4: The Analytic Phase

The quantitative data gathered in the empirical phase are not reported to consumers in raw form. They are subjected to various types of analysis and interpretation, which occurs in the fourth major phase of the project.

Step 13: Analyzing the Data

The data themselves do not answer the research questions. Ordinarily, the amount of data collected in a study is too extensive to be reliably described by mere perusal. To answer the research questions meaningfully, the data must be processed and analyzed in some orderly, coherent fashion so patterns and relationships can be discerned. Quantitative data are analyzed through statistical procedures. **Statistical analyses** cover a broad range of techniques, including some simple procedures as well as complex and sophisticated methods. The underlying logic of statistical tests, however, is relatively simple.

Step 14: Interpreting the Results

Before the results of a study can be communicated effectively, they must be organized and interpreted in a systematic fashion. **Interpretation** refers to the process of making sense of the results and examining the implications of the findings within a broader context. The process of interpretation in quantitative studies is essentially the researcher's attempt to explain the findings in light of what is known about theory and previous findings in the area, and in light of the adequacy of the methods used in the investigation.

Phase 5: The Dissemination Phase

In the previous (analytic) phase, the researcher comes full circle: the questions posed in the first phase of the project are answered. The researcher's job is not completed, however, until the results of the study are disseminated.

Step 15: Communicating the Findings
The results of a research investigation are of little use if they are not communicated to others. Even the most compelling hypothesis, the most careful and thorough study, or the most dramatic results are of no value to the nursing community if they are not disseminated. Another—and often final—task of a research project, therefore, is the preparation of a **research report** that can be shared with others. We discuss research reports in a subsequent section of this chapter.

Step 16: Utilizing the Findings
Many interesting studies have been conducted by nurses without having any effect on nursing practice or nursing education. Ideally, the concluding step of a high-quality study is to plan for its utilization in the real world. Although nurse researchers are not always in a position to implement a plan for utilizing research findings, they can contribute to the process by including in their research reports recommendations regarding how the results of the study could be incorporated into the practice of nursing.

▨ ACTIVITIES IN A QUALITATIVE STUDY

As we have just seen, quantitative research involves a fairly linear progression of tasks (*i.e.,* the researcher lays out in advance the steps to be taken to maximize the integrity of the study, and then follows those steps as faithfully as possible). In a qualitative study, by contrast, the progression is closer to a circle than to a straight line—the qualitative researcher is continually examining and interpreting data and making decisions about how to proceed based on what has already been discovered.

Because the qualitative researcher has a flexible approach to the collection and analysis of data, it is impossible to precisely define the flow of activities—the flow varies from one study to another and researchers do not know ahead of time exactly how the study will proceed. However, we try to give a feel for how a qualitative study is conducted by describing some major activities and indicating how and when they might be performed.

Conceptualizing and Planning a Qualitative Study

Like quantitative researchers, qualitative researchers generally begin with a broad topic area to be studied. However, qualitative researchers are usually interested in an aspect of a topic that is poorly understood and about which little is known. Therefore, they do not develop hypotheses or pose highly refined research questions before going into the field. The general topic area may be narrowed and clarified on the basis of self-reflection and discussion with colleagues (or clients), but usually the researcher proceeds with a fairly broad research question that allows the focus to be sharpened and more clearly delineated once the study is underway. Initially, the qualitative researcher places few boundaries or delimitations on the research question.

There are conflicting ideas among qualitative researchers regarding the performance of a literature review at the outset of the study. At one extreme are those who believe that the researcher should not consult the literature at all before collecting any data. The concern is that prior studies might exert an undue influence on the researcher's conceptualization of the phenomena under study. According to this view, the phenomena should be elucidated based on the participants' viewpoints rather than on any prior information. Others feel that the researcher should conduct at least a cursory up-front literature review to obtain some possible guidance (including guidance in identifying the kinds of biases that have emerged in studying the topic). In any event, qualitative researchers typically find a relatively small body of relevant previous work because of the nature of the questions they ask.

During the planning phase, the qualitative researcher must also identify a **site** for the data collection. Before entering the field, the researcher must select a site that is consistent with the topic under study. For example, if the topic is the health care beliefs of the urban poor, an inner-city neighborhood with a high percentage of low-income residents must be identified. The researcher may have to further identify the types of **setting** within the site where data collection will occur (*e.g.,* in homes, clinics, the workplace, and so on). In many cases, the researcher needs to make preliminary contacts with key actors in the selected site to ensure cooperation and access to informants (*i.e.,* the researcher needs to **gain entrée** into the setting).

Before going into the field, the qualitative researcher also has to arrange for and test any equipment that might be needed. For example, most qualitative studies involve audiotaping (in some cases videotaping) interviews with informants.

Conducting the Qualitative Study

In a qualitative study, the activities of sampling, data collection, data analysis, and interpretation take place in an iterative fashion. The qualitative researcher begins by talking with and/or observing a few people who have first-hand experience with the phenomenon under study. The discussions and observations are loosely structured, allowing for a full range of beliefs, feelings, and behaviors to be expressed. Analysis and interpretation are ongoing, concurrent activities used to guide the kinds of people to sample next and the types of questions to ask or observations to make. The actual process of data analysis involves clustering together related types of narrative information into a coherent scheme. The analysis of qualitative data is a very intensive, time-consuming activity.

As analysis and interpretation progress, the researcher begins to identify themes and categories, which are used to build a descriptive theory of the phenomenon. The kinds of data obtained and the people selected as participants tend to become increasingly focused and purposeful as a theory emerges. Theory development and verification shape the sampling process—as the theory develops, the researcher seeks participants who can confirm and enrich the theoretical understandings, as well as participants who can potentially challenge them and lead to further theoretical development.

A quantitative researcher decides in advance how many subjects to include in the study, but a qualitative researcher's sampling decisions are guided by the data. Many qualitative researchers use the principle of **saturation,** which occurs when themes and categories in the data become repetitive and redundant, such that no new information can be gleaned by further data collection.

In a quantitative study, the researcher seeks to collect high-quality data by selecting in advance methods and measuring instruments that have been previously demonstrated to be accurate and rigorous. The qualitative researcher, by contrast, must take steps to demonstrate the trustworthiness of the data while in the field. The central feature of these efforts is to confirm that the findings accurately reflect the experiences and viewpoints of the participants, rather than the perceptions of the researcher. For example, one confirmatory activity involves going back to participants and sharing preliminary interpretations with them so they can evaluate whether the researcher's thematic analysis is consistent with their experiences.

Disseminating Qualitative Findings

Qualitative nursing researchers also strive to share their findings with other nurses and other health-care specialists. Qualitative research reports are increasingly being published in the nursing literature. Qualitative findings, because of their depth and richness, also lend themselves more readily to book-length manuscripts than do quantitative ones. It should be noted that, regardless of the researcher's position about when a literature review should be conducted, qualitative researchers usually include a summary of prior research in their reports as a means of providing context for the study.

Quantitative reports almost never contain any **raw data**—data exactly in the form they were collected, which are numeric values. Qualitative reports, by contrast, are generally filled with rich verbatim passages directly from the participants. The excerpts are used in an evidentiary fashion to support or illustrate the researcher's interpretations and theoretical formulations.

Like quantitative researchers, qualitative nurse researchers want to see their findings used by other nurses. Qualitative findings often are used as the basis for the formulation of hypotheses that are tested by quantitative researchers. Qualitative findings are especially useful in the development of assessment tools used for both research and clinical purposes. Most importantly, qualitative studies help to shape nurses' perceptions of a problem or situation, and their conceptualization of potential solutions.

▧ READING RESEARCH REPORTS

The findings and interpretations of a research investigation, together with a description of all the major methodologic decisions, are communicated to the nursing community through research reports. Research reports—especially reports for a quantitative study—are often daunting to those without research training. We believe a few tips will help to make research reports more accessible to you even before you learn about the methods researchers use to conduct their research.

There are several types of research reports, the most common of which are the following:

- *Theses and dissertations.* Most doctoral degrees and many master's degrees are granted on the successful completion of an empirical research project, which is described in a thesis or dissertation.
- *Reports to funders.* When researchers obtain financial support to do research, they normally submit a final report that summarizes their research to the funder.
- *Books.* Sometimes research is reported in books, in many cases as a chapter in anthologies on a specific topic.
- *Presentations at conferences.* Institutions and professional organizations sponsor conferences that provide a forum for describing studies orally or in visual displays called **poster sessions.**
- *Journal articles.* Many nursing journals publish articles that summarize the results of a research investigation.

Students are most likely to encounter research results in professional journals. Therefore, much of this section is devoted to a discussion of journal articles.

What Are Research Journal Articles?

Research **journal articles** are reports that summarize the highlights of an investigation. Their major intent is to communicate the contribution that a study has made to knowledge. Because the competition for journal space is keen, the typical research article is relatively brief—generally only 10 to 25 typewritten double-spaced pages. This means that the researcher must condense a lot of information about the purpose of the study, the methods used, the findings, and the interpretation into a short report.

Research reports are accepted by journals on a competitive basis. Usually research articles are reviewed by two or three **peer reviewers** (*i.e.,* by other researchers doing work in the field) who make a recommendation about whether the article should be accepted, rejected, or revised and reviewed again. These are usually **"blind" reviews** (*i.e.,* the reviewers are not told the names of the researchers, and the researchers are not informed about the identity of the reviewers).

In most major nursing research journals, the rate of acceptance is relatively low—it can be as low as 5% of all submitted articles. Thus, consumers of research journal articles have some assurance that these research reports have already been scrutinized for their merit and nursing relevance by other nurse researchers. Nevertheless, the publication of an article does not mean that the research findings can be uncritically accepted. The validity of the findings depends to a large degree on how the study was conducted. Research methods courses help consumers to understand the strengths and limitations of studies reported in professional journals.

Several nursing journals accept research articles for publication. *Nursing Research* is the oldest—and remains one of the major—communication outlets for research in the field of nursing. Other nursing journals that focus primarily on publishing reports of studies include *Advances in Nursing Science, Applied Nursing Research, Clinical Nursing Research, Qualitative Health Research, Research in Nursing and Health,* and the *Western Journal of Nursing Research.* Many other clinical specialty journals, such as *Heart & Lung, Public Health Nursing, Oncology Nursing Forum,* and the *Journal of Obstetric, Gynecologic, and Neonatal Nursing,* also accept research reports for publication.

Research reports in journals tend to follow a certain format for the presentation of material and tend to be written in a particular style. The next two sections discuss the content and style of research reports for quantitative and qualitative studies.

The Content of Research Reports

Research reports in professional journals often consist of six major sections: an abstract, an introduction, a method section, a results section, a discussion section, and references. These sections are briefly described below to provide you with some guidelines for what to look for and expect in a research report.

The Abstract

The **abstract** is a brief description of the study placed at the beginning of the journal article. The abstract answers, in about 100 to 200 words, the following questions: What were the research questions? What methods did the researcher use to address those questions? and What did the researcher discover? Readers can readily review an abstract to assess whether the entire report should be read.

Because researchers know that many people will read only the abstract, they normally strive to communicate only that which is essential for readers to grasp what the study was all about. Box 2–3 presents abstracts from two actual studies—one quantitative and the other qualitative.

The Introduction

The purpose of the introductory section of a research report is to acquaint readers with the research problem and with the context within which it was formulated. The introduction often is not specifically labeled "Introduction," but rather follows immediately after the abstract. The introductory section may contain the following elements:

- *The central phenomena, concepts, or variables under study.* The key topic under investigation is identified.

Examples of Abstracts from Published Research

Box 2–3

Quantitative Study

Combined mother–infant postnatal nursing care was compared with traditional, separate postpartum and newborn care in two studies. In Study I, self-administered questionnaires were completed by 408 mothers and 63 staff nurses. Data were collected both before and after mother–infant care was implemented. Benefits of the new system included increased maternal competence and satisfaction with parent education, parent–infant contact, and the nurse–client relationship, increased staff satisfaction, with no increase in operational cost. There were no breastfeeding differences, but ways to improve duration were implied by reasons for stopping. These findings were replicated in a separate setting with similar sample sizes. However, in the latter case, low staff ratios appeared to limit the benefits of mother–infant care to multiparas rather than primiparas. (Watters & Kristiansen, 1995)

Qualitative Study

The purpose of this study was to explore the process of managing disease-related information through various developmental stages from the inside perspective of those who lived with a long-term health condition. The retrospective, longitudinal, life-history method was used to generate a descriptive theory from accounts constructed with 21 informants: 10 adolescents and young adults with cystic fibrosis aged 16 to 25 years, and 11 of their significant family members. People chose a specific telling strategy according to the perceived ability of the audience to deal with the information and the situational context. Four strategies of managing disease-related information emerged: visibility, direct telling, silent telling, and concealment. The informants frequently chose information management strategies that enabled an ordinary style of living. These strategies neither reflect feelings of shame nor of pride, as it is suggested in the existing literature. Implications for theory, health care practice, and further research are discussed. (Admi, 1995)

- *The statement of purpose, research questions, and/or hypotheses to be tested.* The reader is usually told what the researcher set out to accomplish.
- *A review of the related literature.* Current knowledge relating to the study problem is often briefly described so readers can understand how the study fits in with previous findings and can assess the contribution of the new study.
- *The theoretical framework.* In quantitative studies designed to test a theory, the framework is usually presented in the introduction.
- *The significance of and need for the study.* The introduction to most research reports includes an explanation of why the study is important and how it can contribute to the existing base of knowledge or improve nursing practice.

In summary, the purpose of the introduction is to set the stage for a description of what the researcher did and what the researcher discovered.

The Method Section

The purpose of the method section is to communicate to readers what the researcher did to solve the research problem or to answer the research questions. The method section tells readers about major methodologic decisions, and often offers rationales for those decisions. For example, a report for a qualitative study often explains why a qualitative approach was considered to be especially appropriate and fruitful.

In a quantitative study, the method section usually describes the following, which are often presented as subsections:

- *The subjects.* Quantitative research reports generally describe the population under study, specifying the criteria by which the researcher decided whether a person would be eligible for the study. The method section also describes the actual research sample, indicating how people were selected or recruited and the number of participants in the sample.
- *The research design.* A description of the research design focuses on the overall plan for the collection data, often including the steps the researcher took to minimize biases and enhance the interpretability of the results by instituting various controls.
- *Instruments and data collection.* An important component of the methods section is the discussion of the methods used to collect the data. The researcher describes how the critical research variables were operationalized and the specific instruments used to measure the variables. The researcher may also present information concerning the quality of the measuring tools.
- *Study procedures.* The methods section usually contains a description of the procedures used during the conduct of the study. For example, if a nursing intervention is being evaluated, then that intervention is fully described. Procedures for data collection are also summarized. The re-

searcher's efforts to protect the rights of human subjects may also be documented in the methods section.

In a qualitative report, the researcher discusses many of the same issues as in a quantitative one, although often with different emphases. For example, a qualitative study generally provides much more information about the research setting and the context of the study, and less information on sampling design. Also, because formal instruments are generally not used to collect data in qualitative studies, there is little discussion about the specific data collection methods, but there may be more information on data collection procedures. Increasingly, reports of qualitative studies are including descriptions of efforts the researcher made to ensure high-quality data. Many qualitative reports also have a subsection on data analysis. Whereas there are fairly standard ways of analyzing quantitative data, such standardization does not exist for qualitative data, so there is often a need for qualitative researchers to briefly describe their analytic approach.

The Results Section

The results section presents the **research findings** (*i.e.,* the results obtained in the analyses of the data). The text summarizes the findings, often accompanied by tables or figures that highlight the most noteworthy results.

Virtually all results sections contain some basic descriptive information, including a description of the study participants (*e.g.,* the average age or the percentage male versus female). In quantitative studies, the researcher provides basic descriptive information for the key variables, using simple statistics. For example, in a study of the effect of prenatal drug exposure on the birth outcomes of infants, the results section might begin by describing the average birth weights and Apgar scores of the infants, or the percentage who were low-birth-weight (under 2500 g).

In quantitative studies, the results section typically reports the following additional types of information relating to the statistical analyses performed:

- *The name of any statistical tests used.* A **statistical test** is, simply, a procedure for evaluating the believability of the findings. For example, if the percentage of low-birth-weight infants in the sample of drug-exposed infants is computed, how likely is it that the percentage is accurate? If the researcher finds that the average birth weight of drug-exposed infants in the sample is lower than the birth weight of infants in the sample who were not exposed to drugs, how probable is it that the same would be true for other infants not in the sample? That is, is the relationship between prenatal drug exposure and infant birth weight in the sample *real* and likely to be replicated with a new sample of infants? Statistical tests provide answers to questions such as these. Dozens of statistical tests exist, but they are all based on common principles; readers do not have to know the names of all statistical tests to comprehend the findings.
- *The value of the calculated statistic.* Computers are used almost universally to process the research data and compute a value for the particular

statistical test used. The value allows the researchers to draw conclusions about the meaning of the results. The actual numeric value of the statistic, however, is not inherently meaningful and need not concern readers of research reports.

- *The significance.* The most important information in the results section is whether the results of the statistical tests were significant (not to be confused with important). If a researcher reports that the results are **statistically significant,** it means that, according to the statistical test, the findings are likely to be valid and replicable with a completely new sample of subjects. Research reports also indicate the **level of significance,** which is an index of how probable it is that the findings are reliable. For example, if a report indicates that a finding was significant at the .05 level, this means that only 5 times out of 100 would the obtained result be spurious or haphazard. In other words, 95 times out of 100, similar results would be obtained, and the researcher can therefore have a high degree of confidence that the findings are reliable.

In a qualitative report, the researcher usually organizes the findings according to the major **themes** that emerged directly from the data. The results section of qualitative reports typically has several subsections, the headings of which correspond to the researcher's labels for the themes. For example, Jarrett and Lethbridge (1994) studied women's experience with waning fertility during midlife and identified the central process as "Looking Forward, Looking Back." Within this overall process were three main themes that were used as headings for the results subsections: Reflecting on Childbearing Years, Doing a Midlife Review, and Anticipating Getting Older. In qualitative studies, excerpts from the actual data are included in the report to support and provide a rich description of the thematic analysis. The results sections of qualitative studies may also present the researcher's emerging theory about the phenomenon under study, although this may also appear in the concluding section of the report.

The Discussion Section

The discussion section of a journal article draws conclusions about the meanings and implications of the study. This section tries to unravel what the results mean and why things turned out the way they did. The discussion in both qualitative and quantitative reports may incorporate the following elements:

- *An interpretation of the results.* The interpretation involves the translation of findings into practical, conceptual, and/or theoretical meaning.
- *Implications.* Researchers may offer suggestions for how their findings could be used to improve nursing, and they may also make recommendations on how best to advance knowledge in the area through additional research.
- *Study limitations.* The researcher often is in the best position possible to discuss study limitations, such as sample deficiencies, design problems,

weaknesses in data collection, and so forth. A discussion section that presents these limitations demonstrates to readers that the author was aware of these limitations and probably took them into account in interpreting the findings.

The References

Research journal articles conclude with a list of the books, reports, and other journal articles that were referenced in the text of the report. For those interested in pursuing additional reading on a substantive topic, the reference list of a current research study is an excellent place to begin.

The Style of Research Reports

Research reports tell a story. However, the style in which many research journal articles are written—especially reports of quantitative studies—makes it difficult for beginning research consumers to become interested in the story the researcher is communicating. To unaccustomed audiences, research reports may sound stuffy and pedantic. Four factors—only the first two of which are relevant to qualitative research reports—contribute to this impression:

- *Compactness.* As mentioned above, journal space is limited, so authors must try to compress many ideas and concepts into the short space available. Some of the interesting, personalized aspects of the investigation often cannot be reported.
- *Jargon.* The authors often use research terms that are assumed to be part of the reader's vocabulary. In most cases, the jargon can be translated into everyday terms, but this is at the expense of efficiency and, in some cases, precision.
- *Objectivity.* The writer of a quantitative research report generally strives to present findings in a manner that suggests neutrality and the absence of personal biases. Quantitative researchers normally take pains to avoid any impression of subjectivity and thus research stories are told in a way that makes them sound impersonal. For example, most quantitative research reports are written in the passive voice (*i.e.,* personal pronouns are avoided). Use of the passive voice tends to make a report less inviting and lively than the use of the active voice, and it tends to give the impression that the researcher did not play an active role in conducting the study. (Qualitative reports, by contrast, are more subjective and personal, and written in a more conversational style.)
- *Statistical information.* Numbers and statistical symbols may intimidate readers who do not have strong mathematic interest or training. Most nursing studies are quantitative, and thus most research reports summarize the results of statistical analyses. Indeed, nurse researchers have become

increasingly sophisticated over the past decade and have begun to use more powerful and complex statistical tools.

A major goal of this textbook is to assist nurses in dealing with these issues.

Tips on Reading Research Reports

As you progress through this textbook, you will acquire skills with which to evaluate critically various aspects of research reports. Some preliminary hints on digesting research reports and dealing with the issues described above follow.

- Grow accustomed to the style of research reports by reading them frequently, although you may not yet understand all the technical points. Try to keep the underlying rationale for the style of research reports (as just described) in mind as you are reading.
- We recommend that, at least initially, you read research journal articles rather slowly; it may be useful to first skim the article to get the major points and then read the article more carefully a second time.
- Try not to get bogged down in (or scared away by) the statistical information. Try to grasp the gist of the story without letting formulas and numbers frustrate you.
- Until you become more accustomed to the style and jargon of research journal articles, you may want to mentally translate research articles. You can do this by translating compact paragraphs into looser constructions, by translating jargon into more familiar phrases and terms, by recasting the report into an active voice to get a better sense of the researcher's dynamic role in the research process, and by summarizing the findings with words rather than with numbers. As an example of such a translation, Box 2–4 presents a brief summary of a fictitious study. The top panel is written in the style typically found in research journal articles. The bottom panel presents a translation of the summary that recasts the information into language that is more digestible to students and novice consumers.

◫ GENERAL QUESTIONS IN REVIEWING A RESEARCH STUDY

The remaining chapters of this book contain guidelines to help consumers to evaluate different aspects of a research report critically, focusing primarily on the methodologic decisions that the researcher made in conducting the study. Box 2–5 presents some further suggestions for performing a preliminary overview of a research report, drawing on the concepts explained in this chapter. These guidelines supplement those presented in Chapter 1.

Summary of a Fictitious Study and a Translation

Box 2-4

Original Version

The potentially negative sequelae of having an abortion on the psychological adjustment of adolescents have not been adequately studied. The present study sought to determine whether alternative pregnancy resolution decisions have different long-term effects on the psychological functioning of young women.

Three groups of low-income pregnant teenagers attending an inner-city clinic were the subjects in this study: those who delivered and kept the baby; those who delivered and relinquished the baby for adoption; and those who had an abortion. There were 25 subjects in each group. The study instruments included a self-administered questionnaire and a battery of psychological tests measuring depression, anxiety, and psychosomatic symptoms. The instruments were administered upon entry into the study (when the subjects first came to the clinic) and then 1 year after termination of the pregnancy.

The data were analyzed using analysis of variance (ANOVA). The ANOVA tests indicated that the three groups did not differ significantly in terms of depression, anxiety, or psychosomatic symptoms at the initial testing. At the posttest, however, the abortion group had significantly higher scores on the depression scale, and these girls were significantly more likely than the two delivery groups to report severe tension headaches. There were no significant differences on any of the dependent variables for the two delivery groups.

The results of this study suggest that young women who elect to have an abortion may experience a number of long-term negative consequences. It would appear that appropriate efforts should be made to follow-up abortion patients to determine their need for suitable treatment.

Translated Version

As researchers, we wondered whether young women who had an abortion had any emotional problems in the long run. It seemed to us that not enough research had been done to know whether any actual psychological harm resulted from an abortion.

We decided to study this question ourselves by comparing the experiences of three types of teenager who became pregnant—first, girls who delivered and kept their babies; second, those who delivered the babies but gave them up for adoption; and third, those who elected to have an abortion. All teenagers in the sample were poor, and all were patients at an inner-city clinic. Altogether, we studied 75 girls— 25 in each of the three groups. We evaluated the teenagers' emotional states by asking them to fill out a questionnaire and to take several psychological tests. These tests allowed us to assess things such as the girls' degree of depression and anxiety and whether they had any complaints of a psychosomatic nature. We asked them to fill out the forms twice: once when they came into the clinic, and then again a year after the abortion or the delivery.

We learned that the three groups of teenagers looked pretty much alike in terms of their emotional states when they first filled out the forms. But when we compared how the three groups looked a year later, we found that the teenagers who had abortions were more depressed and were more likely to say they had severe tension headaches than teenagers in the other two groups. The teenagers who kept their babies and those who gave their babies up for adoption looked pretty similar 1

(Continued)

(Continued)

year after their babies were born, at least in terms of depression, anxiety, and psychosomatic complaints.

Thus, it seems that we might be right in having some concerns about the emotional effects of having an abortion. Nurses should be aware of these long-term emotional effects, and it even may be advisable to institute some type of follow-up procedure to find out if these young women need additional help.

RESEARCH EXAMPLES

This section presents brief overviews of a quantitative and a qualitative study. Our overviews deal primarily with the key concepts of the studies and on the organization of the research reports. Use the questions in Box 2–5 as a guide to thinking about these studies. You may wish to consult the full research report in answering these questions and in thinking about the differences in style and content of qualitative and quantitative reports.

Box 2–5

Additional Questions for a Preliminary Overview of a Research Report

1. What is the study all about? What are the main phenomena, concepts, or constructs under investigation?
2. If the study is quantitative, what are the independent and dependent variables?
3. Are they key concepts clearly explained? Are operational definitions provided?
4. What is the nature of the relationship (if any) under study?
5. Does the report have an abstract? Does the abstract communicate concisely what the study was about, how the research was conducted, and what the main findings were?
6. How was the research report organized? Was the structure consistent with the structure discussed in this chapter? Were headings and subheadings used effectively to facilitate reading of the report?

Research Example of a Quantitative Study

Tuten and Gueldner (1991) initiated a study to determine if the patency of the peripheral intermittent intravenous device (PIID) would be maintained as effectively with a sodium chloride solution as with a dilute heparin solution, and if a sodium chloride solution could be used with fewer complications. Two groups of subjects (hospitalized patients) were studied: those whose PIIDs were maintained using sodium chloride solution and those whose PIIDs were maintained using dilute heparin solution. Tuten and Gueldner described their variables as follows: "The type of maintenance solution used was the independent variable, and incidence of device complications (coagulation, infiltration, phlebitis) was the dependent variable." (p. 65).

Staff nurses completed a PIID Complication Assessment Form for 30 patients whose PIIDs were maintained with sodium chloride and 47 patients whose devices were maintained with dilute heparin. The form contained brief descriptions of possible intravenous complications and was used to measure the dependent variable.

Tuten and Gueldner's study began with an unlabeled introduction that presented the study's purpose and the research questions. The report included an explicitly labeled "Literature Review" section. The method section had three subsections: Sample, Instruments, and Data Collection Procedure. The Results section presented both descriptive information (e.g., frequency of device use) and the results of the comparison of the two groups. The findings indicated that there were no differences in device complications in the two groups of patients. The Discussion section discussed the study's implication that sodium chloride may be an effective alternative to dilute heparin for maintenance of patency in PIIDs.

Research Example of a Qualitative Study

Langner (1993) conducted an in-depth study of the process of caring for an elderly relative. Her focus was on the process by which the family member copes with the day-to-day caregiving experience, the dilemmas to which it gives rise, and the coping strategies used to deal with the dilemmas.

Twenty-three primary caregivers of an elderly relative participated in the study. Each participant was interviewed on three separate occasions over a 4-month period, beginning shortly after the older relative was discharged from the hospital. All interviews, which yielded narrative, conversational data, were tape recorded and transcribed. Questions for the interviewing evolved from the ongoing analysis of data. Three major strategies for managing the caregiving process emerged from the analysis. One theme, establishing and maintaining a routine, is exemplified by the following excerpt:

> We have a regular schedule now. I get up at 5:30 every morning, and I'm at work
> between 8:30 and 9:00. I do his sponge bath, breakfast, get all the medicines

ready and put them in little cups for the day. There is a fair amount of planning that you do. I wasn't organized at first . . . But now we have a regular schedule, and we follow that schedule every day as much as we can. I feel like I've got things under better control these days. (p. 586)

Langner's report contained a brief introduction with sections labeled Purpose of the Study, Definition of Terms, and Design, and then the Method section. The Findings section began with a statistical description of the sample (*e.g.,* 47% of the caregivers were married), followed by the substantive results organized within three subsections corresponding to the major themes: Establishing and Maintaining a Routine, "Taking One Day at a Time," and Retelling the Reasons for Caregiving. In the discussion section, the researcher offered an interpretation of the various strategies.

▨ SUMMARY

A research **study** (or **investigation** or **research project**) is undertaken by one or more **researchers** (or **investigators** or **scientists**). The people who provide information to the researchers are referred to as **subjects, study participants,** or **respondents** (in quantitative research) or study participants or **informants** in qualitative research.

Researchers investigate **phenomena and concepts** (or **constructs**), which are abstractions or mental representations inferred from behavior or events. Concepts are the building blocks of **theories,** which are systematic explanations of some aspect of the real world. In quantitative studies, the concepts under investigation are referred to as **variables.** A variable is a characteristic or quality that takes on different values (*i.e.,* a variable is something that varies from one person or object to another). An important distinction is differentiation between the dependent variables and independent variables of a study. The **dependent variable** is the behavior, characteristic, or outcome the researcher is interested in understanding, explaining, predicting, or affecting. The **independent variable** is the presumed cause of, antecedent to, or influence on the dependent variable. In a quantitative study, the variables must be clarified and defined in such a way that they are amenable to observation or measurement. The **operational definition** of a concept is the specification of the procedures and tools required to make the measurements. The term **data** is used to designate the information collected during the course of a study. Data may take the form of narrative information (**qualitative data**) or numeric values (**quantitative data**). Researchers usually are not interested in studying concepts in isolation but rather in learning about the relationship between two or more concepts simultaneously. A **relationship** refers to a bond or connection (or pattern of association) between two phenomena. Quantitative researchers focus on the relationship between the independent variables and dependent variables.

In a quantitative study, the steps involved in the conduct of an investigation are fairly standard, and the researcher progresses in a fairly linear fashion from the posing of a research question to answering it. The conceptual phase involves (1) defining the problem to be studied; (2) doing a **literature review;** (3) developing a theoretical framework; and (4) formulating **hypotheses** to be tested. The design and planning phase includes (5) selecting a **research design;** (6) specifying the **population;** (7) specifying the methods to measure the research variables; (8) selecting a **sample;** (9) finalizing the research plan; and (10) conducting a **pilot study** and making revisions. The empirical phase involves (11) collecting the data and (12) preparing the data for analysis. The analytic phase includes (13) analyzing the data through **statistical analysis** and (14) interpreting the results. The dissemination phase involves (15) communicating the findings and (16) promoting their utilization.

The flow of activities in a qualitative study is more flexible and less linear. The qualitative researcher begins with a broad question regarding the phenomenon of interest, often focusing on a little-studied aspect. The focus is less likely to be sharpened by reviewing the literature than by the actual process of data collection and analysis. In the early phase, the researcher selects a **setting** and then seeks to **gain entrée** into it. Once in the field, the researcher selects informants, collects data, and analyzes and interprets the data in an iterative fashion. Early analysis leads to refinements in sampling and data collection, until **saturation** (redundancy of information) is achieved. The qualitative researcher concludes by writing a research report.

Students are most likely to encounter research findings reported in professional journals. Research **journal articles** provide brief descriptions of research studies and are designed to communicate the contribution the study has made to knowledge. Journal articles often consist of six major sections: the **abstract** (a brief synopsis of the study); the introduction (which explains the study problem and its context); the methods (the strategy the researcher used to address the research problem); the results (the actual study findings); the discussion (the interpretation of the findings); and the references. Qualitative research reports are written in a more inviting, conversational, and personal style than quantitative ones. Beginning research consumers have a more difficult time reading quantitative journal articles because of their conciseness, their use of technical terms, the impersonal style, and the description of **statistical tests.** Students may need to translate the ideas contained in a quantitative research article before trying to digest them.

▧ STUDY SUGGESTIONS

Chapter 2 of the accompanying *Study Guide to Accompany Essentials of Nursing Research,* 4th edition offers various exercises and study suggestions for reinforcing the concepts presented in this chapter.

Suggested Readings

Methodologic References

Kerlinger, F. N. (1986). *Foundations of behavioral research* (3rd ed.). New York: Holt, Rinehart & Winston.

Morse, J. M., & Field, P. A. (1995). *Qualitative research methods for health professionals* (2nd ed.). Thousand Oaks, CA: Sage Publications.

Tornquist, E. M., Funk, S. G., Champagne, M. T., & Wiese, R. A. (1993). Advice on reading research: Overcoming the barriers. *Applied Nursing Research, 6,* 177–183.

Substantive References

Admi, H. (1995). "Nothing to hide and nothing to advertise": Managing disease-related information. *Western Journal of Nursing Research, 17,* 484–501.

Anderson, G. C., Lane, A. E., & Chang, H. P. (1995). Axillary temperature in transitional newborn infants before and after tub bath. *Applied Nursing Research, 8,* 123–128.

Evans, M. L., Dick, M. J., & Clark, A. S. (1995). Sleep during the week before labor: Relationships to labor outcomes. *Clinical Nursing Research, 4,* 238–252.

Fridriksdottir, N., & McCarthy, D. O. (1995). The effect of caloric density on energy intake and body weight in tumor-bearing rats. *Research in Nursing and Health, 18,* 357–363.

Fuller, B. F., & Conner, D. A. (1995). The effect of pain on infant behaviors. *Clinical Nursing Research, 4,* 253–273.

Good, M. (1995). A comparison of the effects of jaw relaxation and music on postoperative pain. *Nursing Research, 44,* 52–57.

Horns, P. N., Ratcliffe, L. P., Leggett, J. C., & Swanson, M. S. (1996). Pregnancy outcomes among active and sedentary primiparous women. *Journal of Obstetric, Gynecologic, and Neonatal Nursing, 25,* 49–54.

Jarrett, M. E., & Lethbridge, D. J. (1994). Looking forward, looking back: Women's experience with waning fertility during midlife. *Qualitative Health Research, 4,* 370–384.

King, S., Collins, C., & Liken, M. (1995). Values and the use of community services. *Qualitative Health Research, 5,* 332–347.

Langner, S. R. (1993). Ways of managing the experience of caregiving to elderly relatives. *Western Journal of Nursing Research, 15,* 582–594.

McDonald, D. D. (1994). Gender and ethnic stereotyping in narcotic analgesic administration. *Research in Nursing and Health, 17,* 45–49.

Narsavage, G. L., & Weaver, T. E. (1994). Physiologic status, coping, and hardiness as predictors of outcomes in chronic obstructive pulmonary disease. *Nursing Research, 43,* 90–94.

Tiller, C. M. (1995). Fathers' parenting attitudes during a child's first year. *Journal of Obstetric, Gynecologic, and Neonatal Nursing, 24,* 508–516.

Tuten, S. H. & Gueldner, S. H. (1991). Efficacy of sodium chloride versus dilute heparin for maintenance of peripheral intermittent intravenous devices. *Applied Nursing Research, 4,* 63–71.

Watters, N. E., & Kristiansen, C. M. (1995). Two evaluations of combined mother-infant versus separate postnatal nursing care. *Research in Nursing and Health, 18,* 17–26.

Preliminary Steps in the Research Process

PART II

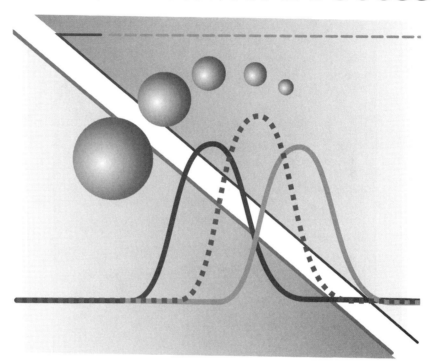

Research Problems, Research Questions, and Hypotheses

Student Objectives

On completion of this chapter, the student will be able to:

- cite five different sources of ideas for a research problem
- describe the process of developing and refining a research problem
- evaluate the compatibility of a research problem and a paradigm
- evaluate a research problem in terms of its significance, researchability, and feasibility
- distinguish the functions and forms of statements of purpose and research questions for quantitative and qualitative studies
- describe the function and characteristics of research hypotheses
- distinguish different types of hypotheses (*e.g.,* simple versus complex, directional versus nondirectional, research versus null)
- locate statements of purpose, research questions, and/or hypotheses in research reports
- critique statements of purpose, research questions, and/or hypotheses in research reports with respect to their placement, clarity, and wording
- define new terms in the chapter

New Terms

Complex hypothesis
Directional hypothesis
Hypothesis
Multivariate hypothesis
Nondirectional hypothesis
Null hypothesis
Objective
Problem statement

Research aim
Research hypothesis
Research problem
Research question
Simple hypothesis
Statement of purpose
Statistical hypothesis

A research study begins as a problem that a researcher would like to solve or as a question (or set of questions) that a researcher would like to answer. Often the question or problem evolves from a broad topic area, and researchers usually find it necessary to devote some time to delimiting and explicating the problem. Quantitative researchers, in particular, are apt to formulate a refined and specific research question or hypothesis that guides the development of a research design and the plan for the collection and analysis of data. This chapter discusses the formulation and evaluation of research questions and hypotheses. We begin by clarifying some related terms.

At the most general level, a researcher is interested in a **topic,** which is sometimes referred to as the **focus** of the research. Examples of research topics are adolescent smoking, patient compliance, coping with disability, and pain management. Within each of these broad topic areas are many potential research questions or research problems.

A **research problem** is a situation involving an enigmatic, perplexing, or conflictful condition. Both qualitative and quantitative researchers identify a research problem within a broad topic area of interest. The purpose of disciplined research is to "solve" the problem—or to contribute to its solution—by accumulating sufficient information to lead to understanding or explanation. A **research question** is a statement of the specific query the researcher wants to answer, to address the research problem. The research question or questions guide the types of data to be collected in the study. Research questions are sometimes referred to as formal **problem statements,** especially in quantitative studies. If a researcher makes a specific prediction regarding the answers to the research questions, he or she poses a **hypothesis** that is tested empirically.

In a research report, consumers are also likely to encounter other related terms. For example, many reports include a **statement of purpose** (or purpose statement), which is the researcher's summary of the overall goal of a study. A researcher might also identify several specific **research aims** or **objectives**—the specific accomplishments the researcher hopes to achieve by conducting the study. The objectives include obtaining answers to the research questions or testing the research hypotheses, but may also encompass some broader aims (*e.g.,* to develop recommendations for changes to nursing practice based on the study results).

These various terms are not always consistently defined in research methods textbooks, and differences between the terms are often subtle. Table 3–1 illustrates the interrelationships among the terms as we have defined them.

RESEARCH PROBLEMS

Sources of Research Problems

Students are sometimes puzzled about the origins of research problems. Where do ideas for research problems come from? How does a researcher identify a topic area and develop research questions? At the most basic level, topics for disciplined research originate with the interests of the researcher. Because research is a time-consuming enterprise, curiosity about and interest in a topic are essential to the success of the project. Explicit sources that might fuel the researcher's curiosity include experience, the nursing literature, social issues, theories, and ideas from others.

Experience. The nurse's everyday experience provides a rich supply of problems for investigation. Problems that are in need of immediate solution or that excite the curiosity are relevant and have high potential for clinical signifi-

Table 3–1. Example of Terms Relating to Research Problems

Term	Example
Topic/focus	Side effects in chemotherapy patients
Research problem	Nausea and vomiting are common side effects among chemotherapy patients. What intervention can reduce or prevent these side effects?
Statement of purpose	The purpose of the study is to test an intervention to reduce chemotherapy-induced side effects—specifically, to compare the effectiveness of patient-controlled and nurse-administered antiemetic therapy for controlling nausea and vomiting in chemotherapy patients.
Research question (Problem statement)	What is the relative effectiveness of patient-controlled antiemetic therapy versus nurse-controlled antiemetic therapy with regard to (a) medication consumption and (b) control of nausea and vomiting in chemotherapy patients?
Hypotheses	(1) Subjects receiving antiemetic therapy by way of a patient-controlled pump will report less nausea than subjects receiving the therapy by way of nurse-administration; (2) Subjects receiving antiemetic therapy by way of a patient-controlled pump will vomit less than subjects receiving the therapy by way of nurse-administration; (3) Subjects receiving antiemetic therapy by way of a patient-controlled pump will consume less medication than subjects receiving the therapy by way of nurse-administration.
Aims/objectives	This study seeks to accomplish the following objectives: (1) to develop and implement two alternative procedures for administering antiemetic therapy for patients receiving moderate emetogenic chemotherapy (patient-controlled versus nurse-controlled); (2) to test three hypotheses concerning the relative effectiveness of the alternative procedures on medication consumption and control of side effects; and (3) to use the findings to develop recommendations for possible changes to therapeutic procedures.

cance. Nurses may ask such questions as: I wonder what would happen if . . . ? Why are things done this way? What approach would work better? What is really going on? Nurses who pose such questions about areas of interest to them may well be on their way to identifying a researchable problem for a nursing study.

Nursing Literature. Ideas for research projects often come from reading the nursing literature, including published research reports as well as opinion articles, anecdotes, and discussions of clinical issues. Published research reports may suggest problem areas indirectly by stimulating the reader's imagination and directly by explicitly stating the types of additional research that are needed. Inconsistencies or gaps in the reported findings of studies sometimes generate new ideas for research studies. Thus, a familiarity with existing research or with problematic and controversial nursing issues is an important route to developing a research topic.

Social Issues. Sometimes topics are suggested by more global contemporary social or political issues of relevance to the health-care community. For example, the feminist movement has raised questions about such topics as gender equity, sexual harassment, and domestic violence. The civil rights movement has led to research on minority health problems, access to health care, and other relevant topics.

Theories. The fourth major source of problems lies in the theoretical schemes and conceptual frameworks that have been developed in nursing and other related disciplines. A researcher sometimes works from a theory of interest to a research problem, through a process of deduction. Essentially, the researcher asks: If this theory is correct, what are the implications for people's behaviors, states, or feelings in certain situations or under certain conditions?

Ideas From External Sources. External sources can sometimes provide the impetus for a research idea. In some cases (*e.g.,* in a research course), a research topic may be given to students as a direct suggestion. In other cases, ideas for studies may emerge as a result of a brainstorming session or from discussions with other nurses, researchers, or nursing faculty.

Development and Refinement of Research Problems

The development of a research problem is essentially a creative process, dependent on imagination and insight. Researchers often begin with an interest in some broad topic area, such as anxiety in hospitalized children, postpartum depression, postoperative loss of orientation, and so on. Once a broad topic is identified, the researcher must transform the topic into a more specific researchable problem. It is impossible for any researcher to study all aspects of a topic.

Let us consider an example of the refinement process. Suppose a nurse working on a medical unit observed that some patients always complained about having to wait for pain medication when certain nurses were assigned to them. The nurse wonders why this phenomenon occurs. The general research problem is discrepancy in complaints from patients regarding pain medications administered by different nurses. The nurse might ask, What accounts for this discrepancy? or, How could this situation be altered? These questions are not the final research questions because they are too broad and vague. They may, however, lead the nurse to other questions, such as, How do the two groups of nurses differ?, or What characteristics do the complaining patients share? At this point, the nurse may observe that the cultural background of the patients and nurses appears to be a relevant factor. This may direct the nurse to a review of the literature for studies concerning ethnic subcultures and their relationship to nursing behaviors, or it may provoke a discussion of these observations with peers. The result of these efforts may be several researchable problems, such as the following:

- What is the essence of patient complaints among patients of different ethnic backgrounds?
- How do complaints by patients of different ethnic backgrounds get expressed by patients and perceived by nurses?
- How do the interactions between nurses and patients differ among nurses and patients with same or dissimilar ethnic backgrounds?
- Is the ethnic background of nurses related to the frequency with which they dispense pain medication?
- Is the ethnic background of patients related to the frequency and intensity of their complaints of having to wait for pain medication?
- Does the number of patient complaints increase when the patients are of dissimilar ethnic backgrounds as opposed to when they are of the same ethnic background as the nurse?
- Do nurses' dispensing behaviors change as a function of the similarity between their own ethnic background and that of the patients?

All these questions stem from the same general problem, yet each would be studied in a different manner. Some suggest a qualitative approach and others suggest a quantitative one. Researchers choose the final problem to be studied based on several factors, including its inherent interest to them and its compatibility with a paradigm of preference.

Research Problems and Paradigms

Although there is some overlap in the type of research problems that can be addressed within the context of the two major paradigms, there are certain problems that are better suited for qualitative and quantitative studies. Quantitative studies usually involve concepts that are fairly well developed, about which there is an existing body of literature, and for which reliable methods of measurement have been developed. In our example of patient complaints about waiting for medications, a quantitative researcher might become curious about nurses' dispensing behaviors, based on some interesting evidence in the literature regarding ethnic differences. Both ethnicity and nurses' dispensing behaviors are variables that can be measured in a straightforward and reliable manner. Generally, a quantitative researcher is likely to pursue a research problem that has been previously explored but has yielded results that need verification, clarification, or extension.

Qualitative studies are often undertaken because some aspect of a concept is poorly understood, and the researcher wants to develop a rich, comprehensive, and context-bound understanding of a phenomenon. In our example, a qualitative researcher who noticed differences in patient complaints would likely be more interested in understanding the *essence* of the complaints, the patients' *experience* of frustration, the *process* by which the problem got resolved, or the full *nature* of the nurse–patient interactions vis-à-vis the dispensing of medications. These are aspects of the research problem that would be difficult to measure quantitatively.

In evaluating a research report, an important consideration is whether the research problem fits the chosen paradigm and its associated methods. Other factors to take into account are discussed next.

Significance, Researchability, and Feasibility of Research Problems

Whether you are developing your own research study or critiquing someone else's, several considerations should be kept in mind in assessing the value of a research problem. A key issue in evaluating a nursing research problem is its significance to nursing. Answers to the research questions should have the potential of contributing to nursing knowledge in a meaningful way. The following issues are relevant:

- Is the problem an important one? Are there practical applications that might stem from the research?
- Does the possibility exist that patients, nurses, or the broader health-care community will benefit by the knowledge produced?
- Can the findings potentially help to improve nursing practice?
- Will more knowledge about the problem make a difference that matters?
- Will the findings contribute to nursing theory?

If the answer to all these questions is no, the worth of the research problem is probably low.

Another consideration in evaluating a problem is its researchability. Not all questions are amenable to study through disciplined research. Problems or issues of a moral or ethical nature, although provocative, are not researchable. An example of such a question is, Should nurses join unions? The answer to this question is ultimately based on a person's values. There are no right or wrong answers, only points of view. The question as stated is more suitable to a debate than to scientific research.

In addition to the significance and researchability of a problem, its feasibility needs to be considered. Although most factors that determine the feasibility of studying a problem are relevant primarily to producers of research, consumers should be cognizant of these factors to better appreciate the challenges of conducting disciplined research. The primary factors include the following:

Time. The problem must be one that can be adequately studied within the available time. Qualitative studies are often especially time-consuming.

Cooperation of participants and others. In any study involving human beings, the researcher needs to consider whether prospective participants will be available and willing to cooperate. It is usually necessary to obtain the cooperation of others as well. For example, in institutional settings (*e.g.,* hospitals, clinics, public schools), access to clients or records usually requires administrative approval. In many qualitative studies, a critical requirement is gaining entrée into an appropriate community or institutional setting.

Facilities, equipment, and other resources. Researchers need to consider what facilities and equipment will be required and whether these facilities will be available.

Experience of the researcher. The problem should be one about which the investigator has some experience, knowledge, and personal interest. Moreover, the problem should be one that is compatible with the investigator's research skills (*e.g.,* a researcher trained in quantitative methods may not be sufficiently skilled in qualitative methods to do in-depth field research.)

Ethical considerations. A research problem may not be feasible if a study addressing the problem would pose unfair or unethical demands on the participants. Ethical considerations are discussed in Chapter 5.

COMMUNICATING THE RESEARCH PROBLEM

As suggested in the introduction to this chapter, researchers communicate their research problems in various ways in research reports. The general topic or focus of the research is almost always communicated in the title, the abstract, and/or in the first paragraph of the report. The nature of the research problem, and its background and significance, are usually described in the introduction to the report. Many reports also include both an explicit statement of purpose *and* research questions or hypotheses. (Research objectives as we have defined them are less frequently articulated in research reports, but are almost always found in written research proposals that describe plans for a study before its undertaking.) This section discusses the wording of purpose statements and research questions, and the following major section discusses hypotheses.

Statements of Purpose

Many researchers first state their research problem formally as a broad statement of purpose. The statement captures—usually in one or two sentences—the essence of the study. The purpose statement establishes the general direction of the inquiry and provides a synopsis of its overall goal. The words *purpose* or *goal* usually appear in a purpose statement (The purpose of this study was . . . or The goal of this study was . . .), but sometimes the words *intent, aim,* or *objective* are used instead.

In a quantitative study, the statement of purpose should identify the key study variables and their possible interrelationships, as well as the nature of the population of interest, as in the following example: The purpose of this research was to investigate the effect of renal transplant patients' dependency level on their rate of recovery. This statement indicates the population of interest (renal transplant patients), the independent variable (the patients' dependency level), and the dependent variable (rate of recovery).

In qualitative studies, the statement of purpose indicates the nature of the inquiry, the key concept or phenomenon under investigation, and the group, community, or setting under study, as in the following example: The purpose of this study is to describe the decision-making process of adult children with regard to the placement of elderly parents in nursing homes. This statement indicates that the central phenomenon of interest is the decision-making process relating to nursing home placements, and the group under study is adult children with parents in need of care.

The statement of purpose communicates more than just the nature of the problem. Through the researcher's selection of verbs, a statement of purpose suggests the manner in which the researcher sought to solve the problem or the state of knowledge on the topic. That is, a study whose purpose is to *explore* or *describe* some phenomenon is likely to be an investigation of a little-researched topic; such a study often involves a qualitative approach. A statement of purpose for a qualitative study may also imply a flexible design through the use of verbs such as *understand, discover,* and *develop.* By contrast, a purpose statement indicating that the purpose is to *test* the effectiveness of some intervention or to *compare* two alternative nursing strategies suggests a study with a better established knowledge base, using a quantitative approach and perhaps a design with tight scientific controls. Note that the researcher's choice of verbs in a statement of purpose should connote a certain degree of objectivity. A statement of purpose indicating that the intent of the study was to *prove, demonstrate,* or *show* something suggests a bias on the part of the researcher. Some examples of well-worded statements of purpose from quantitative and qualitative nursing research studies are presented in Table 3–2.

Research Questions

Research questions are, in some cases, direct rewordings of statements of purpose, phrased interrogatively rather than declaratively, as in the following examples:

- What is the relationship between the dependency level of renal transplant patients and their rate of recovery?
- What is the process by which adult children make decisions regarding the placement of their elderly parents in nursing homes?

The question form has the advantage of simplicity and directness. Questions invite an answer and help to focus the researcher's and the reader's attention on the kinds of data that would have to be collected to provide that answer. Some research reports thus omit a statement of purpose and state only the research question.

Other researchers use a set of research questions to clarify or lend greater specificity to the purpose statement. For example, the statement of purpose might

Table 3–2. Examples of Statements of Purpose
From the Nursing Research Literature

Statement of Purpose	Key Concepts/ Variables*	Population/Study Group
Quantitative Studies		
The purpose of this study was to examine the effects of a computer network on decision-making confidence and skill for caregivers of persons with Alzheimer's disease. (Brennan, Moore, & Smyth, 1995)	Computer network intervention (IV) Decision-making confidence and skill (DV)	Caregivers of Alzheimer disease patients
The purpose of this study was to compare deaf parents' perceptions of their family's functioning with hearing parents' perceptions of their family functioning. (Jones, 1995)	Deafness status of child (IV) Perceptions of family functioning (DV)	Parents of deaf and hearing children
Qualitative Studies		
The purpose of this study was to examine whether reciprocity as a dimension of social support exists in the social network of caregivers. (Neufeld & Harrison, 1995)	Reciprocity	Caregivers
The purpose of this exploratory study is to understand and develop the concept of empowerment from a theoretical and practical perspective with a particular focus on women's perception of the meaning of empowerment in their lives. (Shields, 1995)	Empowerment	Women

*Independent variable (IV); dependent variable (DV).

be the following: The purpose of this research was to study psychosocial functioning among married couples experiencing a fertility problem. Some specific research questions stemming from this overall purpose might be as follows:

- What percentage of husbands and wives in infertile couples experience depression and depressive symptoms?
- Do husbands in infertile couples differ from wives with respect to their levels of depression?
- What are the coping strategies used by husbands and wives to deal with their infertility?

• Does infertility treatment lead to lower levels of depression among married people with a fertility problem?

In a quantitative study, research questions identify the key variables (most often, the independent and dependent variable), the relationships among them if a relationship is being studied, and the population under study. If a set of questions is used to elaborate upon a broad statement of purpose, the research question would delineate, in fairly specific terms, the measurable research variables (*e.g.,* level of depression).

In qualitative studies, the research questions often evolve and change over the course of the study. At the outset, the research question is fairly broad, giving the researcher the flexibility to explore the phenomenon in depth, to narrow (or even redirect) the focus of the inquiry in the field, and to evolve in more than one direction. The qualitative researcher ideally begins with a question that provides a general starting point but does not prohibit discovery. Thus, at the beginning, the qualitative research question may be little more than a broad query regarding the study focus (*e.g.,* Why do some patients complain about waiting for pain medications?) As the researcher collects and analyzes data, the research question becomes progressively more focused (*e.g.,* What is the essence of patient complaints and how are these complaints expressed by patients of different ethnic backgrounds?). In a research report, only the final research question is usually presented.

Some examples of research questions from the quantitative and qualitative nursing studies are presented in Table 3–3.

THE RESEARCH HYPOTHESIS

What Is a Research Hypothesis?

In quantitative studies, researchers often present a statement of purpose and then one or more hypotheses. A hypothesis is a tentative prediction or explanation of the relationship between two or more variables; a hypothesis thus translates a research question into a precise prediction of expected outcomes. In a qualitative study, the researcher does not begin with a hypothesis, in part because there is generally too little known about the topic to justify a hypothesis, and in part because qualitative researchers want their inquiry to be guided by participants' viewpoints rather than by their own. Thus, our discussion here focuses on hypotheses used to guide the inquiry in quantitative research.

Research questions, as we have seen, are queries about how phenomena are related and interact. Hypotheses, on the other hand, are tentative solutions or answers to these research queries. For instance, the research question might ask: Does room temperature affect the optimal placement time of rectal temperature measurements in adults? As a tentative solution to this problem, the researcher might predict the following: Cooler room temperatures require longer placement

Table 3–3. Examples of Research Questions
From the Nursing Research Literature

Research Question	Variables*/Concept
Quantitative Studies	
Among patients with some form of cardiovascular disease, are older patients less likely than younger ones to return to precardiovascular disease levels of sexual activity? (Quandagno et al., 1995)	Patient's age (IV) Resumption of sexual activities (DV)
Do obese pregnant women develop more obstetric complications than nonobese pregnant women? (Morin, 1995)	Obesity status (IV) Obstetric complications (DV)
Qualitative Studies	
How do adults view the prospective loss of their parents? (Fitzgerald, 1994)	Views about parental loss
How do elders survive in the midst of "drug warfare" in an inner-city community known for its dangerous streets and public spaces? (Kauffman, 1995)	Elder survival in a dangerous environment

*Independent variable (IV); dependent variable (DV).

times for rectal temperature measurements in adults than warmer room temperatures.

Hypotheses sometimes follow directly from a theoretical framework. The scientist reasons from theories to hypotheses and tests those hypotheses in the real world. The validity of a theory is never examined directly. Rather, it is through hypotheses that the worth of a theory can be evaluated. Let us take as an example the general theory of reinforcement. This theory maintains that behavior or activity that is positively reinforced (rewarded) tends to be learned or repeated. Because nurses play an important teaching and guiding role in hospitals or clinical settings, there are many opportunities for this general theory to be incorporated into the context of nursing practice. The theory is too abstract to be put to an empirical test. Nevertheless, if the theory is valid, then it should be possible to make predictions (hypotheses) about certain kinds of behavior in hospitals. For example, the following hypotheses have been deduced from reinforcement theory: (1) Elderly patients who are praised (reinforced) by nursing personnel for self-feeding require less assistance in feeding than patients who are not praised; and (2) Pediatric patients who are given a reward (*e.g.*, cookies or permission to watch television) when they cooperate during nursing procedures tend to be more compliant during those procedures than nonrewarded peers. Both of these propositions can be put to a test in the real world. If the hypotheses are confirmed, the theory is supported, and we can place more confidence in it.

Not all hypotheses are derived from theory. Even in the absence of a theoretical underpinning, well-conceived hypotheses can offer direction and suggest explanations in a quantitative study. Perhaps an example will clarify this point. Suppose we hypothesized that nurses who have received a baccalaureate education are more likely to experience stress in their first nursing job than nurses with a diploma-school education. We could justify our speculation on the grounds of a theory (*e.g.,* role conflict theory, cognitive dissonance theory), on the basis of earlier studies, as a result of personal observations, or on the basis of some combination of these.

> *The development of predictions in and of itself forces the researcher to think logically, to exercise critical judgment, and to tie together earlier research findings.*

Now let us suppose the above hypothesis is not confirmed by the evidence collected; that is, we find that baccalaureate and diploma nurses demonstrate an equal amount of stress in their first nursing assignment.

> *The failure of data to support a prediction forces the investigator to critically analyze theory or previous research, to carefully review the limitations of the study's methods, and to explore alternative explanations for the findings.*

The use of hypotheses in quantitative studies tends to induce critical thinking and, hence, to facilitate understanding and interpretation of the data.

To further illustrate the utility of hypotheses, suppose we conducted the investigation guided only by the research question, Is there a relationship between a nurse's basic preparation and the degree of stress experienced on the first job? The investigator without a hypothesis is, apparently, prepared to accept any results. The problem is that it is almost always possible to explain something superficially after the fact, no matter what the findings are. Hypotheses guard against superficiality and minimize the possibility that spurious results will be misconstrued.

Characteristics of Workable Hypotheses

An essential characteristic of a workable research hypothesis is that it states the relationship between two or more measurable variables. The variables related to one another through the hypothesis are the independent variable (the presumed cause or antecedent) and the dependent variable (the presumed effect or phenomenon of primary interest). Unfortunately, researchers occasionally present hypotheses that fail to make a relational statement. The following prediction is not an acceptable research hypothesis: Pregnant women who receive prenatal instruction by a nurse regarding the immediate postpartum experience are not likely to experience postpartum depression. This statement expresses no anticipated relationship; in fact, there is only one variable (postpartum depression), and a relationship by definition requires at least two variables. This prediction, however, can be altered to make it a suitable hypothesis with an independent variable and dependent variable: Pregnant women who receive prenatal instruction are less likely to experience postpartum depression than pregnant women with no prenatal instruction. Here the dependent variable is the women's depression and the independent variable is their status with respect to prenatal instruction—some will have received it and others will not have received it.

The relational aspect of the prediction is embodied in the phrase *less than.* If a hypothesis lacks a phrase such as more than, less than, greater than, different from, related to, associated with, or something similar, it is not amenable to testing in a quantitative study. As an example of why this is so, consider the original prediction: Pregnant women who receive prenatal instruction are not likely to experience postpartum depression. How would we know whether this hypothesis was supported—what absolute standard could be used to decide whether to accept or reject the hypothesis? To illustrate the problem more concretely, suppose we asked a group of mothers who have been given instructional sessions on the postpartum experience the following question 1 month after delivery: On the whole, how depressed have you been since you gave birth—would you say:

1. Extremely depressed,
2. Moderately depressed,
3. Somewhat depressed, or
4. Not at all depressed?

Based on this question, how could we compare the actual outcome with the predicted outcome? Would *all* the women in the sample have to say they were not at all depressed? Would the prediction be supported if 51% of the women said they were not at all depressed *or* only somewhat depressed? There is no adequate way of testing the accuracy of the prediction. A test is simple, however, if we modify the prediction, as suggested above, to: Pregnant women who receive prenatal instruction are less likely to experience postpartum depression than those with no prenatal instruction. We could simply ask two groups of women with different prenatal instruction experiences to respond to the question and then compare the responses of the two groups. The absolute degree of depression of either group would not be at issue.

Hypotheses, ideally, should be based on sound, justifiable rationales. The most defensible hypotheses follow from previous research findings or are deduced from a theory. When a relatively new area is being investigated, the researcher may have to turn to logical reasoning or personal experience to justify the predictions.

Wording of the Hypothesis

Hypotheses state the expected relationship between the independent variables and dependent variables. When there is a single independent variable and a single dependent variable, the hypothesis is referred to as a **simple** (or univariate) **hypothesis. A complex** (or **multivariate**) **hypothesis** is one that predicts a relationship between two or more independent variables or two or more dependent variables. Complex hypotheses offer the advantage of allowing researchers to mirror the complexity of the real world in their research problems. Table 3–4 presents some examples of simple and complex hypotheses. Each of these hypotheses is potentially testable, and each delineates a predicted relationship. Novice research students should carefully scrutinize this table to familiarize themselves with the language and style of research hypotheses.

Although researchers adopt a certain style in the phrasing of hypotheses, there is some degree of flexibility. The same hypothesis can be stated in a variety of ways as long as the researcher specifies or implies the relationship that will be tested. As an example of how a hypothesis can be reworded, let us state the first hypothesis from Table 3–4 in several ways:

1. Older patients are more at risk of experiencing a fall than younger patients.
2. There is a relationship between the age of a patient and the risk of falling.
3. The older the patient, the greater the risk that she or he will fall.
4. Older patients differ from younger ones with respect to their risk of falling.
5. Younger patients tend to be less at risk of a fall than older ones.
6. The risk of falling increases with the age of the patient.

Other variations are also possible. The important point to remember is that the hypothesis should specify the independent variables and dependent variables and the anticipated relationship between them.

Hypotheses can be described as being either directional or nondirectional. A

Table 3–4. Examples of Simple and Complex Hypotheses

Hypothesis	Independent Variable	Dependent Variable	Simple or Complex
Older patients are more at risk of experiencing a fall than younger patients.	Age of patients	Falling behavior	Simple
Infants born to heroin-addicted mothers have lower birth weights than infants with nonaddicted mothers.	Addiction versus nonaddiction of mother	Birth weight of infant	Simple
Structured preoperative support is more effective in reducing surgical patients' perceptions of pain and requests for analgesics than structured postoperative support.	Timing of nursing intervention	Patients' pain perceptions; requests for analgesics	Complex
Positive health practices are favorably affected by high self-esteem and greater amounts of social support.	Self-esteem; social support	Health practices	Complex

directional hypothesis is one that specifies the expected direction of the relationship between variables. That is, the researcher predicts not only the existence of a relationship, but also the nature of the relationship. In the six versions of the same hypothesis above, versions 1, 3, 5, and 6 are all directional because there is an explicit expectation that older patients are at greater risk of falling than younger ones.

A **nondirectional hypothesis,** by contrast, does not stipulate the direction of the relationship. Such a hypothesis predicts that two or more variables are related but makes no projections about the exact nature of the association. Versions 2 and 4 in the example illustrate the wording of nondirectional hypotheses. These hypotheses state the prediction that a patient's age and the risk of falling are related; they do not stipulate, however, whether the researcher thinks that older patients or younger patients are at greater risk.

Hypotheses derived from theory almost always are directional because theories attempt to explain phenomena and, hence, provide a rationale for expecting variables to behave in certain ways. Existing studies also supply a basis for specifying directional hypotheses. When there is no theory or related research, when the findings of prior studies are contradictory, or when the researcher's own experience results in ambivalent expectations, the investigator may use nondirectional hypotheses. Some people argue, in fact, that nondirectional hypotheses are preferable because they connote a degree of impartiality or objectivity. Directional hypotheses, it is said, carry the implication that the researcher is intellectually committed to a certain outcome, and such a commitment might lead to bias. This argument fails to recognize that researchers typically *do* have specific expectations or hunches about the outcomes, whether they state those expectations explicitly or not. We prefer directional hypotheses—when there is a reasonable basis for them—because they demonstrate that the researcher has thought critically and carefully about the phenomena under investigation and because they make clear to the readers of a research report the framework within which the study was conducted.

One further distinction should be noted, and that is the difference between research and statistical hypotheses. **Research hypotheses** (also referred to as substantive, declarative, or scientific hypotheses) are statements of expected relationships between variables. All the hypotheses in Table 3–4 are research hypotheses. Such hypotheses indicate what the researcher expects to find as a result of conducting a study.

The logic of statistical inference, which is used in hypothesis testing, operates on principles that are somewhat confusing to many students. This logic requires that, for the purposes of the statistical analysis, hypotheses be expressed as though no relationship were expected. **Null hypotheses** or **statistical hypotheses** state that there is no relationship between the independent variables and dependent variables. The null form of hypothesis 2 in Table 3–4 would be: Infants born to heroin-addicted mothers have the same birth weight as infants born to nonaddicted mothers. The null hypothesis might be compared to the assumption of innocence of an accused criminal in our system of justice; the variables are assumed to be "innocent" of any relationship until they can be shown to be "guilty" through appropriate statistical procedures. The null hypothesis represents the formal statement of this assumption of innocence.

The researcher typically is concerned only with the research hypotheses. Although some research reports express the hypotheses in null form, it is more desirable to state the researcher's actual expectations. When statistical tests are performed, the underlying null hypotheses are usually assumed without being explicitly stated.

Hypothesis Testing and Quantitative Research

The testing of the hypotheses constitutes the heart of most quantitative studies. After the hypotheses are formulated, the researcher must select a research design, identify the appropriate population and sample, develop or choose data collection instruments, gather the data, and analyze the results. Strictly speaking, the statistical analysis performs the test of the hypothesis, but the steps leading up to the analysis are such an integral part of the research process that they may also be considered as operations designed to test the hypotheses.

It must be emphasized, however, that neither theories nor hypotheses are ever proved in an ultimate sense through hypothesis testing. It is inappropriate to say that the data proved the validity of the hypothesis or that the conclusions proved the worthiness of the theory. Findings are always considered tentative. Certainly, if the same results are replicated in a large number of investigations, then greater confidence can be placed in the conclusions. Hypotheses, then, come to be increasingly accepted or believed with mounting evidence, but ultimate proof is never possible.

◩ ASSISTANCE TO CONSUMERS OF NURSING RESEARCH

What to Expect in the Research Literature

One of the first things a reader of a research report needs to know is what the researcher was attempting to accomplish (*i.e.,* what were the research problem, research questions, and/or hypotheses?). Here is what consumers should keep in mind when approaching research reports:

- Although the desirability of having a clearly worded statement of the problem is evident, some research reports fail to state unambiguously the research probelm or questions under investigation. In some studies, therefore, the reader has to infer the research questions from several sources, such as the title of the report and information in the abstract and introduction.
- Many research methods textbooks advise researchers to state their research

questions or purpose early in research reports, preferably in the first or second paragraph, but relatively few research reports adhere to this advice. Researchers most often state their purpose at the end of the introduction or immediately after the review of the literature. (In some respects, this organization has some logic; the author builds a case for doing a new study by reviewing the limitations of earlier research or by indicating the need for new research). Sometimes a separate section of a research report—typically located just before the methods section—is devoted to formally stating the research problem and might be labeled "Purpose," "Statement of Purpose," or "Research Questions."

- Some quantitative research reports explicitly state the research hypotheses that guided the investigation, but most do not. In some cases, the absence of a hypothesis is appropriate, but often, the absence of a hypothesis is an indication that the researcher has failed to consider critically the implications of theory or the existing knowledge base, or has failed to disclose the hunches that may have influenced the design of the study.

- If the researcher used any statistical tests (and most quantitative studies do use them), it usually means that there are underlying hypotheses—whether the researcher explicitly stated them or not—because most statistical tests are designed to test hypotheses.

- If a research report includes the researcher's hypotheses, they usually appear at the end of the introduction, just before the methods section. Hypotheses are typically fairly easy to find and identify because the researcher makes a statement such as, The study tested the following hypotheses . . ., or It was hypothesized that. . . . Table 3–5 presents a few examples of hypotheses from actual nursing studies and indicates their placement in the research reports.

Critiquing Research Problems, Research Questions, and Hypotheses

In critiquing research reports, you will need to evaluate the extent to which the researcher has adequately communicated the research problem. The researcher's description of the problem and statement of the study purpose and research questions set the stage for the description of what was done and what was learned by the researcher. Ideally, you should not have to dig too deeply to decipher the research problem or to discover the questions.

A critique of the actual research problem involves multiple dimensions. One dimension is substantive or theoretical. That is, you should consider whether the substance of the problem has merit for a research investigation. The study's relevance to the advancement of nursing knowledge, practice, and theory needs to be carefully evaluated. A second dimension concerns methodologic issues—in particular, whether the research problem is compatible with the chosen research paradigm

Table 3–5. Examples of Hypotheses From the Nursing Research Literature

Hypothesis	Variables*	Location in Report
Men and women will differ with respect to reported frequency and type of behaviors that could lead to the transmission of HIV (Jadack, Hyde & Keller, 1995)	Gender (IV); behaviors affecting HIV transmission (DV)	At the end of the introduction
Endotracheal suctioning using room temperature normal saline will result in a greater decline in PaO₂ and heart rate alterations than body temperature normal saline. (Gunderson & Stoeckle, 1995)	Temperature of saline (IV); arterial blood gases; heart rate (DVs)	In a separate section just before method section, labeled "Hypothesis"
Optimism will be associated with less delay and less anxiety in seeking care for breast cancer symptoms. (Lauver & Tak, 1995)	Level of optimism (IV) amount of delay; amount of anxiety (DVs)	At the end of the introduction
Nursing home residents exposed to a combined behavior management and mutual goal-setting condition will perform more self-care tasks than those in a behavior management or mutual goal-setting condition alone. (Blair, 1995)	Treatment condition (IV); self-care task performance (DV)	In a separate section after introduction, labeled "Hypotheses"
The availability of adequate self-care resources is directly related to the emotional well-being of caregivers of cognitively impaired adults. (Irvin & Acton, 1996)	Availability of self care resources (IV); emotional well-being of caregivers (DV)	At end of section labeled "Theoretical Framework"

* Independent variable (IV); dependent variable (DV).

and its associated methods. You should also evaluate whether the statement of purpose or research questions have been properly worded.

In a quantitative study, you should determine whether the research report contains explicit hypotheses and, if not, whether their absence is justified. A critique of the actual hypotheses has multiple elements. From a substantive point of view, it is clear that the hypotheses should be logically connected to the research problem and should be consistent with available knowledge or relevant theory. In some cases, this requirement may be difficult to satisfy, as, for example, when findings from previous research on a topic are inconsistent. In such instances, the research report should provide the researcher's rationale for the stated prediction. For example, the researcher may have decided that certain incongruent findings could be discounted because of flaws in the designs of those studies.

The hypothesis is a valid guidepost to scientific inquiry only if it is testable. To be testable, the hypothesis must contain a prediction about the relationship between two or more variables that can be measured. The hypothesis must imply the criteria by which it could be rejected or accepted through the collection of empirical data.

Specific guidelines for critiquing research problems, research questions, and hypotheses are presented in Box 3–1.

� RESEARCH EXAMPLES

This section describes the method in which the research problem and research questions were communicated in two nursing studies, one quantitative and one qualitative. The guidelines in Box 3–1 may be useful in evaluating these aspects of the study.

Research Example of a Quantitative Study

Matthews (1991) was interested in studying maternal satisfaction with breastfeeding during the early postpartum period. Matthews noted that other researchers identified the first few days after birth as a critical period in the breastfeeding relationship but that few studies concentrated on the effect of the neonate's early feeding behavior on the mother's perception of, and satisfaction with, breastfeeding. Matthews' statement of purpose appeared in a section with the heading "Purpose of the Study," which was placed after the literature review and just before the methods section. It stated: "The purpose of this study was to determine how and to what degree the mothers' satisfaction with breastfeeding was influenced by the breastfeeding competence of their neonate" (p. 50).

Guidelines for Critiquing Research Problems, Research Questions, and Hypotheses

Box 3-1

1. What is the research problem? Has the researcher appropriately delimited the scope of the problem?
2. Does the problem have significance for the nursing profession? How will the research contribute to nursing practice, nursing administration, or nursing education?
3. Is there a good match between the research problem and the paradigm within which the research was conducted?
4. Is the problem to be addressed formally stated as a statement of purpose, research question, and/or hypothesis to be tested? Is this information communicated clearly and concisely, and is it placed in a logical and easy-to-find location in the report?
5. Are the purpose statements and/or research questions worded appropriately (*e.g.*, are key concepts/variables identified and the study group/population of interest specified)?
6. If the report does not formally state any hpotheses, is their absence justifiable?
7. Do the hypotheses (if any) flow from a theory or from previous research? If not, what is the basis for the researcher's predictions?
8. Are hypotheses (if any) properly worded (*i.e.*, do they state a predicted relationship between two or more variables)?
9. Are hypotheses directional or nondirectional? Is there a rationale for the manner in which they were stated?
10. Are hypotheses stated as research hypotheses or null hypotheses?

Matthews included four specific research questions: (1) What percentage offeedings are perceived by mothers to be less than satisfactory in the early initiation period of breastfeeding? (2) What is the relationship, if any, between the quality of the breastfeeding performance of the neonate and the mother's pleasure and satisfaction with the feeding? (3) Is there a significant difference between different groups of mothers? and (4) What other effects, if any, did either positive or negative neonatal feeding behaviors have on the mothers?

In the same section of the report, Matthews also presented the following hypothesis: "Mothers whose neonates are having difficulties with breastfeeding, as evidenced by low scores on the Infant Breastfeeding Assessment Tool, will be less pleased with their neonates' feeding behaviors than mothers whose neonates have high scores and are feeding well" (p. 50).

Matthews collected quantitative data from 56 healthy breastfeeding mothers to test this hypothesis and to address the research questions.

Research Example of a Qualitative Study

Artinian (1995) focused on the topic of the helping relationship, a central concept in the practice of nursing. She noted that the helping relationship has various forms, ranging from the minimal involvement of neutrality to the intense involvement of a "special relationship." Artinian was especially interested in studying involvement at the intense end of the spectrum in the context of caring for cancer patients. She noted that existing research had not provided a systematic examination of the *process* of developing special relationships. Her statement of purpose, which was located in the first paragraph of her report, was stated as follows: "The purpose of this study was to explore and describe the process of how nurses form special relationships with cancer patients" (p. 292).

Artinian elaborated upon her statement of purpose by posing four specific research questions (p. 293):

1. Under what conditions do special nurse–patient relationships form?
2. What are the activities that characterize a special relationship? How are these different from the activities of other relationships?
3. What strategies do nurses use to foster or limit special relationships?
4. What are the consequences of special relationships?

To address these questions, Artinian conducted in-depth interviews with 32 oncology nurses who had worked for more than 6 months on cancer units.

▧ SUMMARY

A **research problem** is a perplexing or enigmatic situation that a researcher wants to address through disciplined inquiry. The most common sources of ideas for nursing research problems are experience, relevant literature, social issues, theory, and external sources, such as peers and advisors. The researcher usually begins a research project by identifying a broad **topic** or **focus** of interest. After a topic has been tentatively selected, the researcher must begin the task of narrowing the scope of the problem and identifying questions that are consistent with a paradigm of choice.

A number of criteria should be considered in assessing the value of a research problem. First, the problem should be significant—the research question should contribute to nursing practice or nursing theory in a meaningful way. Second, the problem should be researchable; questions of a moral or ethical nature are inappropriate. Third, a problem may have to be abandoned if the investigation is not feasible. Feasibility involves the issues of time, cooperation of study participants and other people, availability of facilities and equipment, experience of the researcher, and ethical considerations.

Researchers communicate their research problems in research reports as statements of purpose, research questions, and/or hypotheses. A **statement of purpose** is a summary of the overall goal of the study. In both qualitative and quantitative studies, the purpose statement identifies the key concepts (variables) and the study group or population. The purpose statement usually communicates, through the researcher's selection of verbs, the status of knowledge on the topic and the overall approach to the problem. A **research question** (sometimes referred to as a formal **problem statement**) states the specific query the researcher wants to answer to address the research problem.

Quantitative studies may also present one or more hypotheses. A **hypothesis** is a statement of predicted relationships between two or more variables. A workable hypothesis states the anticipated association between the independent and dependent variables. A hypothesis that projects a result for only one variable is essentially untestable because there is typically no criterion for assessing absolute, as opposed to relative, outcomes. A good hypothesis also should be justifiable; it should be consistent with existing theory or knowledge (or with the researcher's own experiences) and with logical reasoning.

Hypotheses can be classified according to various characteristics. **Simple hypotheses** express a predicted relationship between one independent variable and one dependent variable, whereas **complex hypotheses** state an anticipated relationship between two or more independent variables and two or more dependent variables. A **directional hypothesis** specifies the expected direction or nature of a hypothesized relationship. **Nondirectional hypotheses** denote a relationship but do not stipulate the precise form that the relationship will take. Another distinction is between research and statistical hypotheses. **Research hypotheses** predict the existence of relationships; **statistical** or **null hypotheses** express the absence of any relationship. After hypotheses are developed and refined in a quantitative study, they are subjected to an empirical test through the collection, analysis, and interpretation of data. Hypotheses are never proved or disproved in an ultimate sense—they are accepted or rejected, supported or not supported by the data. Through replication of studies, hypotheses and theories can gain increasing acceptance, but scientists, who are essentially skeptics, avoid the use of the word *proof.*

▨ STUDY SUGGESTIONS

Chapter 3 of the accompanying *Study Guide to Accompany Essentials of Nursing Research,* 4th edition offers various exercises and study suggestions for reinforcing the concepts presented in this chapter.

Suggested Readings

Methodologic References

Kerlinger, F. N. (1986). *Foundations of behavioral research.* (3rd ed.). New York: Holt, Rinehart and Winston.
Moody, L., Vera, H., Blanks, C., & Visscher, M. (1989). Developing questions of substance for nursing science. *Western Journal of Nursing Research, 11,* 393–404.

Polit, D. F., & Hungler, B. P. (1995). *Nursing research: Principles and methods* (5th ed.). Philadelphia: J. B. Lippincott.

Substantive References

Artinian, B. M. (1995). Risking involvement with cancer patients. *Western Journal of Nursing Research, 17,* 292–304.

Blair, C. E. (1995). Combining behavior management and mutual goal setting to reduce physical dependency in nursing home residents. *Nursing Research, 44,* 160–165.

Brennan, P. F., Moore, S. M., & Smyth, K. A. (1995). The effects of a special computer network on caregivers of persons with Alzheimer's disease. *Nursing Research, 44,* 166–172.

Fitzgerald, M. (1994). Adults' anticipation of the loss of their parents. *Qualitative Nursing Research, 4,* 463–479.

Gunderson, L. P., & Stoeckle, M. L. (1995). Endotracheal suctioning of the newborn piglet. *Western Journal of Nursing Research, 17,* 20–31.

Irvin, B. L., & Acton, G. J. (1996). Stress mediation in caregivers of cognitively impaired adults: Theoretical model testing. *Nursing Research, 45,* 160–166.

Jadack, R. A., Hyde, J. S., & Keller, M. L. (1995). Gender and knowledge about HIV, risky sexual behavior, and safer sex practices. *Research in Nursing and Health, 18,* 313–324.

Jones, E. G. (1995). Deaf and hearing parents' perceptions of family functioning. *Nursing Research, 44,* 102–105.

Kauffman, K. S. (1995). Center as haven: Findings of an urban ethnography. *Nursing Research, 44,* 231–236.

Lauver, D., & Tak, Y. (1995). Optimism and coping with a breast cancer symptom. *Nursing Research, 44,* 202–207.

Matthews. M. K. (1991). Mothers' satisfaction with their neonates' breastfeeding behaviors. *Journal of Obstetric, Gynecologic, and Neonatal Nursing, 20,* 49–55.

Morin, K. H. (1995). Obese and nonobese postpartum women: Complications, body image, and perceptions of the intrapartal experience. *Applied Nursing Research, 8,* 81–87.

Neufeld, A., & Harrison, M. J. (1995). Reciprocity and social support in caregivers' relationships: Variations and consequences. *Qualitative Health Research, 5,* 348–365.

Quandagno, D., Nation, A. J., Johnson, D., Waitley, C., Waitley, N., Epstein, D., & Satterwhite, A. (1995). Cardiovascular disease and sexual functioning. *Applied Nursing Research, 8,* 143–146.

Shields, L. E. (1995). Women's experiences of the meaning of empowerment. *Qualitative Health Research, 5,* 15–35.

4

Conceptual Contexts for Research Problems: Literature Reviews and Theoretical Frameworks

Student Objectives

On completion of this chapter, the student will be able to:

- describe several purposes of a literature review
- identify several bibliographic aids for retrieving nursing research reports
- locate appropriate references for a research topic
- select appropriate information to include in a review of the literature
- explain the difference between a primary and secondary source
- evaluate the adequacy of the types of information (*e.g.,* research findings versus anecdotes; primary versus secondary sources) included in a written literature review
- evaluate the organization, content, and style of a written review
- identify the major purposes and characteristics of theories
- distinguish between theories, conceptual models, and frameworks
- describe how theory is linked to research in quantitative and qualitative studies
- identify the four concepts included in most conceptual models of nursing
- identify several conceptual models of nursing and several other conceptual models frequently used by nurse researchers
- determine whether a research study was based on a conceptual model or theory and, if it was, identify that model
- discuss the limitations of a study that does not have a theoretical basis or a study whose link to a conceptual framework is artificially contrived
- define new terms in the chapter

New Terms

Abstract journal
Azjen-Fishbein Theory of Reasoned
    Action
Becker's Health Belief Model (HBM)
Borrowed theory
CD-ROM
CINAHL database
Conceptual definition
Conceptual framework
Conceptual map
Conceptual model
Descriptive theory
Electronic database
End-user system
Framework
Grand theory

Grounded theory
Key words
Lazarus and Folkman's Theory of
    Stress and Coping
Literature review
Macro-theory
Mapping
Middle-range theory
Mishel's Uncertainty in Illness Theory
Model
On-line catalog system
On-line search
Orem's Model of Self-Care
Pender's Health Promotion Model
    (HPM)
Primary source

Print index
Schematic model
Secondary source
Statistical model

Subject search
Textword search
Theoretical framework
Theory

Research is usually conducted within a rich context of world views, prior knowledge, and theory relating to the phenomena under study. The link between a research project and its conceptual and knowledge context can take several forms. In this chapter, we discuss two important types of linkages—literature reviews and theoretical frameworks.

◣ LITERATURE REVIEWS

There are two ways in which the term **literature review** is used in research circles. The first refers to the activities involved in searching for information on a topic and developing a comprehensive picture of the state of knowledge on that topic. A nurse may say he or she is doing a literature review before recommending some change in nursing practice. The term is also used to designate a written report that summarizes the state of knowledge on a research problem.

For the person engaged in a research project, becoming acquainted with relevant research literature is usually a critical early task—although, as previously noted, some qualitative researchers deliberately avoid an in-depth literature search before entering the field to avoid having their inquiries guided by prior thought on the topic. However, in most cases, an up-front review of existing research can provide an important context for the study. For instance, a review of work conducted in an area of general interest can help the researcher in the formulation or clarification of a research question. A scrutiny of previous work also acquaints the researcher with what has been done in a field, thereby minimizing the possibility of unintentional duplication and increasing the probability that a new study will make a distinctive contribution to knowledge. Finally—especially in quantitative studies—the review can be highly useful in acquainting the researcher with relevant theory and pointing out the research strategies and specific procedures and instruments that might be productive in addressing the research question.

Researchers usually summarize the literature relevant to their own studies in the introductory section of research reports, regardless of *when* they perform the literature search. The written literature review provides readers with a background for understanding what has already been learned on a topic and illuminates the significance of the new study. Written literature reviews thus serve an integrative function and facilitate the accumulation of knowledge.

Written research reviews are not prepared solely in the context of doing a research study. For example, they may be prepared by nurses who are interested primarily in utilizing research (*e.g.,* in planning an innovative practice or a research-based intervention). Students also prepare written reviews to demonstrate their expertise on a particular topic. Thus, we include information on actually performing a literature review in this book because consumers are frequently expected to locate and summarize information on a research topic. Both consumers and producers of nursing research need to acquire the skills for preparing written summaries of the state of current knowledge on a given problem. This section on literature reviews describes how to locate research literature, how to prepare a written review, and how to critique reviews that appear in research reports.

Locating Relevant Literature for a Research Review

The ability to identify and locate documents on a research topic is an important skill that is worth cultivating. It is also a skill that requires adaptability—rapid technological changes, such as the expanding use of the Internet, are making manual methods of finding information from print resources obsolete, and more sophisticated methods of searching the literature are being introduced continuously. Because the changes are ongoing and the risk of our presenting outdated information is high, we present only a brief glimpse of currently available resources for locating research literature. We urge you to consult with librarians at your institution, who are knowledgeable about the literature, literature retrieval tools, and services in their own libraries.

Electronic Literature Searches

Most college and university libraries now offer students the capability of performing their own searches of **electronic databases** (*i.e.,* huge bibliographic files that can be accessed by computer). Although electronic literature retrieval has been available since the 1970s, it was initially necessary to have the search performed by a librarian, usually at considerable cost. The expanding development of **end-user systems** has made it possible for those without specialized computer expertise to conduct their own electronic search on a terminal or personal computer in a library—or even in their own homes, dorm rooms, or offices.

Access to the various databases is made possible through special software programs distributed by several competing vendors. Currently, the most widely used programs are offered by Aries Knowledge Finder, Ovid, PaperChase, and SilverPlatter. All of these programs are designed to be user-friendly—they are menu-driven with on-screen support, so retrieval usually can proceed with fairly minimal instruction.

Several electronic databases of particular interest to the nursing community can be accessed either through an **on-line search** (*i.e.,* by directly communicating with a host computer over telephone lines) or by way of **CD-ROM** (compact disks that store the bibliographic information). The databases most likely to contain references on nursing research include the following:

- CINAHL (**C**umulative **I**ndex to **N**ursing and **A**llied **H**ealth **L**iterature)
- MEDLINE (**Med**ical Literature On-**Line**)
- PsycLIT (**Psyc**hology **Lit**erature)
- ERIC (**E**ducational **R**esources **I**nformation **C**enter)
- AIDSLINE (**AIDS** Literature On-**Line**)
- CancerLit (**Cancer Lit**erature)
- Health (**Health** Planning and Administration)
- Current Contents

Libraries subscribe to different databases, so not all of these resources are universally available. Most libraries at institutions with a school of nursing do, however, subscribe to CINAHL, one of the most useful databases for nurses.

Before describing the CINAHL database in greater detail, we should also note that the books and other holdings of libraries can almost always be scanned electronically using **on-line catalog systems.** Moreover, through the Internet, the catalog holdings of libraries across the country can be reviewed.

The CINAHL Database

This section illustrates some of the features of an electronic search, through the use of the **CINAHL database,** the most important electronic database for nurses. Our illustrated example relied on the Ovid Search Software for CD-ROM, but similar features are available through other software programs.

CINAHL's database covers references to virtually all English-language and many foreign-language nursing journals, as well as to books, book chapters, nursing dissertations, and selected conference proceedings in nursing and allied health fields. The database covers materials dating from 1982 to the present. In addition to providing bibliographic information (*i.e.,* the author, title, journal, year of publication, volume, and page numbers of a reference), abstracts are available for over 300 journals. Supplementary information such as names of data collection instruments and references cited in the source document are available for many records in the database.

Most searches are likely to begin with a **subject search** (*i.e.,* a search for references relating to a specific topic). After selecting the search command from the main menu, you would type in a single word or phrase that captures the essence of the topic, and the computer would then proceed with the search. Fortunately, CINAHL is a database with **mapping** capabilities, which means you do not have to enter a term that is exactly the same as the CINAHL subject heading. The software translates (maps) the topic you type in to thc most plausible CINAHL subject heading. An important alternative to a subject search is a **textword search** that looks for your topic in text fields of each record, including the title and the abstract.

After you have typed in your topic, the computer will give you feedback on how many "hits" there are in the database (*i.e.,* matches against your topic). In most cases, the number of hits initially will be rather large, and you will want to constrain the search to ensure that you retrieve only the most appropriate references. You can limit your search in a number of ways. For example, you can restrict the search to those for which your topic is the main focus of the document. For most subject headings, you also can select from a number of subheadings specific to the topic you are searching. You might also want only references published in nursing journals; only those that are for research investigations; only those published in certain years (*e.g.,* after 1990); or only those dealing with study participants in certain age groups (*e.g.,* infants).

To illustrate with a concrete example, suppose we were interested in recent research on drug treatments for postoperative pain, and we began our subject search by typing in *postoperative pain.* In the CINAHL database, there are 11 subheadings for this topic, one of which relates to drug therapy. Here is an example of how many hits there were on successive restrictions to the search, using the CINAHL database current to September 1995:

Search Topic/Restriction	*Hits*
Postoperative pain	601
Restrict to main focus	497
Restrict to drug therapy subheading	269
Limit to nursing journals	213
Limit to research reports	58
Limit to 1990–1995 publications	43

This narrowing of the search—from 601 initial references on postoperative pain to 43 references for recent nursing research reports on drug therapies for postoperative pain—took under a minute to perform. Next, we would view the titles of the 43 references on the computer monitor, and we could then display (and print) full bibliographic information for those titles that appeared especially promising. An example of one of the CINAHL record entries for a study identified through this search on postoperative pain treatments is presented in Figure 4–1. Each entry shows an accession number, which is the unique identifier for each record in the database. Then the authors and title of the study are displayed, followed by source information. The source indicates the following:

- Name of the journal (*JOGNN*)
- Volume (23)
- Issue (2)
- Page numbers (99–103)
- Year and month of publication (1994 Feb.)
- Number of cited references (17 ref.)

The printout shows all the CINAHL subject headings for the entry, any one of which could have been used to retrieve this reference through a subject search.

Accession Number

1994186349.

Authors

Gordon SC. Gaines SK. Hauber RP.

Title

Self-administered versus nurse-administered epidural analgesia after cesarean section.

Source

JOGNN—Journal of Obstetric, Gynecologic, & Neonatal Nursing. 23(2):99–103, 1994 Feb. (17 ref).

Cinahl Subject Headings

Adult	Patient Satisfaction
*Analgesia, Epidural	*Patient-Controlled Analgesia
*Cesarean Section/nu [Nursing]	*Postnatal Care
Chi Square Test	*Postoperative Pain/dt [Drug Therapy]
Convenience Sample	Pregnancy
Female	Quasi-Experimental Studies
*Fentanyl/ad [Administration and Dosage]	Research Instruments
Inpatients	T-Tests
	Visual Analog Scaling

Instrumentation

Inventory of Functional Status After Childbirth (IFSAC) (Fawcett).

Abstract

Objective: To compare two methods of administering analgesia by the epidural route after cesarean sections. Design: Quasi-experimental. Setting: The postpartum area of a large community hospital. Participants: Fifty women undergoing planned cesarean sections with epidural anesthesia. Interventions: The control group received continuous epidural analgesia with nurse-administered boluses and the experimental group with self-administered boluses. Main Outcome Measures: Pain control, side effects from medication, amount of medication required, postoperative activity levels, and patient satisfaction. Results: Subjects receiving continuous epidural analgesia with self-administered boluses of analgesic used significantly less fentanyl and fewer supplemental intravenous pain medications than subjects receiving continuous epidural analgesia with nurse-administered boluses of analgesic. Conclusions: Subjects in self-administered group required less pain medication than subjects in nurse-administered group. (17 ref)

Figure 4–1. Example of a printout from a CINAHL search.

Note that the subject headings include both substantive/topical ones (*e.g.,* patient-controlled analgesia, pregnancy) and methodologic ones (*e.g.,* convenience sample, quasi-experimental studies). Next, when formal, named instruments are used in the study, these are printed under Instrumentation. Finally, the abstract for the study is presented. Based on the abstract, we would then decide whether this study was pertinent to our review. Once relevant references are identified, the full research reports can be obtained and read.

Print Resources

Print-based resources that must be manually searched are rapidly being overshadowed by electronic databases, but their availability should not be ignored—especially because smaller libraries (such as hospital libraries) sometimes rely on these print resources due to cost constraints. Moreover, it is sometimes necessary to refer to print resources to perform a thorough search that includes early literature on a topic. For example, the CINAHL database does not include references to research reports published before 1982.

Print indexes are books used to locate research reports in journals and periodicals, books, dissertations, publications of professional organizations, and government documents. Indexes that are particularly useful to nurses are the *International Nursing Index, Cumulative Index to Nursing and Allied Health Literature* (the "red books"), *Nursing Studies Index, Index Medicus,* and *Hospital Literature Index.* Indexes are published periodically throughout the year (*e.g.,* quarterly), with an annual cumulative index. When using a print index, you usually need to first identify the appropriate subject heading. Subject headings can be located in the index's thesaurus, which lists commonly used terms or **key words.** Once the proper subject heading is determined, you can proceed to the subject section of the index, which lists the actual references.

Abstract journals summarize articles that have appeared in other journals. Abstracting services are generally more useful than indexes because they provide a summary of a study rather than just a title. Two important abstract sources for the nursing literature are *Nursing Abstracts* and *Psychological Abstracts.*

Tips on Locating Research Reports

Locating all relevant information on a research question is a bit like being a detective. The various electronic and print literature retrieval tools are a tremendous aid, but there inevitably needs to be some digging for, and a lot of sifting and sorting of, the clues to knowledge on a topic. Here are a few suggestions:

- If you are interested in identifying all major research reports on a topic, you need to be flexible and to think broadly about the key words and subject headings that could be related to the topic in which you are interested. For example, if you are interested in anorexia nervosa in adolescents, you should look under *anorexia, eating disorders,* and *weight loss,* and perhaps under *appetite, eating behavior, nutrition, bulimia, body weight changes,* and *body image.*

- If the topic of interest includes independent and dependent variables, you may need to do separate searches for both. For example, if you were interested in learning about the effect of daily stress on the health beliefs of acquired immunodeficiency syndrome (AIDS) patients, you might want to read about the effects of stress (in general) and about people's health beliefs (in general). Moreover, you might also want to learn something generally about AIDS patients and their problems. If you are searching for references electronically, you can also combine searches, so that the references for two independent searches can be linked (*e.g.,* the computer can identify those references that have both stress and health beliefs as subject headings).

- If you are doing a completely manual search, it is a wise practice to begin the search for relevant references with the most recent issue of the index or abstract journal and then to proceed backward. (Most electronic databases are organized chronologically, with the most recent references appearing at the beginning of a listing.)

- It is rarely possible to identify all relevant studies if you rely on literature retrieval mechanisms exclusively. An excellent method of identifying additional research reports is to find several recently published relevant studies and examine the references at the end. Researchers who are conducting studies on a topic are usually knowledgeable about other research on that topic and refer to major relevant studies as a means of providing a context for their own investigations.

Preparing Written Literature Reviews

The task of identifying references for the literature review, using the guidelines and tools described in the previous section, is the first step in preparing a written review of research literature. Subsequent steps are summarized in Figure 4–2.

Screening References

As Figure 4–2 shows, after identifying potential references, you will need to locate and screen them for relevance and appropriateness. The relevance of the reference concerns the extent to which the reference bears on the research question or topic of interest. You can usually judge the relevance of a reference fairly quickly based on the abstract or a brief perusal of the introduction.

Not all the references identified in a literature search will be appropriate for a research review. The most important type of information for a research review comes from research reports that describe the findings of empirical investigations. As noted in Chapter 2, research reports are published in nursing journals, but they can also be found in books, dissertations, and conference proceedings. You should rely primarily on **primary source** research reports, which are descriptions of studies written by the researchers who conducted them. **Secondary source** research articles are descriptions of studies prepared by someone other than the original

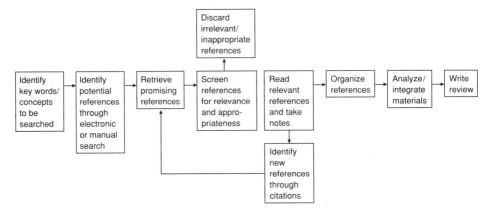

Figure 4–2. Flow of tasks in preparing a written research review.

researcher. For example, literature review articles are secondary sources. Review articles, if they are recent, are an especially good place to begin a literature review because they orient you to what is known and because their list of references is a good source for tracking down the original research reports. However, secondary descriptions of studies should not be considered substitutes for the primary sources.

For some topics, it is also important to include references from the conceptual literature (*i.e.,* references on a theory or conceptual model). Descriptions of theory are useful in providing a conceptual context for a problem, as we discuss later in this chapter. In the conceptual literature, a primary source is a description of a theory written by the developer of the theory, and a secondary source is a discussion or critique of the theory.

In addition to empirical and conceptual references, two other types of references may be identified through the literature search: (1) articles presenting opinions, beliefs, or points of view on the topic of interest; and (2) articles describing anecdotes, clinical impressions, or narrations of incidents and situations. There are numerous papers and articles that focus on an author's opinions or attitudes on a given topic area. These articles are inherently subjective, presenting the suggestions and views of the author. There are also many reports of an anecdotal nature that appear frequently in nursing, medical, and health-related literature, such as in nursing specialty journals. These articles relate the experiences and clinical impressions of the authors.

Opinion articles and anecdotal or other types of nonresearch articles may serve to broaden your understanding of a research problem. These sources may also illustrate a point or demonstrate a need for rigorous research. Thus, these last two sources may play important roles in formulating research ideas, but they generally have limited utility in written research reviews because of their subjective nature and because they do not address the central question of written reviews: What is the current state of knowledge on this research problem? You thus should avoid relying heavily on opinion and anecdotal references in written reviews of the research literature. This is not to say that these materials are uninteresting or unimportant. Generally, however, they are inappropriate in summarizing scientific knowledge about a research question.

Abstracting and Recording Notes

Once a reference has been retrieved and is considered useful, the entire report should be read critically, using guidelines that are provided throughout this book. Notes should be taken as a reminder of the content of the report and its strengths and limitations. The following kinds of information should usually be noted: the full citation, the research question or hypothesis, the methods and procedures, and the results and conclusions. If the article is not a research report, the main points of the author's presentation should be abstracted, together with any collaborating or supportive evidence.

Organizing the Review

Organization of the gathered information is a critical task in preparing a written review. Several devices may help in the successful accomplishment of this task. When the literature on a topic is extensive, it is sometimes useful to organize the findings from studies in a summary table. The table could include columns with headings such as Author, Type of Study (Qualitative versus Quantitative), Number of Participants, Type of Design, Data Collection Approach, and Key Findings. Such a table provides a quick overview that allows the reviewer to make sense of a large mass of information. As an example, Tuten and Gueldner (1991), in the introduction to their study of the effectiveness of sodium chloride versus dilute heparin for maintenance of peripheral intermittent intravenous devices, present an excellent table summarizing earlier research.

Most writers find it helpful to work from an outline. If the review is lengthy and complex, it is useful to write down the outline. For short reviews, a mental outline may be sufficient. The important point is to sit back before starting to write and work out a structure so the presentation has a meaningful flow. Lack of organization is a common weakness in first attempts to write a research review.

Some research reviews can be organized in a chronologic fashion by summarizing the history of research on a topic, but this is likely to prove useful only if clear trends over time can be discerned (*e.g.*, early research on factors associated with adolescent pregnancy focused primarily on knowledge of and access to contraception, but recent research has examined more complex social and psychological factors such as poverty, family functioning, and perceived life options). Another approach is to provide an overview of research on the dependent variable, the independent variable, and then the two combined, followed by research on factors that affect the relationship between the two. Although the specifics of the organization differ from topic to topic, the overall goal is to structure the review in such a way that the presentation is logical, demonstrates meaningful integration, and leads to a conclusion of what is known and not known about the topic.

Once the main topics and their order of presentation have been determined, a review of the notes (or the summary table) is in order. This not only helps refresh your memory about material read earlier but also lays the groundwork for decisions about where a particular reference fits in the outline. If certain references do not seem to fit anywhere, the outline may need to be revised or the references discarded. You should avoid the temptation to force a reference into the review if it does not make a contribution. The number of references used in the review is much less important than the relevance of the references, the quality of the summary, and the overall organization.

Content of a Written Review

A review of the literature should be neither a series of quotes nor a series of abstracts. The central task is to summarize the references so they reveal the current state of knowledge on the selected topic. The review should point out both consistencies and contradictions in the literature as well as offer possible explanations for the inconsistencies (*e.g.,* different conceptualizations or data collection methods).

Studies that are especially important should be described in some detail, including information about the study design, findings, and conclusions. It is neither necessary nor desirable, however, to provide such extensive coverage for every reference. Reports that result in comparable findings can usually be grouped together and briefly summarized, as in the following fictitious example:

> A number of studies have found that the incidence of phlebitis is directly related to the method of administering intravenous infusions and to certain parameters of materials used in the infusions (Wells & Brown, 1996; Yepsen, 1995; Bristol & Wardlaw, 1996).

It is important to summarize a report in your own words. The review should demonstrate that thoughtful consideration has been given to the cumulative significance of the body of research. Stringing together quotes from various documents fails to show that previous research and thought on the topic have been assimilated and understood.

Another point to bear in mind is that the review should be as objective as possible. Studies that fail to support your hypotheses or that conflict with personal values should not be omitted. It is not unusual to find studies with conflicting results. The review should not deliberately ignore a study simply because its findings contradict other studies. Inconsistent results should be analyzed and the supporting evidence evaluated objectively.

The literature review should conclude with a summary or overview of the state-of-the-art position of the problem under consideration. Not only should the summary point out what has been studied and how adequate the investigations have been, it should also make note of any gaps or areas of research inactivity. In other words, the summary requires some critical judgment about the extensiveness and dependability of information on a topic.

As you progress through this book, you will become increasingly proficient in critically evaluating the research literature. We hope you will understand the mechanics of writing a research review once you have completed this chapter, but we do not expect that you will be in a position to write a state-of-the-art review until you have acquired more skills in research methods.

Style of a Research Review

One of the most frequent problems for students preparing a written research review for the first time is adjusting to the style of writing that is used in research reviews. For example, students tend to accept research results without criticism or reservation. This tendency reflects, in part, a common misunderstanding about the degree of conclusiveness that can be achieved through empirical research. You should keep in mind that no hypothesis or theory can be definitively proved or disproved by empirical testing, and no research question can be definitely answered in a single study.

Every study has some limitations, the severity of which depends on the researcher's methodologic decisions. The fact that theories and hypotheses cannot ultimately be proved or disproved does not, of course, mean that we must disregard evidence or challenge every idea we encounter. The problem is partly a semantic one: hypotheses are not proved, but they are *supported* by research findings; theories are not *verified,* but they may be tentatively *accepted* if there is a substantial body of evidence demonstrating their legitimacy. You should learn to adopt this language of tentativeness in writing a review of the literature.

A related stylistic problem is the inclination of novice reviewers to intersperse opinions liberally (their own or someone else's) with the findings of research investigations. The review should use statements of opinions sparingly and should be explicit about the source of the opinion. A description of the point of view of a knowledgeable or influential person may be useful in establishing the need to investigate the problem or in providing a perspective on the topic, but it should occupy a relatively small section of a research review. The researcher's own opinions generally do not belong in a review section, with the exception of an assessment of the quality of existing studies.

The left-hand column of Table 4–1 presents several examples of the kinds of stylistic difficulties we have been discussing in this section. The right-hand column offers some recommendations for rewording the sentences to conform to a more acceptable form for a research literature review. Many alternative wordings are possible.

⬙ ASSISTANCE IN READING AND CRITIQUING LITERATURE REVIEWS

Many nurses may never prepare a written review of research literature. Most nurses, however, do read research reports and, therefore, should be able to evaluate written research reviews carefully and critically. This section provides some assistance to consumers of literature reviews.

Table 4–1. Examples of Stylistic Difficulties for Research Reviews

Inappropriate Style or Wording	Recommended Change
1. It is known that unmet expectations engender anxiety.	Several experts (Abraham, 1996; Lawrence, 1995) have asserted that unmet expectations engender anxiety.
2. The woman who does not participate in childbirth preparation classes tends to manifest a high degree of stress during labor.	Previous studies have indicated that women who participate in preparation for childbirth classes manifest less stress during labor than those who do not (Klotz, 1996; McTygue, 1995).
3. Studies have proved that doctors and nurses do not fully understand the psychobiologic dynamics of recovery from a myocardial infarction.	The studies by O'Hara (1995) and Carson (1996) suggest that doctors and nurses do not fully under the psychobiologic dynamics of recovery from a myocardial infarction.
4. Attitudes cannot be changed overnight.	Attitudes have been found to be relatively enduring attributes that cannot be changed overnight (O'Connell, 1995; Valentine, 1996).
5. Responsibility is an intrinsic stressor.	According to Doctor A. Cassard, an authority on stress, responsibility is an intrinsic stressor (Cassard, 1994, 1995).

NOTE: All references are fictitious.

What to Expect in the Research Literature

Most research reports contain a literature review. Here are a few tips on what to expect:

- Because of space limitations in journal articles, most literature reviews that appear in research reports are fairly brief. The main functions of literature reviews that appear in research reports are to demonstrate the need for the new study and to provide a context for the research questions or hypotheses.
- Sometimes there is a separate review section that is explicitly labeled "Review of the Literature," "Related Literature," or "Background." More often, however, the review is simply integrated into the introduction.
- Some qualitative researchers summarize research literature in their discussion section rather than in the introduction. In such a situation, the researchers use prior studies as the basis for comparing and contrasting research findings.
- Occasionally, an entire journal article is devoted to a research literature review. For example, Bauer (1994) published an integrated review of the research on psychoneuroimmunology in relation to cancer.

Critiquing a Research Review

It is frequently difficult to critique a research review because the reader usually is less familiar with the topic than the writer. Therefore, the reader may not be in a good position to judge whether the author has included all or most of the relevant literature on the topic and may not be able to tell whether the review does a good job of summarizing the state of knowledge on that topic. Many aspects of a research review, however, are amenable to evaluation by readers who are not experts on the topic being reviewed, including aspects discussed earlier in this chapter. Some specific suggestions for evaluating written literature reviews are presented in Box 4–1.

In assessing a written literature review, the overarching question is whether the review adequately summarizes knowledge. If the review is written as part of an original research report, an equally important question is whether the review lays a solid foundation for the new study.

EXAMPLES OF RESEARCH LITERATURE REVIEWS

The best way to learn about the style, content, and organization of a research literature review is to read several reviews that appear in the nursing literature. We present two excerpts from reviews here and urge you to read other reviews on a topic of interest to you.

Guidelines for Critiquing Research Literature Reviews

Box 4–1

1. Does the coverage of the literature seem thorough? Does it appear that the review includes all or most of the major studies that have been conducted on the topic of interest? Is recent literature cited?
2. Does the review rely on appropriate materials (*e.g.,* primarily on research reports, using primary sources)?
3. Is the review organized in such a way that the development of ideas is clear? If the review is part of a research report for a new study, does the review document the need for the new research? Does the review conclude with a synopsis of the state-of-the-art knowledge on the topic?
4. Is the style of the review appropriate? Does the review appear unbiased? Does the reviewer use appropriately tentative language?

Literature Review From a Quantitative Research Report

Holditch-Davis, Barham, O'Hale, and Tucker (1995) conducted a quantitative study to examine the effects of standardized rest periods on the sleep–wake states of preterm infants who are convalescing. The following excerpt represents essentially the entire literature review section of their research report, which appeared in the *Journal of Obstetric, Gynecologic, and Neonatal Nursing.*[1]

> One of the most difficult problems for neonatal nurses is modifying the neonatal intensive-care unit environment so that it provides appropriate stimulation for the growth and development of preterm infants. Preterm infants are adapted to the uterus, a warm, dark environment that provides kinesthetic stimulation and complex hormonal support. By contrast, the neonatal intensive-care unit is a bright and noisy environment with limited diurnal variation, frequent technical procedures, and little positive handling (Duxbury et al., 1984; Gottfried & Gaiter, 1985). Sick infants lack the physiologic reserves to cope with this environment. Critically ill infants become hypoxic in response to such stimulation as noise (Long et al., 1980), technical procedures (Evans, 1991; Peters, 1992), and social touches (Gorski et al., 1983). Even spontaneous changes in sleep–wake states can result in decreased oxygenation (Brazy, 1988; Gabriel et al., 1980).
>
> The intermediate care environment is similar to that of intensive care. Light levels and number of technical procedures are decreased, but preterm infants still experience limited diurnal variation and few social interactions (Blackburn & Barnard, 1985; Gaiter, 1985; Gottfried, 1985). Responses to infant cues are inconsistent. Gottfried (1985) found that nurses responded to fewer than half the cries of premature infants in intermediate or convalescent care.
>
> The sleeping and waking states of preterm infants in particular are affected by the environment. Infants have identifiable sleep–wake states that develop during the preterm period (Curzi-Dascalova et al., 1988; Holditch-Davis, 1990a). Their sleep–wake states are influenced by aspects of the intermediate care environment, such as handling for routine nursing care (Duxbury et al., 1984; Holditch-Davis, 1990b), high levels of light (Moseley et al., 1988), painful procedures (Field & Goldson, 1984; Holditch-Davis & Calhoon, 1989), and interactions between the infants and their parents (Miller & Holditch-Davis, 1992; Minde et al., 1975). However, not all the effects of the intermediate nursery environment are detrimental. For example, interactions with parents appear to decrease arousal and to increase social behaviors (Miller & Holditch-Davis, 1992; Minde et al., 1975). Therefore, determining how the intermediate care nursery (ICN) environment affects sleep–wake states is essential to provide optimal nursing care for preterm infants who are convalescing.
>
> Studies have examined the effects that changes in the ICN have on the sleep–wake states of infants. Gabriel et al. (1981) clustered routine nursing

[1] Reprinted from Holditch-Davis, D., Barham, L. N., O'Hale, A., & Tucker, B. (1995). Effect of standard rest periods on convalescent preterm infants. *Journal of Obstetric, Gynecologic, and Neonatal Nursing, 24,* 424–432, with permission. The reader is referred to this source for the full article and the references cited in the literature review.

care. Strauch et al. (1993) reduced noise levels for 1 hour on each nursing shift. Fajardo et al. (1990) developed a special nursery with diurnal cycles, reduced noise, demand feedings, and responsive nursing care. Other researchers provided greater day–night differentiation by reducing light and/or noise levels at night (Blackburn & Patteson, 1991; Mann et al., 1986). Modifications of the environment to meet the needs of individual infants also have been examined (Als et al., 1986; Becker et al., 1991). Preterm infants benefitted from these changes, but the nature of the benefits differed between studies. Some of the environmental changes resulted in infants experiencing more sleep and fewer state changes (Fajardo et al., 1990; Gabriel et al., 1981; Strauch et al., 1993); decreased activity levels (Blackburn & Patteson, 1991; Fajardo et al., 1990); or less time on mechanical ventilation and earlier bottle feedings (Als et al., 1986; Becker et al., 1991).

The findings of these studies must be interpreted cautiously because most of the studies have small samples (fewer than 15 per group) (Als et al, 1986; Fajardo et al., 1990; Gabriel et al, 1981; Strauch et al., 1993). Control and experimental groups sometimes were not well matched (Fajardo et al., 1990). Often, experimental groups were studied after control groups (Als et al., 1986; Becker et al., 1991; Gabriel et al., 1981). Yet outcomes for infants studied at later time should be better than those studied at an earlier time, even if a special intervention had no effect, because neonatal care is constantly improving. These studies all modified multiple aspects of the environment, and it is impossible to determine whether all the modifications were necessary for the beneficial effects.

The purpose of this study was to determine whether modifying a single aspect of the intermediate care environment alters the sleep–wake patterns of preterm infants. (pp. 424–425)

Literature Review From a Qualitative Research Report

Brodsky (1995) conducted a qualitative study that explored survivors' perceptions of the psychosocial impact of testicular cancer.[2] Brodsky's introduction, all of which is presented below, contained a brief review that was used to frame the study and highlight the need for in-depth research:

Testicular cancer is the most common malignancy in men aged 15–34 (Ganong & Markovitz, 1987) and incidence rates have risen in the United States in recent decades (Schottenfeld et al., 1980). However, there is still a dearth of information pertaining to the male's experience with testicular cancer and its treatment. This is evident in a review of the literature that reveals only two first-person accounts of men who have had testicular cancer (Fiore, 1979; Moreland, 1982), one survey that focused on the psychological aspects of testicular cancer

---

[2] Reprinted from Brodsky, M. S. (1995). Testicular cancer survivors' impressions of the impact of the disease on their lives. *Qualitative Health Research, 5,* 78–96, with permission. The reader is referred to this source for the full article and the references cited in the review.

(Schover & von Eschenbach, 1984), and research that focused on the psychological response of patients cured of advanced cancer (Kennedy et al., 1976).

This lack of information may be due to the fact that in the recent past, few patients ever survived the disease. However, new developments in medical technology have led to increased survival rates. These developments have benefitted patients by keeping them alive, but new problems have been created. These problems pertain to the rehabilitation of patients following treatment. Thus, surviving testicular cancer is a new phenomenon (Donohue et al., 1978; Einhorn, 1987). As a result of its novelty, we do not yet understand the impact of survival on men's sense of self (Gorzynski & Holland, 1979). We are now at the point where we can begin to explore the nature of the phenomenon. Therefore, the focus of this research was to examine changes in one's sense of self due to the experience of having had testicular cancer. (pp. 78–79)

In the discussion section of Brodsky's report, the findings from the research are compared to those from other studies. Here is an excerpt that helps to provide additional context for Brodsky's research:

Others who have made observations about the impact of trauma have uncovered similar findings to those of the researcher. In her qualitative study of people and bereavement, Kessler (1987) found that bereavement, much like the experience of testicular cancer, can help many to "appreciate the preciousness of life and discover inner sources of strength."

Similar findings are supported by Kennedy et al. (1976) who concluded "Patients with advanced cancer apparently cured of the disease have a greater appreciation of time, life, people, and interpersonal reactions. . . ."

Findings also support those of Liss-Levinson (1982) and Farrell (1974). Liss-Levinson recognized males' difficulty with dependency and loss of control. This was verified for almost one half of the respondents in the present study. Farrell (1974) spoke of the men's problems communicating with others on an emotional level. This was reflected in the study by the decision of so few respondents to seek psychiatric assistance in identifying feelings and communicating them to others. . . . Findings by Schover and von Eschenbach (1984) and Cash et al. (1986) concerning the relationship between body image and psychological well-being were also confirmed. (pp. 93–94)

◻ THEORETICAL CONTEXTS

Although a synthesis of existing knowledge is an important task in a study, a literature review in and of itself does not integrate research findings into an orderly, coherent system. Theories and conceptual models are the primary mechanisms by which researchers organize findings into a broader conceptual context.

Theories, Models, and Frameworks

Many different terms are used in connection with conceptual contexts for research, including *theories, models, frameworks, schemes,* and *maps.* There is considerable overlap in how these terms are used, caused in part by the fact that they are used differently by different writers. We offer some guidance in distinguishing these terms, but note that there is often a blurring of these terms in the literature, and that our definitions are not universal.

Theories

The term *theory* is used in many ways. For example, nursing instructors and students frequently use the term to refer to the content covered in classrooms, as opposed to the actual practice of performing nursing activities. In both lay and scientific language, the term *theory* connotes an abstraction or generalization.

Even within research circles, the term *theory* has been defined in various ways. Classically, scientists have used **theory** to refer to an abstract generalization that presents a systematic explanation about how phenomena are interrelated. Thus, the traditional definition requires that a theory embody at least two concepts that are related to one another in a manner that the theory purports to explain.

However, others use the term *theory* less restrictively to refer to a broad characterization of some phenomenon. According to this less restrictive definition, a theory can account for (*i.e.,* thoroughly describe) a single phenomenon. Some authors specifically refer to this type of theory as **descriptive theory.** For example, Fawcett and Downs (1992) define descriptive theories as empirically driven theories that "describe or classify specific dimensions or characteristics of individuals, groups, situations, or events by summarizing commonalities found in discrete observations" (p. 7). Descriptive theory plays an especially important role in qualitative studies. The uses of theory in qualitative and quantitative studies are described later in this chapter.

Regardless of the discipline, theory serves essentially the same functions in disciplined inquiries. *The overall purpose of theory is to make research findings meaningful and interpretable.* Theories allow researchers to knit together observations and facts into an orderly system. The linkage of findings into a coherent structure makes the body of accumulated knowledge more accessible and, thus, more useful both to practitioners who seek to implement findings and to researchers who seek to extend the knowledge base. In addition to summarizing, theories serve to explain research findings. Theory guides the researcher's understanding of not only the *what* of natural phenomena but also the *why* of their occurrence. Finally, theories help to stimulate research and the extension of knowledge by providing both direction and impetus.

Concepts are the basic ingredients of a theory. Examples of nursing concepts are health, interaction, stress, and adaptation. As classically defined, theories also consist of a set of statements or propositions, each of which indicates a relationship. Relationships are denoted by such phrases as *is associated with, varies directly with,* and *is contingent on.* In theories, the propositions form a logically interrelated deductive system. This means that the theory must provide a mechanism for logically arriving at new statements from the original propositions.

We use again a simple illustration of a theory, also referred to as the theory of reinforcement. As we discussed in Chapter 3, this theory posits that behavior that is reinforced (*i.e.,* that is rewarded) tends to be repeated and therefore learned. This theory consists of broad concepts (reinforcement and learning) and a proposition stating the relationship between those concepts. The proposition readily lends itself to deductive hypothesis generation. For example, if the theory of reinforcement is valid, then we could deduce that hyperactive children who are praised or rewarded when they are engaged in quiet play will exhibit less acting-out behaviors than similar children who are not praised. This prediction, as well as many others based on the theory of reinforcement, could then be tested in a study.

It should be noted that theories are abstractions that are created and invented by humans. The building of a theory depends not only on the observable facts in our environment but also on the theorist's ingenuity in pulling those facts together and making sense of them. Because theories are not just "out there" waiting to be discovered or revealed, it follows that theories should be considered tentative. Ultimately, a theory can never be proved—a theory simply represents a theorist's best efforts to describe and explain phenomena. Today's successful theory may be relegated to tomorrow's intellectual junk yard.

Theories have been categorized in a number of different ways. As we have seen, descriptive theory is sometimes distinguished from explanatory or predictive theory. Theories are sometimes classified in terms of their level of generality. **Grand theories** (also known as **macro-theories**) purport to describe and explain large segments of the human experience. Some learning theorists, such as Clark Hull, or sociologists, such as Talcott Parsons, have developed highly general theoretical systems that claim to account for broad classes of behavior and social functioning. Within nursing and fields such as psychology, sociology, and education, theories are usually somewhat restricted in scope, focusing only on a narrow range of phenomena. Theories that focus on only a piece of reality or human experience and that incorporate a selected number of concepts are sometimes referred to as **middle-range theories.** For example, there are middle-range theories that attempt to explain such phenomena as decision-making behavior, infant attachment, and stress. This limited scope is consistent with the state of scientific developments in many fields dealing with human behavior and is, therefore, appropriate and realistic. In the physical sciences, macrotheories such as the theory of mechanics are feasible and provide a goal toward which the younger social and applied sciences may aspire (but may never achieve because of the complexity of human behavior).

Models

Conceptual models represent a less formal and less well-developed mechanism for organizing phenomena than theories. As the name implies, conceptual models deal with abstractions (concepts) that are assembled by virtue of their relevance to a common theme. Conceptual models provide a conceptual perspective regarding interrelated phenomena. However, conceptual models are generally even more abstract and more loosely structured than theories. A conceptual model broadly presents an understanding of the phenomenon of interest and reflects the assumptions and philosophical views of the model's designer. As we discuss later in this chapter, there are many conceptual models of nursing that offer broad explanations of the nursing process. Conceptual models are not directly testable by researchers in the same way that theories are. However, conceptual models, like theories, can serve as important springboards for the generation of hypotheses to be tested.

Some writers use the term **model** to designate a mechanism for representing phenomena with a minimal use of words. Language can sometimes pose problems because a word or phrase that designates a concept can convey different meanings to different people. A visual or symbolic representation of a phenomenon can help to express abstract ideas in a more readily understandable or precise form than the original conceptualization. Two types of model of relevance here are schematic models and statistical models, both of which can be found in the research literature.

Statistical models, not elaborated on here, are mathematic equations that express the nature and magnitude of relationships among variables. A **schematic model** (also referred to as a **conceptual map**) represents a phenomenon of interest figuratively. Concepts and the linkages between them are represented diagrammatically through the use of boxes, arrows, or other symbols. An example of a schematic model is presented in Figure 4–3. This model, known as the **Pender's Health Promotion Model (HPM),** is described by its designer as "a multivariate paradigm for explaining and predicting the health-promotion component of lifestyle" (Pender, Walker, Sechrist & Frank-Stromborg, 1990, p. 326). Schematic models of this type can be useful in the research process in clarifying concepts and their associations, in enabling researchers to place a specific problem into an appropriate context, and in revealing areas of inquiry.

Frameworks

A **framework** is the conceptual underpinnings of a study. Not every study is based on a theory or conceptual model, but every study has a framework. In a study based on a theory, the framework is referred to as the **theoretical framework;** in a study that has its roots in a specified conceptual model, the framework is often called the **conceptual framework** (although the terms *conceptual framework* and *theoretical framework* are often used interchangeably).

In many cases, the framework for a study is implicit (*i.e.,* not formally acknowledged or described by the researcher). The concepts in which a researcher is interested are, by definition, abstractions of observable phenomena, and our world view (and views on nursing) shape how those concepts are defined and operationalized. What often happens, however, is that researchers fail to clarify the conceptual underpinnings of their research variables, thereby making it more difficult to integrate research findings. Consider, for example, the concept of *caring.* Caring can be conceptualized as a human trait, a moral ideal, an affect, an interaction, or an intervention (Morse et al., 1990). A researcher undertaking a study concerned with caring should make clear what **conceptual definition** of caring he or she has adopted (*i.e.,* what the framework for the study is).

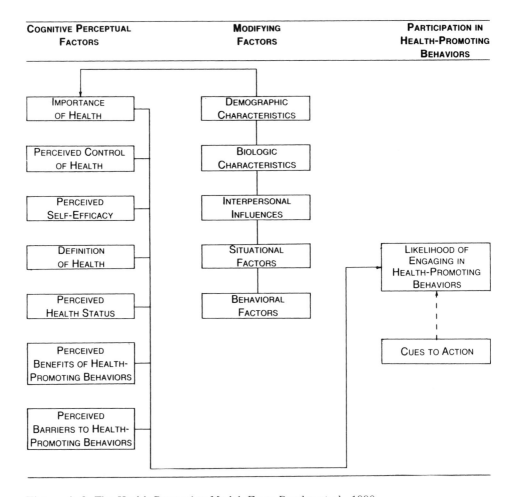

Figure 4–3. The Health Promotion Model. From Pender et al., 1990.

Developing and Testing Theory Through Research

The relationship between theory and research is a reciprocal and mutually beneficial one. Theories and conceptual models are built inductively from observations, and one source for those observations is disciplined research. Concepts and relations that are validated empirically become the foundation for theory development. The theory, in turn, must be tested by subjecting deductions from it (hypotheses) to further scientific inquiry. Thus, research plays a dual and continuing role in theory building and testing. Theory can guide and generate ideas for research; research can assess the worth of the theory and provides a foundation for new ones. While prior research can be used as the basis for theory development, an alternative approach is to conduct qualitative research.

Developing Theory Through Qualitative Research

Qualitative researchers often strive to develop a conceptualization of the phenomena under study that is grounded in the actual observations made by the researcher. As we discuss in Chapter 7, these researchers seek to develop what is referred to as a **grounded theory**—an empirically based conceptualization for integrating and making sense of a process or phenomenon.

Theory development in a qualitative study is primarily an inductive process. The qualitative researcher seeks to identify patterns, commonalities, and relationships through the scrutiny of specific instances and events. During the ongoing analysis of data, the qualitative researcher moves from specific pieces of data to abstractions that synthesize and give structure to the observed phenomenon. The goal is to use the data, grounded in reality, to provide an explanation of events as they occur in reality—not as they have been conceptualized in preexisting theories.

It should be noted that not all qualitative studies have theory development as a goal. Moreover, some qualitative researchers acknowledge an explicit conceptual model as a framework for their study. For example, a number of qualitative nurse researchers acknowledge that the philosophical roots of their studies lie in such conceptual models of nursing as those developed by Rosemarie Parse (1987) or Martha Rogers (1986).

Testing Theory Through Quantitative Research

There are several ways in which quantitative researchers link research to a theory, but the most common approach is to test hypotheses deduced from a previously proposed theory. Usually the theory (or conceptual model) was developed on the basis of cumulated research evidence, but sometimes the theory is the product of a qualitative inquiry. For example, Duffy (1994) conducted a rigorous quantitative study to test a theory (Theory of Transcending Options) developed in a grounded theory study of health behaviors.

The process of theory testing typically begins when a researcher tries to imagine what the implications of the theory or conceptual framework are for some problem of interest. Essentially, the researcher asks the following questions: (1) If this theory or model is correct, what kinds of behavior would I expect to find in specified situations or under certain conditions? and (2) What kinds of evidence could be found to support this theory? Through such questioning, the researcher deduces the implications of the theory in the form of research hypotheses. These hypotheses are predictions about the manner in which the variables would be related, if the theory were correct. For example, a researcher might deduce from reinforcement theory that verbal support and encouragement during primipara's attempts at breastfeeding would result in higher rates of successful continuation with breastfeeding. It should be noted that theories are never tested directly. It is the hypotheses deduced from theories that are subjected to testing. Comparisons between the observed outcomes of research and the relationship predicted by the hypotheses are the major focus of the testing process.

Another situation arises when a researcher uses a theoretical framework in a new study in an effort to explain findings from previous research. For example, suppose that several researchers discovered that nursing home patients demonstrate greater levels of depression, anxiety, and noncompliance with nursing staff around bedtime than at other times of the day. These descriptive findings are interesting and important, but they shed no light on the underlying cause of the problem, and consequently suggest no way to ameliorate it. Several explanations, rooted in such theories as social learning theory, Lazarus' stress and coping model, or one or more of the models of nursing, may be relevant in helping us to understand the behavior and moods of the nursing home patients. By directly testing the theory in a new study of nursing home residents (*i.e.,* deducing hypotheses derived from the theory), a researcher could gain some understanding of *why* bedtime is a vulnerable period for the elderly in nursing homes.

A few nurse researchers have begun to adopt an interesting strategy for furthering knowledge; this involves the direct testing of two competing theories within a single investigation. Almost all phenomena can be explained in alternative ways. The researcher who directly tests alternative explanations, using a single sample of subjects, is in a position to make powerful comparisons about the utility of the competing theories to explain specific phenomena. As an example, Mahon and Yarcheski (1992) tested two explanations for loneliness in adolescents: an explanation dependent on situational factors, and one linking loneliness to characterologic or personality traits. The findings suggested that the situational explanation had more support for older, but not younger, adolescents.

Conceptual Models and Theories Used by Nurse Researchers

Nurse researchers have used both nursing and nonnursing frameworks to provide a conceptual context for their studies. This section briefly discusses frameworks that have appeared in the nursing research literature.

Conceptual Models of Nursing

In the past few decades, nurses have formulated a number of conceptual models of nursing and for nursing practice. These models constitute formal explanations of what the nursing discipline is, according to the developer's point of view. As Fawcett (1989) has noted, four concepts are central to models of nursing: *Person, environment, health, and nursing.* The various nursing models define these concepts differently, link them in diverse ways, and give different emphasis to the relationships among them. Moreover, different models emphasize different processes as being central to nursing. For example, Sister Calista Roy's Adaptation Model identifies adaptation of patients as a critical phenomenon (Roy & Andrews,

1991). Martha Rogers (1986), by contrast, emphasizes the centrality of the individual as a unified whole, and her model views nursing as a process in which individuals are aided in achieving maximum well-being within their potential.

Nurse researchers increasingly are turning toward these conceptual models for their inspiration and conceptual frameworks in formulating research questions and hypotheses. Table 4–2 lists eight conceptual models of nursing, together with a study for each that claimed the model as its framework.

Let us consider one conceptual model of nursing that has received particular attention among nurse researchers in greater detail—**Orem's Model of Self-Care.** Orem's (1985) model focuses on each person's ability to perform self-care, defined as "the practice of activities that individuals initiate and perform on their own behalf in maintaining life, health, and well-being" (p. 35). One's ability to care for oneself is referred to as *self-care agency,* and the ability to care for others is referred to as *dependent-care agency.* In Orem's model, the goal of nursing is to help people meet their own therapeutic self-care demands. Orem's Self-Care Model has been cited as

Table 4–2. Examples of Studies Linked to Conceptual Models of Nursing

Conceptual Model	Research Question
King's Open System Model	What is the effect of a nurse–client transactional intervention on female adolescents' oral contraceptive adherence? (Hanna, 1993)
Levine's Conservation Model	What are the dimensions of fatigue as experienced by patients with congestive heart failure? (Schaefer & Potylycki, 1993)
Neuman's Health Care Systems Model	What factors influence weaning from mechanical ventilation? (Lowry & Anderson, 1993)
Orem's Self-Care Model	What are the self-care practices of healthy adolescents, and how does self-concept affect those practices? (McCaleb & Edgil, 1994)
Parse's Theory of Human Becoming	What is the experience of laughing at oneself as described by older couples? (Malinski, 1991)
Peplau's Interpersonal Relations Model	What nurse factors and client factors are predictive of the therapeutic relationship? (Forchuk, 1994)
Rogers' Science of Unitary Human Beings	What is the effect of therapeutic touch on pain and the need for analgesic medication (Meehan, 1993)
Roy's Adaptation Model	What are the differences in hope and functional status in elderly people with and without cancer? (McGill & Paul, 1993)

the conceptual framework by many researchers. For example, Jirovec and Kasno (1993) studied the predictors of self-care abilities among the institutionalized elderly. Monsen (1992) compared the autonomy, coping styles, and self-care agency of healthy adolescents and adolescents with spina bifida. Hartweg (1993) studied the self-care actions that healthy middle-aged women perform to promote well-being.

In addition to conceptual models that are designed to describe and characterize the entire nursing process, nurses have developed other models and theories that focus on more specific phenomena of interest to nurses. An important example is Nola Pender's Health Promotion Model (1987), a conceptual map for which was presented in Figure 4–3. We present a detailed research example of a study based on Pender's model at the end of the chapter. Another example is **Mishel's Uncertainty in Illness Theory** (1988), which focuses on the concept of uncertainty—the inability of a person to determine the meaning of illness-related events. According to this theory, a situation appraised as uncertain will mobilize individuals to use their resources to adapt to the situation. Mishel's conceptualization of uncertainty has been used as a framework for both qualitative and quantitative studies. For example, Baier (1995) conducted an in-depth qualitative study focusing on uncertainty in illness of persons with schizophrenia. Lemaire and Lenz's (1995) quantitative study was designed to identify predictors of uncertainty among menopausal women.

Other Models Used by Nurse Researchers

Many of the phenomena in which nurse researchers are interested involve concepts that are not unique to nurses, and therefore nursing studies are sometimes linked to conceptual frameworks that are not models of nursing. Three conceptual models that have been used frequently in nursing research investigations are as follows:

- *Becker's Health Belief Model (HBM).* The HBM is a framework for explaining people's health-related behavior, such as health-care use and compliance with a medical regimen. According to the model, health-related behavior is influenced by a person's perception of a threat posed by a health problem as well as by the value associated with actions aimed at reducing the threat (Becker, 1978). Nurse researchers have used the HBM in connection with studies of women's practice of breast self-examination and use of mammography (Douglass, Bartolucci, Waterbor, & Sirles, 1995; Champion, 1994); parent's involvement in a drug and alcohol prevention program (Hahn, 1995); and gender differences in leisure-time physical exercise (Hawkes & Holm, 1993).
- *Lazarus and Folkman's Theory of Stress and Coping.* This model represents an effort to explain people's methods of dealing with stress (*i.e.,* environmental and internal demands that tax or exceed people's resources and endanger their well-being). The model posits that coping strategies are learned, deliberate responses to stressors that are used to adapt to or change the stressors. According to this model, people's perception of mental and physical health is related to the ways they evaluate and cope with the

stresses of living (Lazarus & Folkman, 1984). Many nurses have conducted research within the context of this model, including studies of coping and psychological well-being in elderly patients with arthritis (Downe-Wamboldt & Melanson, 1995), effective coping with stroke disability (DeSepulveda & Chang, 1994), and stress and coping among family members responsible for a nursing home placement (Kammer, 1994).

- *Azjen-Fishbein Theory of Reasoned Action (TRA).* The TRA is a model that provides a framework for understanding the relationships among a person's attitudes, intentions, and behaviors. According to the TRA, behavioral intentions are the best predictor of a person's behavior, and behavioral intentions are a function of attitude toward performing the behavior and the subjective norm, which is the person's perception of whether relevant others think the behavior should be performed (Azjen & Fishbein, 1980). The TRA has been used as a framework for nurse researchers in studies of nurses' behaviors regarding the conduct of pain assessment (Nash, Edwards, & Nebauer, 1993), nurses' intended care behavior with patients who are HIV positive (Laschinger & Goldenberg, 1993), and hypertensive patients' regimen compliance behavior (Miller, Wikoff, & Hiatt, 1992).

The use of theories and conceptual models developed within other disciplines such as physiology or psychology (sometimes referred to as **borrowed theories**) has not been without controversy—some commentators advocate the development of unique nursing theories. However, nursing research is likely to continue on its current path of conducting studies within a multidisciplinary and multitheoretical perspective.

◻ ASSISTANCE IN READING ABOUT THEORIES AND FRAMEWORKS

What to Expect in the Research Literature

Students who are gaining skills in reading nursing studies should be prepared to find references to theories and conceptual frameworks in some of the studies they read. Here is what nursing research consumers are likely to encounter in published research reports:

- In most nursing studies, the research problem is *not* linked to a specific theory or conceptual model. Thus, students may read many studies before finding a study with an explicit theoretical underpinning.
- When a quantitative study is based on a theory or conceptual model, the research report generally states this fact fairly early—often in the first paragraph, or even in the title. Many studies also have a subsection of the introduction called "Conceptual Framework" or "Theoretical Framework." The report

usually includes a brief overview of the theory so that even readers with no theoretical background can understand, in a general way, the conceptual context of the study. Readers can obtain more detailed information on the theory by consulting the theoretical references cited in the report.

- When a quantitative nursing study is linked to a conceptual model or theory, it is about as likely to be a model not unique to nursing as it is to be an explicit model of nursing. Among the models of nursing, those of Orem, Rogers, and Roy are especially likely to be used as the basis for research.

- Some studies (in nursing as in any other discipline) claim a theoretical linkage that is not really justified. This is most likely to occur when researchers first formulate the research problem, design the study, and *then* find a theoretical context to fit it. Although an after-the-fact linkage of theory to a research question *may* prove useful, it is usually problematic. This is true because there are many different theories that could potentially fit any given research question and because the researcher will not have taken the nuances of the theory into consideration in designing the study. Artificially linking a problem to a theory is not the route to scientific usefulness. If a conceptual framework really is linked to a research problem, then the design of the study, the measurement of key constructs, and the analysis and interpretation of data will flow from that conceptualization.

Critiquing Conceptual and Theoretical Frameworks

It is often difficult to critique the theoretical context of a published research report. In a qualitative study in which a grounded theory is presented, the reader rarely has enough information for challenging the proposed descriptive theory: the only evidence presented to readers is that which supports the theoretical conceptualization. However, you can determine whether the theory seems logical, whether the conceptualization seems insightful, and whether the evidence is solid and convincing.

Critiquing a theoretical framework in a quantitative report is also difficult for students. Most of you are not familiar with the range of available models in nursing and other related disciplines. Furthermore, the whole notion of theoretical frameworks, precisely because they are so abstract, is often anxiety provoking. Some suggestions for evaluating the conceptual basis of a quantitative research project are offered in the following discussion and in Box 4–2 in the hope of lessening some of that anxiety.

The first task is to determine whether the study does, in fact, have a theoretical or conceptual framework. If there is no mention of a theory or conceptual model, you should consider whether the contribution that the study is likely to make to knowledge is diminished by the absence of such a framework. Nursing has been criticized for producing many pieces of isolated research that are difficult to integrate because of the absence of a theoretical foundation, but, in many cases, the research may be so pragmatic in nature that it does not really need a theory to

Guidelines for Critiquing Theoretical/Conceptual Frameworks

Box 4-2

1. Does the research report describe an explicit theoretical or conceptual framework for the study? (If not, does the absence of an explicit framework detract from the usefulness or significance of the research?)
2. Does the report adequately describe the major features of the framework so that readers can understand the conceptual basis of the study?
3. Does the research problem and hypotheses naturally flow from the framework, or does the purported link between the problem and the framework seem contrived?
4. Are conceptual definitions of the concepts in the study provided—and are the definitions consistent with the framework?
5. Does the researcher tie the findings of the study back to the framework at the end of the report? How do the findings support or undermine the framework?

enhance its usefulness. For example, research designed to determine the optimal frequency of turning patients has a utilitarian goal; it is difficult to see how placing the problem in a theoretical context would enhance the value of the findings.

If the study does involve an explicit framework, you must then ask whether this particular framework is appropriate. You may not be able to challenge the researcher's use of a particular theory or model or to recommend an alternative because that would require a solid theoretical grounding. (Advanced students, of course, should do this whenever possible.) However, you can evaluate the logic of using a particular framework and assess whether the link between the problem and the theory is genuine. Does the particular framework make sense for the given research problem? Does the researcher present a sufficiently convincing rationale for the framework used? Do the hypotheses seem to flow from the theory? Is there a correspondence between the underlying philosophy or world view inherent in the framework and that of the research problem and hypotheses? Will the answers to the research questions really contribute to the validation of the theory? Does the researcher interpret the findings within the context of the framework? If the answer to such questions is no, then students may have grounds for criticizing the study's framework, even though they may not be in a position to clearly articulate how the conceptual basis of the study could be improved.

RESEARCH EXAMPLES OF THEORETICAL CONTEXTS

This section presents two examples of the linkages between theory and research from the nursing research literature—one from a quantitative study and the other from a qualitative study.

Research Example
From a Quantitative Study:
Testing the Health Promotion Model

Pender's Health Promotion Model (HPM) has been used as the conceptual framework in numerous studies. For example, Gillis (1994) studied the determinants of health-promoting lifestyles in adolescent females. Stuifbergen and Becker (1994) studied the predictors of health-promoting lifestyles in persons with disabilities. Here we describe in some detail a study conducted by Pender herself.

Pender, Walker, Sechrist, and Frank-Stromborg (1990) used Pender's HPM to predict health-promoting lifestyles among employees enrolled in six employer-sponsored health-promotion programs. The researchers noted that when workplace health-promotion programs are initially introduced, employee enrollment tends to be high. However, over time, erratic participation and a high dropout rate tend to characterize many such programs.

Pender and her coresearchers indicated that most studies of the determinants of healthy lifestyles have used a prevention-oriented model in which fear of the consequences of illness are viewed as the primary motivation for health-related behavior. In contrast, these researchers used a wellness-oriented framework, the HPM, in their investigation. The model tested by this team of researchers is shown in Figure 4–3. The arrows in this figure denote the hypothesized direction of causal influences. The model includes seven Cognitive/ Perceptual Factors that are hypothesized to be influenced by five Modifying Factors. The Cognitive/Perceptual Factors, which are viewed as directly affecting participation in health-promoting behaviors, are considered to be amenable to change—an important feature with respect to the design of interventions to promote healthy lifestyles. These seven factors are as follows:

- *Importance of Health*—the value placed on health in relation to other personal values
- *Perceived Control of Health*—perception of whether health is self-determined, influenced by powerful others, and/or is the result of chance factors
- *Perceived Self-Efficacy*—the belief that one has the competence and skills to carry out specific actions
- *Definition of Health*—the personal meaning of health to each individual
- *Perceived Health Status*—the self-evaluation of current health as a subjective state
- *Perceived Benefits of Health-Promoting Behavior*—the perceived desirability of behavioral outcomes
- *Perceived Barriers to Health-Promoting Behaviors*—perceived hindrances to taking action.

Pender and her colleagues tested the utility of the HPM in explaining health-promoting lifestyles among employees who had enrolled in a workplace health-promotion program (thereby suggesting an intent to change their health habits) but who varied greatly in their level of participation in the program. With a sample of nearly 600 subjects, the researchers assessed each of the Cognitive/ Perceptual Factors, as well as several of the Modifying Factors. The dependent variable, participation in health-promoting behaviors, was measured by the Health-Promoting Lifestyle Profile (HPLP), a 48-question scale focusing on such behaviors as health responsibility, exercise, nutrition, and stress management.

The findings provided some support for the HPM model. In particular, perceptions of control of health, personal efficacy, definition of health, and health status emerged as a constellation of HPM constructs most closely associated with health-promoting lifestyle behaviors among employees enrolled in a worksite health-promotion program. However, other hypothesized factors (*e.g.,* valuing health) was not a significant determinant of a health-promoting lifestyle.

Research Example From a Qualitative Study: Development of a Theory of Caring

As noted earlier in this chapter, many qualitative studies have theory development as an explicit goal. Here we describe the efforts of a qualitative researcher who developed a middle-range theory of caring on the basis of three separate qualitative inquiries.

Swanson (1991) developed an empirically driven descriptive theory of caring. Using data from three separate qualitative investigations, Swanson inductively derived and then refined a theory of the caring process.

Swanson studied caring in three separate perinatal contexts: as experienced by women who miscarried, as provided by parents and professionals in the newborn intensive care unit, and as recalled by at-risk mothers who had received a long-term public health nursing intervention. Data were gathered through in-depth interviews with study participants and also through observations of care provision. Data from the first study led to the identification and preliminary definition of five caring processes. The outcome of the second study was confirmation of the five processes and refinement of their definitions. In the third study, Swanson confirmed the five processes, redefined one of them, developed subdimensions of each process, and derived a definition of the overall concept of caring: *"Caring is a nurturing way of relating to a valued other toward whom one feels a personal sense of commitment and responsibility"* (p. 165).

According to Swanson's theory, the five caring processes are as follows:

- *Knowing*—Striving to understand an event as it has meaning in the life of the other
- *Being With*—Being emotionally present to the other
- *Doing For*—Doing for the other as he/she would do for the self if it were at all possible
- *Enabling*—Facilitating the other's passage through life transitions and unfamiliar events
- *Maintaining Belief*—Sustaining faith in the other's capacity to get through an event or transition and face a future with meaning

In presenting her theory, Swanson described the five processes, supporting each with rich excerpts from her in-depth interviews. Here is an example of the excerpt illustrating the process of knowing:

> When things weren't right, I could say that things were fine and it was only a matter of time. I mean the nurse would ask certain questions and there would be no way that I could be consistent without telling the truth. And then we would talk, and pretty soon instead of saying it was fine, I would start out with what was really wrong. (p. 163)

Swanson noted that her theory of caring was being used in the development and testing of a caring-based nurse counseling program for women who miscarry. Her theory was also used as a conceptual framework for a qualitative study that examined the interactions of AIDS family caregivers and professional health-care providers (Powell-Cope, 1994).

▧ SUMMARY

Contexts for research investigations are provided through literature reviews and theoretical/conceptual frameworks. The term **literature review** is used to refer to both the activities involved in searching for information on a topic as well as the actual written report that summarizes the state of the existing knowledge on a research problem. Both researchers and research consumers prepare written research reviews.

For those preparing a literature review, the first steps are to identify the key concepts and to locate appropriate references. An important bibliographic development to emerge in recent years is the increasing availability of various **electronic databases,** many of which can be accessed through an **on-line search** or by way of **CD-ROM.** For nurses, the **CINAHL database** is especially useful. Because of the **mapping** capabilities of this database, users can perform a **subject search** without knowing the exact subject heading used by CINAHL. Although electronic information retrieval is now widespread and growing, print resources such as **print**

indexes and **abstract journals** are also available, and are especially useful for locating references published before 1982.

In writing a research review, the reviewer should carefully organize the relevant materials, which should consist primarily of **primary source** research reports. The review should not be a succession of quotes or abstracts. The role of the reviewer is to point out what has been studied to date, how adequate and dependable those studies are, and what gaps there are in the existing body of research. The reviewer should present facts and findings in the tentative language that befits scientific inquiry and should remember to identify the source of opinions, points of view, and generalizations. These guidelines should be kept in mind both in producing literature reviews and in critiquing those of others.

Theories and conceptual models are the primary means of providing a conceptual context for a study. In its least restrictive definition, a **theory** is a broad and abstract characterization of some phenomenon; this definition encompasses **descriptive theory** that thoroughly describes a phenomenon. As classically defined, a theory is an abstract generalization that systematically explains the relationships among phenomena. The overall objective of theory is to make scientific findings meaningful and generalizable. In addition, theories help to summarize existing knowledge into coherent systems, stimulate new research by providing both direction and impetus, and explain the nature of relationships between or among variables. The basic components of a theory are concepts; classically defined theories consist of a set of statements about the interrelationships among concepts, arranged in a logically interrelated system that permits new statements to be derived from them.

Conceptual models are less formal mechanisms for organizing phenomena than theories. As in the case of theories, concepts are the basic elements of a conceptual framework; however, the concepts are not linked to one another in a logically ordered, deductive system. **Schematic models** (sometimes referred to as **conceptual maps**) are symbolic representations of phenomena that depict a theory or conceptual model through the use of symbols or diagrams. A **framework** is the conceptual underpinnings of a study. In many studies, the framework is implicit and not fully explicated, but nurse researchers are increasingly using theories and conceptual models as their frameworks.

The link between research and theory is a mutually beneficial one. Qualitative studies are often used to develop inductively derived theories. Some qualitative researchers specifically seek to develop **grounded theories,** data-driven explanations to account for phenomena under study. Quantitative studies are more likely to test hypotheses developed on the basis of an existing theory or conceptual model.

A number of conceptual models of nursing have evolved and have been used in nursing research. **Orem's Self-Care Model**, for example, has been used as the conceptual framework for numerous studies. **Pender's Health Promotion Model**, which is a model to explain healthy lifestyles, has also had considerable research attention. Three nonnursing models frequently used by nurse researchers are **Becker's Health Belief Model, Lazarus and Folkman's Theory of Stress and Cop-**

ing, and **Azjen-Fishbein's Theory of Reasoned Action**. Unfortunately, researchers sometimes develop a problem, design a study, and *then* look for a conceptual framework in which to place it; such an after-the-fact selection of a framework usually is less compelling than the systematic testing of a particular theory. In many nursing studies, the absence of a formal theoretical framework is appropriate.

STUDY SUGGESTIONS

Chapter 4 of the accompanying *Study Guide to Accompany Essentials of Nursing Research,* 4th edition offers various exercises and study suggestions for reinforcing the concepts presented in this chapter.

Suggested Readings

Methodologic References

Azjen, I., & Fishbein, M. (1980). *Understanding attitudes and predicting social behavior.* Englewood Cliffs, NJ: Prentice-Hall.

Becker, M. (1978). The Health Belief Model and sick role behavior. *Nursing Digest, 6,* 35–40.

Fawcett, J. (1989). *Analysis and evaluation of conceptual models of nursing* (2nd ed.). Philadelphia: F. A. Davis.

Fawcett, J., & Downs, F. (1992). *The relationship between theory and research.* (2nd ed.) Philadelphia: F.A. Davis.

Lazarus, R. S., & Folkman, S. (1984). *Stress, appraisal, and coping.* New York: Springer.

Mishel, M. H. (1988). Uncertainty in illness. *Image: Journal of Nursing Scholarship, 20,* 225–232.

Morse, J. M., Solberg, S. M., Neander, W. L., Bottorff, J. L., & Johnson, J. L. (1990). Concepts of caring and caring as a concept. *Advances in Nursing Science, 13,* 1–14.

Orem, D. E. (1985). *Concepts of practice* (3rd ed.). New York: McGraw-Hill.

Parse, R. R. (1987). *Nursing science: Major paradigms, theories, and critiques.* Philadelphia: W. B. Saunders.

Pender, N. (1987). *Health promotion in nursing practice* (2nd ed.). Norwalk, CT: Appleton and Lange.

Rogers, M. E. (1986). Science of unitary human beings. In V. Malinski (Ed.), *Explorations on Martha Rogers' science of unitary human-beings.* Norwalk, CT: Appleton-Century-Crofts.

Roy, Sr., C., & Andrews, H. (1991). *The Roy adaptation model: The definitive statement.* Norwalk, CT: Appleton and Lange.

Substantive References

Baier, M. (1995). Uncertainty in illness for persons with schizophrenia. *Issues in Mental Health Nursing, 16,* 201–212.

Bauer, S. M. (1994). Psychoneuroimmunology and cancer: An integrated review. *Journal of Advanced Nursing, 19,* 1114–1120.

Brodsky, M. S. (1995). Testicular cancer survivors' impressions of the impact of the disease on their lives. *Qualitative Health Research, 5,* 78–96.

Champion, V. L. (1994), Beliefs about breast cancer and mammography by behavioral stage. *Oncology Nursing Forum, 21,* 1009–1014.

DeSepulveda, L. I., & Chang, B. (1994). Effective coping with stroke disability in a community setting. *Journal of Neuroscience Nursing, 26,* 193–203.

Douglass, M., Bartolucci, A., Waterbor, J., & Sirles, A. (1995). Breast cancer early detection: Differences between African American and white women's health beliefs and detection practices. *Oncology Nursing Forum, 22,* 835–837.

Downe-Wamboldt, B. L., & Melanson, P. M. (1995). Emotions, coping, and psychological well-being in elderly people with arthritis. *Western Journal of Nursing Research, 17,* 250–265.

Duffy, M. E. (1994). Testing the Theory of Transcending Options: Health behavior of single parents. *Scholarly Inquiry for Nursing Practice, 8,* 191–205.

Forchuk, C. (1994). The orientation phase of the nurse-client relationship: Testing Peplau's theory. *Journal of Advanced Nursing, 20,* 532–537.

Gillis, A. J. (1994). Determinants of health-promoting lifestyles in adolescent females. *Canadian Journal of Nursing Research, 26,* 13–28.

Hahn, E. J. (1995). Predicting Head Start parent involvement in an alcohol and other drug prevention program. *Nursing Research, 44,* 45–51.

Hanna, K. M. (1993). Effect of nurse-client transaction on female adolescents' oral contraceptive adherence. *Image—the Journal of Nursing Scholarship, 25,* 285–290.

Hartweg, D. L. (1993). Self-care actions of healthy middle-aged women to promote well-being. *Nursing Research, 42,* 221–227.

Hawkes, J. M., & Holm, K. (1993). Gender differences in exercise determinants. *Nursing Research, 42,* 166–172.

Holditch-Davis, D., Barham, L. N., O'Hale, A., & Tucker, B. (1995). Effect of standard rest periods on convalescent preterm infants. *Journal of Obstetric, Gynecologic, and Neonatal Nursing, 24,* 424–432,

Jirovec, M. M., & Kasno, J. (1993). Predictors of self-care abilities among the institutionalized elderly. *Western Journal of Nursing Research, 15,* 314–323.

Kammer, C. H. (1994). Stress and coping of family members responsible for nursing home placement. *Research in Nursing and Health, 17,* 89–98.

Laschinger, H. K. S., & Goldenberg, D. (1993). Attitudes of practicing nurses as predictors of intended care behavior with persons who are HIV positive. *Research in Nursing and Health, 16,* 441–450.

Lemaire, G. S., & Lenz, E. R. (1995). Perceived uncertainty about menopause in women attending an educational program. *International Journal of Nursing Studies, 32,* 39–48.

Lowry, L. W., & Anderson, B. (1993). Neuman's framework and ventilator dependency. *Nursing Science Quarterly, 6,* 195–200.

Mahon, N. E., & Yarcheski, A. (1992). Alternative explanations of loneliness in adolescents: A replication and extension study. *Nursing Research, 41,* 151–156.

Malinksi, V. M. (1991). The experience of laughing at oneself in older couples. *Nursing Science Quarterly, 4,* 69–75.

McCaleb, A., & Edgil, A. (1994). Self-concept and self-care practices of healthy adolescents. *Journal of Pediatric Nursing, 9,* 233–238.

McGill, J. S., & Paul, P. B. (1993). Functional status and hope in elderly people with and without cancer. *Oncology Nursing Forum, 20,* 1207–1213.

Meehan, T. C. (1993). Therapeutic touch and postoperative pain: A Rogerian research study. *Nursing Science Quarterly, 6,* 69–78.

Miller, P., Wikoff, R., & Hiatt, A. (1992). Fishbein's Model of Reasoned Action and compliance behavior of hypertensive patients. *Nursing Research, 41,* 104–109.

Monsen, R. B. (1992). Autonomy, coping, and self-care agency in healthy adolescents and in adolescents with spina bifida. *Journal of Pediatric Nursing, 7,* 9–13.

Nash, R., Edwards, H., & Nebauer, M. (1993). Effect of attitudes, subjective norms, and perceived control on nurses' intention to assess patients' pain. *Journal of Advanced Nursing, 18,* 941–947.

Pender, N. J., Walker, S. N., Sechrist, K. R., & Frank-Stromborg, M. (1990). Predicting health-promoting lifestyles in the workplace. *Nursing Research, 39,* 326–332.

Powell-Cope, G. M. (1994). Family caregivers of people with AIDS: Negotiating partnerships with professional health care providers. *Nursing Research, 43,* 324–330.

Schaefer, K. M., & Potylycki, M. J. S. (1993). Fatigue associated with congestive heart failure: Use of Levine's Conservation Model. *Journal of Advanced Nursing, 18,* 260–268.

Stuifbergen, A. K., & Becker, H. A. (1994). Predictors of health-promoting lifestyles in persons with disabilities. *Research in Nursing and Health, 17,* 3–13.

Swanson, K. M. (1991). Empirical development of a middle range theory of caring. *Nursing Research, 40,* 161–166.

Tuten, S. H., & Gueldner, S. H. (1991). Efficacy of sodium chloride versus dilute heparin for maintenance of peripheral intermittent intravenous devices. *Applied Nursing Research, 4,* 63–71.

5

The Ethical Context of Nursing Research

Student Objectives

On completion of this chapter, the student will be able to:

- discuss the historical background that led to the creation of various codes of ethics
- understand the nature of the conflict, in certain situations, between ethics and research demands and provide some examples of ethical dilemmas
- identify the three primary ethical principles articulated in the *Belmont Report* and the important dimensions encompassed by each
- identify some of the salient costs and benefits of participating in a study from a participant's point of view
- describe informed consent and process consent
- identify steps that researchers should undertake to safeguard the confidentiality of participants
- describe the concept of vulnerable subjects and identify several relevant groups
- describe the role of Institutional Review Boards (IRBs) in the review of research plans
- given sufficient information, evaluate the ethical dimensions of a research report
- define new terms in the chapter

New Terms

Anonymity
Belmont Report
Beneficence
Code of ethics
Coercion
Concealment
Confidentiality
Consent form
Covert data collection
Debriefing
Deception
Declaration of Helsinki
Ethical dilemmas
Full disclosure

Human subjects committees
Identification number
Implied consent
Informed consent
Institutional Review Board
Minimal risk
Nuremberg Code
Process consent
Research advisory panels
Risk/benefit ratio
Self-determination
Stipend
Vulnerable subjects

Nurses continually face **ethical dilemmas** in their practice: the prolongation of life by artificial means, the institution of tube feedings when patients are unable to sustain oral nourishment, and the testing of new products to monitor care are but a few examples. Dilemmas such as these have led to an increasing number of discussions and debates concerning ethical issues in the delivery of nursing care.

The rapid increase of research involving humans has led to similar ethical concerns and debates regarding the protection of the rights of people who participate in nursing research. Ethical concerns are especially prominent in the field of nursing because the line of demarcation between what constitutes the expected practice of nursing and the collection of research information has become less distinct as research by nurses increases. Furthermore, ethics poses particular problems to nurse researchers in some situations because ethical requirements sometimes conflict with methodologic considerations. This chapter discusses some of the major ethical principles that should be considered in reviewing (as well as in designing) research studies.

THE NEED FOR ETHICAL GUIDELINES

When humans are used as the study participants in research—as they usually are in nursing research—great care must be exercised in ensuring that the rights of those humans are protected. The requirement for ethical conduct may strike the reader as so self-evident as to require no further comment, but the fact is that ethical considerations have not always been given adequate attention. In this section, we consider some of the reasons the development of ethical guidelines became imperative.

Historical Background

As modern, civilized people, we might like to think that systematic violations of moral principles within the context of research occurred centuries ago rather than in recent times, but this is not the case. The Nazi medical experiments of the 1930s and 1940s are the most famous example of recent disregard for ethical conduct. The Nazi program of research involved the use of prisoners of war and racial "enemies" in numerous experiments designed to test the limits of human endurance and human reaction to diseases and untested drugs. The studies were unethical not only because they exposed the humans to permanent physical harm and even death but also because the participants were not given an opportunity to refuse participation.

Unfortunately, some recent examples are closer to home. For instance, between 1932 and 1972, a study known as the Tuskegee Syphilis Study, sponsored by the U. S. Public Health Service, investigated the effects of syphilis on 400 men from a poor black community. Medical treatment was deliberately withheld to study the course of the untreated disease. Another well-known case of unethical research involved the injection of live cancer cells into elderly patients at the Jewish Chronic Disease Hospital in Brooklyn without the consent of those patients. Even more recently, it was revealed in 1993 that U. S. federal agencies have sponsored radiation experiments since the 1940s on hundreds of people, many of them prisoners or elderly hospital patients. Many other examples of studies with ethical transgressions—often much more subtle than these examples—have emerged to give ethical concerns the high visibility they have today.

Ethical Dilemmas in Conducting Research

Research that violates ethical principles is rarely done specifically to be cruel or immoral but more typically occurs out of a conviction that knowledge is important and potentially life-saving or beneficial (usually to others) in the long run. There are, unfortunately, situations in which the rights of participants and the demands of the research project are put in direct conflict. Here are some examples of research problems in which the desire for rigor conflicts with ethical considerations:

1. *Research question:* How empathic are nurses in their treatment of patients in intensive care units?

   Ethical dilemma: Ethical research generally involves having participants be fully cognizant of their participation in a study. Yet if the researcher informs the nurses participating in the study that their degree of empathy in treating patients will be scrutinized, will their behavior be "normal"? If the nurses' behavior is altered due to the known presence of research observers, the integrity of the study could be undermined.

2. *Research question:* What are the feelings and coping mechanisms of parents whose children have a terminal illness?

   Ethical dilemma: To answer this question fully, the researcher may need to probe intrusively into the psychological state of the parents at a highly vulnerable time in their lives; such probing could be painful and even traumatic. Yet knowledge of the parents' coping mechanisms could help to design more effective ways of dealing with parents' grief and anger.

3. *Research question:* Does a new medication prolong life in cancer patients?

   Ethical dilemma: The best way to test the effectiveness of an intervention is to administer the intervention to some participants but withhold it from others to see if differences between the groups emerge. However, if the intervention is untested (*e.g.,* a new drug), the group receiving the intervention may be exposed to potentially hazardous side effects. On the other hand, the group *not* receiving the drug may be denied a beneficial treatment.

4. *Research question:* What is the process by which adult children adapt to the day-to-day stresses of caring for a terminally ill parent?

   Ethical dilemma: In a qualitative study, which would be appropriate for this research question, the researcher sometimes becomes so closely involved with the study participants that they become willing to share "secrets" and privileged information, as they would with a friend. Interviews can become confessions—sometimes of unseemly or even illegal or immoral behavior. In this example, suppose a participant admitted to physically abusing their adult parent—how does the researcher respond to that information without undermining a pledge of confidentiality? And, if the researcher divulges the information to appropriate authorities, how can a pledge of confidentiality be given in good faith to other participants?

As these examples suggest, researchers involved with human beings are sometimes in a bind: their goal is to advance knowledge, using the best methods possible, but they must also adhere to the dictates of ethical rules that have been developed to protect the rights of study participants. It is precisely because of such conflicts that **codes of ethics** have been developed to guide the efforts of researchers and to help others evaluate their actions.

Codes of Ethics

Over the past four decades, largely in response to the human rights violations described earlier, various codes of ethics have been developed. One of the first internationally recognized set of ethical standards is referred to as the **Nuremberg Code,** developed after the Nazi atrocities were made public in the Nuremberg trials. Several other international standards have followed, the most notable of which is the **Declaration of Helsinki,** which was adopted in 1964 by the World Medical Assembly and then later revised in 1975.

Most disciplines have established their own **code of ethics.** The American Nurses' Association (1975) has put forth a document entitled *Human Rights Guidelines for Nurses in Clinical and Other Research.* The American Sociological Association published its *Code of Ethics* in 1984. Guidelines for psychologists were published by the American Psychological Association (1982) in *Ethical Principles in the Conduct of Research With Human Participants.* Although there is considerable overlap in the basic principles articulated in these documents, each deals with problems of particular concern to their respective disciplines.

An especially important code of ethics was adopted by the National Commission for the Protection of Human Subjects of Biomedical and Behavioral Research (1978). The Commission, established by the National Research Act (Public Law 93-348), issued a report in 1978 that served as the basis for regulations affecting research sponsored by the federal government. The report, sometimes referred to as the *Belmont Report,* also served as a model for many of the guidelines adopted by specific disciplines.

The *Belmont Report* articulated three primary ethical principles on which standards of ethical conduct in research are based: beneficence, respect for human dignity, and justice.

◪ PRINCIPLE OF BENEFICENCE

One of the most fundamental ethical principles in research is that of **beneficence,** which encompasses the maxim: Above all, do no harm. Most researchers consider that this principle contains multiple dimensions.

Freedom From Harm

Clearly, exposing research participants to experiences that result in serious or permanent harm is unacceptable. An ethical researcher must be prepared at any time during the study to terminate the research if there is reason to suspect that continuation would result in injury, death, disability, or undue distress to study participants. When a new medical procedure or drug is being tested, it is almost always necessary to first experiment with animals or tissue cultures before proceeding to tests with humans.

Although protecting study participants from physical harm is in many cases clearcut, some psychological consequences of participating in a study may be subtle and thus require closer attention and sensitivity. Sometimes, for example, people are asked questions about their personal views, weaknesses, or fears. Such queries might lead people to reveal highly sensitive personal information. The point is not that researchers should refrain from asking questions but rather that it is necessary for them to think carefully about the nature of the intrusion on people's psyches. Researchers strive to avoid inflicting psychological harm by carefully considering the phrasing of questions, by providing **debriefing** sessions after the data collection is completed to permit participants to ask questions or air complaints, and, in some situations, by making referrals to appropriate health, social, or psychological services.

Freedom From Exploitation

Involvement in a research study should not place participants at a disadvantage or expose them to situations for which they have not been explicitly prepared. Participants need to be assured that their participation, or the information they might provide to the researcher, will not be used against them in any way. For example, a person describing his or her economic circumstances to a researcher should not be exposed to the risk of losing Medicaid benefits; the person reporting drug abuse should not fear exposure to criminal authorities.

The study participant enters into a special relationship with the researcher, and it is critical that this relationship not be exploited in any way. Exploitation might be overt and malicious (*e.g.,* sexual exploitation, use of participants' identifying information to create a mailing list, and use of donated blood for the development of a commercial product), but it may also be more subtle. For example, people may agree to participate in a study requiring 30 minutes of their time. The researcher may then decide 1 year later to go back and talk to the participants, to follow their progress or circumstances. Unless the researcher had previously explained to the participants that there might be a follow-up study, the researcher might be accused of not adhering to the agreement previously reached with participants and of exploiting the researcher–participant relationship.

Because nurse researchers may have a nurse–patient (in addition to a researcher–participant) relationship, special care may need to be exercised to avoid exploitation of people's vulnerabilities. Researchers should be cognizant of the fact that patients' consent to participate in a study may result from their understanding of the researcher's role as *nurse,* not as *researcher.*

In qualitative research, the risk of exploitation may become especially acute because the psychological distance between the investigator and the study participant typically diminishes dramatically as the study progresses. The emergence of a pseudotherapeutic relationship between the researcher and participant is not uncommon, and this imposes additional responsibilities on the researcher—and additional risks that exploitation could inadvertently occur. On the other hand, qualitative researchers are typically in a better position than quantitative researchers to *do good,* rather than just to avoid doing any harm, because of the close relationships they often develop with participants. Munhall (1988) has argued that qualitative nurse researchers have the responsibility of ensuring that the "therapeutic imperative of nursing (advocacy) takes precedent over the research imperative (advancing knowledge) if conflict develops" (p. 151).

Risk/Benefit Ratio

Researchers are expected to assess carefully the risks and benefits that would be incurred in the conduct of a study before its inception. Consumers, in their review of studies, should also be cognizant of the direct **risk/benefit ratio** to those participating in the research.

Box 5–1 summarizes some of the more salient costs and benefits to which research participants might be exposed. It has been suggested that researchers can perhaps best evaluate the risk/benefit ratio by considering how comfortable they would feel having family members participate in the study. In your evaluation of the risk/benefit ratio of a research study, you might consider whether you would have felt comfortable being a participant in the study under review.

The risk/benefit ratio should also be considered in terms of whether the risks

Box 5-1

Potential Benefits and Costs of Research to Participants

Major Potential Benefits to Participants

- Access to an intervention to which they otherwise may not have access
- Gratification in being able to discuss their situation or problem with a nonjudgmental and friendly person
- Increased knowledge about themselves or their conditions, either through opportunity for introspection and self-reflection or through direct interaction with the researcher
- Escape from normal routine, excitement of being part of a study, and satisfaction of curiosity about what it is like to participate in a study
- Satisfaction that the information they provide may help others with similar problems or conditions
- Direct monetary or material gains through stipends or other incentives

Major Potential Costs to Participants

- Physical harm, including unanticipated side effects
- Physical discomfort, fatigue, or boredom
- Psychological or emotional distress resulting from self-disclosure, introspection, fear of the unknown or interacting with strangers, fear of eventual repercussions, anger or embarrassment at the type of questions being asked
- Loss of privacy
- Loss of time
- Monetary costs (*e.g.,* for transportation, child care, time lost from work, and so on)

to research participants are commensurate with the benefit to society and the nursing profession in terms of the knowledge produced. The general guideline is that the degree of risk to be taken by those participating in the research should never exceed the potential humanitarian benefits of the knowledge to be gained. Thus, an important question in assessing the overall risk/benefit ratio is whether the study focuses on a significant topic that has the potential to improve patient care.

All research involves some risks, but in many cases the risk is minimal. **Minimal risk,** according to federal guidelines, is identified as anticipated risks that are no greater than those ordinarily encountered in daily life or during the performance of routine physical or psychological tests or procedures. When the risks are not minimal, it is incumbent on the researcher to proceed with great caution, making every effort possible to reduce risks and maximize benefits. Research should never be undertaken when the perceived risks and costs to participants outweigh the anticipated benefits of the research.

PRINCIPLE OF RESPECT FOR HUMAN DIGNITY

Respect for the human dignity of participants is the second ethical principle articulated in the *Belmont Report*. This principle includes the right to self-determination and the right to full disclosure.

Right to Self-Determination

Humans should be treated as autonomous agents, capable of controlling their own activities and destinies. The principle of **self-determination** means that prospective participants have the right to decide voluntarily whether to participate in a study, without the risk of incurring any penalties or prejudicial treatment. It also means that participants have the right to decide at any point to terminate their participation, to refuse to give information, or to ask for clarification about the purpose of the study or specific questions.

A person's right to self-determination includes freedom from coercion of any type. **Coercion** involves explicit or implicit threats of penalty for failing to participate in a study or excessive rewards from agreeing to participate. The obligation to honor and protect potential participants from coercion requires careful consideration when the researcher is in a position of authority, control, or influence over potential participants, as might be the case in a nurse–patient relationship. The issue of coercion may also require scrutiny even when there is not a preestablished relationship. For example, a monetary incentive offered to an economically disadvantaged group—such as the homeless—might be considered mildly coercive; its acceptability might have to be evaluated in terms of the risk/benefit ratio. That is, if risks are high relative to any benefits, and if the study group is vulnerable, monetary incentives (sometimes referred to as **stipends**) may place undue pressure on prospective participants.

Right to Full Disclosure

The principle of respect for human dignity encompasses people's right to make informed voluntary decisions about their participation in a study. Such decisions cannot be made without full disclosure. **Full disclosure** means that the researcher has fully described the nature of the study, the person's right to refuse participation, the researcher's responsibilities, and the likely risks and benefits that would be incurred. The right to self-determination and the right to full disclosure are the two major elements on which informed consent is based.

Although disclosure is normally provided to study participants before they begin the study, there may be a need for further disclosure at a later point, either in debriefing sessions or in written communications. For example, issues that arise during the course of collecting information from participants may need to be clarified, or the participant may want aspects of the study explained again. Many investigators also offer to send participants summaries of the research findings after the data have been analyzed. As we discuss below, in qualitative studies the consent process may require an ongoing negotiation between the researcher and participants.

Informed Consent

Prospective participants who are fully informed about the nature of the research, the demands it will make on them, and potential costs and benefits to be incurred are in a position to make thoughtful decisions regarding participation in the study. **Informed consent** means that participants have adequate information regarding the research; are capable of comprehending the information; and have the power of free choice, enabling them to consent voluntarily to participate in the research or decline participation. In many cases, researchers document the informed consent process by having participants sign a **consent form,** an example of which is presented in Figure 5–1. This form includes information about the study purpose, the specific expectations regarding participation (*e.g.,* how much time will be involved), the voluntary nature of participation, and the potential costs and benefits.

In some qualitative studies, especially those requiring repeated contact with the same participants, it is difficult to obtain a meaningful informed consent at the outset. A qualitative researcher does not always know in advance how the study will evolve. For example, because the research design emerges during the data collection and analysis process, the researcher may not know the exact nature of the data to be collected, what the risks and benefits to participants will be, nor how much of a time commitment they will be expected to make. Thus, in a qualitative study, consent is often viewed as an ongoing, transactional process, referred to as **process consent.** In process consent, the researcher continuously renegotiates the consent, allowing participants to play a collaborative role in the decision-making process regarding their ongoing participation.

Issues Relating to the Principle of Respect

Although most researchers would endorse participants' right to self-determination and full disclosure, there are circumstances that make these standards difficult to adhere to in practice. One issue concerns the inability of certain people to make well-informed judgments about the costs and benefits associated with participation. Children, for example, may be unable to give truly informed consent. The issue of groups that are vulnerable within a research context is discussed in a subsequent section of this chapter. There are other circumstances in which researchers may

In signing this document, I am giving my consent to be interviewed by an employee of Human-alysis, Inc., a nonprofit research organization based in Saratoga Springs, New York. I understand that I will be part of a research study that will focus on the experiences and needs of mothers of young children in the United States. This study, supported by a grant from the U.S. Department of Health and Human Services, will provide some guidance to people who are trying to help mothers and their children.

I understand that I will be interviewed in my home at a time convenient to me. I will be asked some questions about my experiences as a parent, my feelings about how to raise children, the health and characteristics of my oldest child, and my use of community services. I also understand that the interviewer will ask to have my oldest child present during at least some portion of the interview. The interview will take about 1½ to 2 to hours to complete. I also understand that the researcher may contact me for more information in the future.

I understand that I was selected to participate in this study because I was involved in a study of young mothers at the time of my oldest child's birth. At that time, I was recruited into the study, along with about 500 other young mothers, through a hospital or service agency.

This interview was granted freely. I have been informed that the interview is entirely voluntary, and that even after the interview begins I can refuse to answer any specific questions or decide to terminate the interview at any point. I have been told that my answers to questions will not be given to anyone else and no reports of this study will ever identify me in any way. I have also been informed that my participation or nonparticipation or my refusal to answer questions will have no effect on services that I or any member of my family may receive from health or social services providers.

This study will help develop a better understanding of the experiences of young mothers and the services that can be most helpful to them and their children. However, I will receive no direct benefit as a result of participation. As a means of compensating for any fatigue, inconvenience or monetary costs associated with participating in the study, I have received $25 for granting this interview.

I understand that the results of this research will be given to me if I ask for them and that Dr. Denise Polit is the person to contact if I have any questions about the study or about my rights as a study participant. Dr. Polit can be reached through a collect call at (518) 587-3994.

_____   _____
Date   Respondent's Signature

                                               _____
                                               Interviewer's Signature

Figure 5–1. Sample consent form.

feel that the participants' right to full disclosure and self-determination must be compromised. Researchers concerned with the validity of the study findings are sometimes worried that full disclosure might result in two types of biases: (1) the bias resulting from distorted information, and (2) the bias resulting from failure to recruit a good sample.

Let us suppose that a researcher is studying the relationship between high school students' substance abuse and their absenteeism from school. The researcher wants to know if students with a high rate of absenteeism are, as a group, more likely to be substance abusers than students with a good attendance record. If the researcher approached potential participants and fully explained the purpose of the study, some students might refuse to participate. The problem is that nonparticipation would be highly selective; one would expect, in fact, that those least likely to volunteer for such a study would be students who are substance abusers—the very group of primary interest in the research. Moreover, by knowing the specific research question, those who do volunteer to participate might be less inclined to give candid responses. The researcher in such a situation might argue that full disclosure would totally undermine his or her ability to conduct the study productively.

Researchers who feel that full disclosure is incompatible with the aims of their research sometimes use two techniques. The first is **covert data collection** or **concealment,** which means the collection of information without the participants' knowledge and thus without their consent. This might happen, for example, if a researcher wanted to observe people's behavior in a real-world setting and was concerned that doing so openly would result in changes in the very behavior of interest. In such a situation, the researcher might obtain the information through concealed methods, such as by audiotaping or videotaping participants through hidden equipment, observing through a one-way mirror, or observing while pretending to be engaged in other activities. Some people feel that covert data collection is acceptable as long as the risks to the participants are negligible and their right to privacy has not been violated. Covert data collection is least likely to be ethically acceptable if the research is focused on sensitive aspects of the participants' behavior, such as drug use, sexual conduct, or illegal acts.

The second, and more controversial, technique is the researcher's use of **deception.** Deception can involve either deliberately withholding information about the study or providing participants with false information. For example, the researcher studying high school students' use of drugs might describe the research as a study of students' health practices, which is a mild form of misinformation.

The practice of deception and concealment is clearly problematic from an ethical standpoint because it interferes with the participants' right to make a truly informed decision regarding the personal costs and benefits of participation. Some people argue that the use of deception and concealment are *never* justified. Others, however, believe that, if the study involves minimal risk to participants and if there are anticipated benefits to science and society, then deception or concealment may be justified to enhance the validity of the findings.

◪ PRINCIPLE OF JUSTICE

The third broad principle articulated in the *Belmont Report* concerns justice. This principle includes the participants' right to fair treatment and their right to privacy.

Right to Fair Treatment

Participants have the right to fair and equitable treatment before, during, and after their participation in the study. Fair treatment includes the following aspects:

- The fair and nondiscriminatory selection of participants such that any risks or benefits will be equitably shared; selection should be based on research requirements and *not* on the convenience, gullibility, or compromised position of certain types of people
- The nonprejudicial treatment of people who decline to participate or who withdraw from the study after agreeing to participate
- The honoring of all agreements made between the researcher and the participant, including adherence to the procedures described in advance and the payment of any promised stipends
- Participants' access to research personnel at any point in the study to clarify information
- Participants' access to appropriate professional assistance if there is any physical or psychological damage
- Debriefing, if necessary, to divulge information withheld before the study or to clarify issues that arose during the study
- Sensitivity to and respect for the beliefs, habits, and lifestyles of people from different cultures
- Courteous and tactful treatment at all times

Right to Privacy

Virtually all research with humans constitutes some type of intrusion into their personal lives. Researchers should ensure that their research is not more intrusive than it needs to be and that the participants' privacy is maintained throughout the study.

Participants have the right to expect that any data collected during the course of a study will be kept in strictest confidence. This can occur either through anonymity or through other confidentiality procedures. **Anonymity** occurs when even the researcher cannot link a participant with the data for that person. For example, if questionnaires were distributed to a group of nursing home residents and were returned without any identifying information on them, the responses would be considered anonymous. As another example, if a researcher reviewed hospital records from which all identifying information (*e.g.,* name, address, Social Security number, and so forth) had been expunged, anonymity would again protect the participants' right to privacy.

In situations in which anonymity is impossible, researchers should implement appropriate confidentiality procedures. A promise of **confidentiality** to participants is a guarantee that any information the participant provides will not be publicly reported or made accessible to parties other than those involved in the research. This means that research data should never be shared with strangers or with people known to the participants (*e.g.,* family members, counselors, physicians, and other nurses) unless the researcher has been given explicit permission to do so.

Researchers generally develop fairly elaborate procedures for protecting the privacy of research participants. These procedures include securing individual confidentiality statements from all the people involved in collecting or analyzing research data; maintaining information that might divulge the identities of the participants in a locked file to which only one or two people have access; substituting **identification numbers** for participants' names on study records and computer files to prevent any accidental breach of confidentiality; and reporting only aggregate data for groups of participants or taking steps to disguise a person's identity in a research report.

Qualitative researchers sometimes find that extra precautions are needed to safeguard the privacy of their research participants. Anonymity is almost never possible in qualitative research, because the researcher typically is interjected deeply into the lives of those being studied. Moreover, because of the in-depth nature of many qualitative studies, there may be a greater invasion of privacy than is true in quantitative research. Researchers who spend time in the home of a study participant may, for example, have difficulty segregating the public behaviors the study participant is willing to share from the private behaviors that unfold unwittingly during the course of data collection. A final thorny issue many qualitative researchers face is adequately disguising study participants in their research reports. Because the number of respondents is typically small and because rich descriptive information is obtained and presented in a research report, it is sometimes difficult to adequately protect the identities of the participants.

◪ VULNERABLE GROUPS

Adherence to ethical standards such as those discussed thus far may, in most cases, be straightforward. The rights of special vulnerable groups, however, may need to be protected through additional procedures and heightened sensitivity on the part of the researcher. **Vulnerable subjects** (the term used in federal guidelines) may be incapable of giving fully informed consent (*e.g.,* mentally retarded people) or may be at high risk of unintended side effects because of their circumstances (*e.g.,* pregnant women). In general, research with vulnerable groups should be undertaken only when the researcher has determined that the risk/benefit ratio is very low.

Consumers should pay particular attention to the ethical dimensions of a study when people who are vulnerable are involved.

Among the groups that nurse researchers should consider as being especially vulnerable are the following:

- *Children.* Legally and ethically, children do not have the competence to give their informed consent. Generally, the informed consent of children's parents or legal guardians is obtained. If the child is developmentally mature enough to understand the basic information involved in informed consent (*e.g.,* a 12-year-old child), it is advisable for the researcher also to obtain consent from the child as evidence of respect for the child's right to self-determination.
- *Mentally or emotionally disabled people.* People whose disability makes it impossible for them to weigh the risks and benefits of participation and make an informed decision (*e.g.,* people affected by mental retardation, senility, mental illness, unconsciousness, and so on) also cannot legally or ethically be expected to provide informed consent. In such cases, the researcher generally obtains the written consent of the person's legal guardian. As in the case of children, informed consent from prospective participants should be sought to the extent possible as a supplement to consent from the guardian.
- *Physically disabled people.* For certain physical disabilities, special procedures for obtaining consent may be required. For example, with deaf people, the entire consent process may need to be in writing. For people who have a physical impairment preventing them from writing (or for people who cannot read and write), alternative procedures for documenting informed consent (such as audiotaping or videotaping the consent proceedings) can be used.
- *Institutionalized people.* Nurses often conduct studies with hospitalized or institutionalized people. Special care may be required in recruiting such participants because they depend on health-care personnel and may feel pressured into participating or may believe that their treatment would be jeopardized by their failure to cooperate. Inmates of prisons and other correctional facilities, who have lost their autonomy in many spheres of activity, may similarly feel constrained in their ability to give free consent. Researchers studying institutionalized groups need to emphasize the voluntary nature of participation.
- *Pregnant women.* The government has issued stringent requirements governing research with pregnant women. These requirements reflect a desire to safeguard both the pregnant woman, who may be at heightened physical and psychological risk, and the fetus, who cannot give informed consent. The regulations stipulate that a pregnant woman cannot be involved in a study unless the purpose of the research is to meet the health needs of the pregnant woman and unless risks to her and the fetus will be minimized.

▨ INSTITUTIONAL REVIEW BOARDS AND EXTERNAL REVIEWS

It is sometimes difficult for researchers to be objective in their assessment of the risk/benefit ratio or in the development of procedures to protect the rights of study participants. Biases may arise as a result of the researcher's commitment to an area of knowledge and desire to conduct a study with as much methodologic rigor as possible. Because of the risk of a biased evaluation, the ethical dimensions of a study normally should be subjected to external review.

Most hospitals, universities, and other institutions where research is conducted have established formal committees and protocols for reviewing research plans and proposed research procedures. These committees are sometimes called **human subjects committees** or **research advisory panels.** If the institution receives federal funds that help to pay for the costs of research, it is likely that the committee will be an **Institutional Review Board (IRB).**

Studies supported with federal funds are subject to strict guidelines with respect to the treatment of humans (and animals) used in research. Before undertaking such a study, the researcher must submit research plans to the IRB, whose duty it is to ensure that the proposed plans meet the federal requirements for ethical research. An IRB can reject the proposed plans or require that modifications be made. In many cases, the IRB reviews the progress of the study at regular intervals during its conduct to monitor adherence to the approved procedures. The IRB must determine that a study involving human participants is proceeding in accordance with federal regulations, which may be summarized as follows (Code of Federal Regulations, 1983):

- Risks to participants are minimized.
- Risks to participants are reasonable in relation to anticipated benefits, if any, and the importance of the knowledge that may reasonably be expected to result.
- Selection of participants is equitable.
- Informed consent is sought, as required, and appropriately documented.
- Adequate provision is made for monitoring the research to ensure the safety of participants.
- Appropriate provisions are made to protect the privacy of participants and the confidentiality of data.
- When vulnerable subjects are involved, appropriate additional safeguards are included to protect their rights and welfare.

Not all research is subject to federal guidelines, and thus not all studies are reviewed by IRBs or other formal committees. Nevertheless, researchers have a responsibility to ensure that their research plans are ethically acceptable, and it is a good practice for researchers to solicit external advice even when they are not required to do so.

▨ ASSISTANCE TO CONSUMERS OF NURSING RESEARCH

What to Expect in the Research Literature

Consumers of research reports are increasingly expected to make judgments about the ethical aspects of the studies. Here are a few tips on what to expect in the research literature with regard to discussions of the rights of study participants:

- Many of the terms introduced in this chapter rarely are used explicitly in a research report. For example, a report almost never calls to the readers' attention that the participants in the study were vulnerable subjects. Consumers need to be sensitive to the special needs of groups that may be unable to act as their own advocates or to assess adequately the costs and benefits of participating in a study.
- Research reports do not always provide readers with detailed information regarding the degree to which the researcher adhered to the ethical principles described in this chapter because space limitations in professional journals make it impossible to document all aspects of the study. The absence of any mention of procedures to safeguard participants' rights does not necessarily imply that no precautions were taken.
- When information about ethical considerations *is* presented in a research report, it almost always appears in the methods section, typically in the subsection devoted to data collection procedures but sometimes in the subsection describing the sample.
- Research reports, if they discuss ethical procedures, are most likely to mention whether informed consent was obtained and whether the research plans were reviewed by an IRB or similar group. Reports are less likely to provide detailed information about the methods used to protect the privacy of participants, assurances of confidentiality, or safeguards to protect participants from harm when risks are minimal.
- Researchers almost never obtain written informed consent when the primary means of data collection is through a self-administered questionnaire. The researcher generally assumes **implied consent** (*i.e.,* that the return of the completed questionnaire reflects the respondent's voluntary consent to participate). This assumption, however, is not always warranted (*e.g.,* if patients feel that their treatment may be affected by failure to cooperate with the researcher).
- As a means of enhancing both personal and institutional privacy, research reports frequently avoid giving explicit information about the locale of the study. For example, the report might state that data were collected in a 200-bed, private, for-profit nursing home, without mentioning its name.
- The issue of privacy is sometimes trickier to handle in qualitative studies because samples are small and it may be difficult to disguise the study

setting. Furthermore, because direct verbatim quotes from informants are often excerpted in qualitative research reports, the researcher has to be particularly careful to safeguard the informant's identity. This may mean more than simply using a fictitious name—it may also mean withholding information about the characteristics of the informant, such as age and occupation.

Critiquing the Ethics of Research Studies

Guidelines for critiquing the ethical aspects of a study are presented in Box 5–2. A nurse who is asked to serve as a member of an IRB or human subjects committee should be provided with sufficient information to answer *all* these questions. As noted above, however, it may not always be possible to critique thoroughly the ethical aspects of a study based on a published research report. Nevertheless, we offer a few suggestions for considering the ethical aspects of a study.

Many research reports do acknowledge that the study procedures were reviewed by an IRB or human subjects committee of the institution with which the researchers are affiliated. When a research report specifically mentions a formal external review, it is generally safe to assume that a panel of concerned people thoroughly reviewed the ethical issues raised by the study.

You can also come to some conclusions based on a description of the study methods. There is usually sufficient information to judge, for example, whether the study participants were subjected to any physical or psychological harm. Reports do not always specifically state whether informed consent was secured, but you

---

Box 5–2

Guidelines of Critiquing the Ethical Aspects of a Study

1. Were the study participants subjected to any physical harm, discomfort, or psychological distress? Did the researchers take appropriate steps to remove or prevent the harm?
2. Did the benefits to participants outweigh any potential risks or actual discomfort they experienced? Did the benefits to society outweigh the costs to participants?
3. Was any type of coercion or undue influence used in recruiting participants? Were vulnerable subjects used?
4. Were participants deceived in any way? Were they fully aware of participating in a study and did they understand the purpose of the research? Were appropriate consent procedures implemented?
5. Were appropriate steps taken to safeguard the privacy of participants?
6. Was the research approved and monitored by an IRB or other similar ethics review committee?

should be alert to situations in which the data could not have been gathered as described if participation were purely voluntary.

It is often especially difficult to determine by reading research reports whether the privacy of the participants was safeguarded unless the researcher specifically mentions pledges of confidentiality or anonymity. A situation requiring special scrutiny arises when data are collected from two people simultaneously (*e.g.,* a husband and wife who are jointly interviewed); in such situations, the absence of privacy raises not only ethical concerns but also questions regarding the participants' candor.

Finally, we encourage you to pay special attention to the ethical aspects of a study under two circumstances: (1) when the risks are more than minimal or (2) when vulnerable groups are used as participants.

RESEARCH EXAMPLES

Although detailed information about the ethical dimensions of a study is rarely reported, many researchers do indicate certain steps they have taken to protect study participants. Table 5–1 outlines the procedures reported in several recent studies. Two research examples that highlight ethical issues are presented below. Use the guidelines in Box 5–2 to evaluate the ethical aspects of the studies. You may need to review the actual research reports (cited at the end of the chapter) to more fully assess the adequacy of the steps the researchers took to safeguard the participants.

Research Example From a Quantitative Study

Holdcraft and Williamson (1991) studied levels of hope among psychiatric and chemically dependent inpatients, noting that hospitalization for these patients might be a time of crisis or despair. Patients in a large general hospital were asked to participate in the study and complete the Miller Hope Scale. Patients in the mental unit were approached within the first 3 days after admission or transfer to the unit. Patients on the chemical dependency unit were told about the study during their transition from the detoxification phase of their treatment. For both groups, the study was explained, and informed consent was obtained. Subjects who agreed to participate completed the questionnaire and returned it in a sealed envelope. The participants were asked to complete the questionnaire a second time to determine if levels of hope changed over the course of their treatment. The participants received the materials and instructions to complete the second questionnaires at discharge. The participants' names were not used on any study materials, except on the consent forms and on a master list of names and code numbers. Consent

Table 5–1. Examples of Procedures to Protect Study Participants

Principle	Study Question	Procedures
Informed consent IRB review Privacy Risk reduction Exclusion of at-risk people	What are the experiences of hospitalized patients who have resuscitation option discussions with a health-care professional?	Approval for the study was obtained from both the Human Subjects Committee and IRB. Prospective participants were informed about the study purpose before consenting to participate. Interviews were conducted without family members or health-care professionals present. Participants were told to conclude the interview if they experienced angina symptoms. Only alert and oriented patients with stable vital signs were included. (Larson, 1994)
Informed consent of minors	What are the behavior patterns of children with Turner syndrome in comparison to those of children with learning disabilities?	Informed consent was obtained from the parents of 8- to 15-year-old children. The children also consented. (Williams, 1994).
Informed consent IRB review Risk reduction Exclusion of vulnerable subjects	What are the effects of different temperature cooling blankets in humans with fever, in terms of time to cool, shivering, and perceived discomfort?	Participants were informed of the study purpose and signed a consent form. Vulnerable subjects (e.g., pregnant women) were excluded. All equipment was carefully tested before the study. IRB approval was secured. (Caruso, Hadley, Shukla, Frame, & Khoury, 1992)
Informed consent Confidentiality Privacy IRB approval	What are the experiences of gay couples when at least one member has been diagnosed with symptomatic HIV infection or AIDS?	Before the initial interview, informed consent was obtained and confidentiality ensured. All interviews were conducted with partners individually (except for one couple who requested a joint interview). IRB approval was obtained. (Powell-Cope, 1995)

forms and the list of names were filed in a separate office and destroyed at the completion of the study.

Research Example From a Qualitative Study

Kearney, Murphy, Irwin, and Rosenbaum (1995) conducted a study of how pregnant crack cocaine users perceived their social psychological problems and responded to them. In-depth interviews were conducted with 60 women who reported regular crack cocaine use and who were either pregnant or within 6 months postpartum. Women were contacted through flyers posted in urban neighborhoods and through health and social service agencies.

Interviews with eligible women were conducted in the field setting of the women's choice. Although the pregnancy status of the women was confirmed at the interview by a urine test, drug testing was not performed "in the interest of protection of legally and socially vulnerable participants" (p. 209). The participants were encouraged to participate in the safeguarding of their own privacy: they were invited to use pseudonyms and to decline to provide personal information such as addresses. To prevent an ethical dilemma that might arise because of potential criminal liability of the participants in connection with divulged information on drug use, the researchers obtained a Certificate of Confidentiality from the National Institute of Drug Abuse. The certificate *required* the researchers to protect the data from discovery for nonresearch use. The study was reviewed and approved by two IRBs. Informed consent was obtained from each study participant, who was paid a stipend of $40 for cooperating in the study. The researchers were cognizant of the potential for psychological distress: "Due to the emotionally difficult and illicit nature of the interview content, interviewers sought to provide women with maximal control over their disclosures" (p. 209). Interviewers made referrals for drug treatment, health care, and other services to women who requested help.

◩ SUMMARY

Research involving humans requires a careful consideration of the procedures used to protect the rights of human participants. Because research has not always been conducted ethically, and because of the genuine **ethical dilemmas** researchers often face in designing studies that are both ethical and methodologically rigorous, **codes of ethics** have been developed to guide researchers. The three major ethical principles incorporated into most guidelines are beneficence, respect for human dignity, and justice.

Beneficence encompasses the maxim: Above all, do no harm. This principle involves the protection of participants from physical and psychological harm, protection of participants from exploitation, and the performance of some good. In evaluating the **risk/benefit ratio** of a study, consumers should weigh the benefits of participation against the costs to individual participants and should also weigh the risks to the participants against the potential benefits to society.

The principle of **respect for human dignity** includes the participants' right to **self-determination,** which means participants have the freedom to control their own activities, including their voluntary participation in the study. The respect principle also includes the participants' right to full disclosure. **Full disclosure** means the researcher has fully described to prospective participants their rights and the full nature of the study. Because full disclosure can lead to potentially misleading and distorted study findings, researchers sometimes believe this principle can, in certain cases, be relaxed. When full disclosure poses the risk of biased results, researchers sometimes use **covert data collection** or **concealment,** which means the collection of information without the participants' knowledge or consent. In other research situations, researchers have used **deception** (either withholding information from participants or providing false information) to avoid biases. When deception or concealment is necessary, researchers should use extra precautions to minimize risks and protect the other rights of participants.

Most studies involve **informed consent** procedures designed to provide prospective participants with sufficient information to make a reasoned decision about the potential costs and benefits of participation. Informed consent normally involves having the participant sign a **consent form,** which documents the participant's voluntary decision to participate after receiving a full explanation of the research. In qualitative studies, consent may need to be continually renegotiated with participants as the study evolves, through **process consent** procedures.

The third principle, **justice,** includes the right to fair treatment (both in the selection of participants and during the course of the study) and the right to privacy. **Privacy** of participants can be maintained through **anonymity** (wherein not even the researcher knows the identity of the participants) or through formal **confidentiality procedures** that safeguard the information participants provide.

Certain people, sometimes referred to as **vulnerable subjects,** require additional protection as study participants. These people may be vulnerable because they are not competent with regard to making an informed decision about participating in a study (*e.g.,* children or mentally retarded people); because their circumstances make them believe free choice is constrained (*e.g.,* an institutionalized group of people); or because their circumstances heighten their risk for physical or psychological harm (*e.g.,* pregnant women).

External review of the ethical aspects of a study is highly desirable and, in many cases, required by either the agency funding the research or the organization from which participants are recruited. Most institutions have special review committees for such purposes. Research funded through the federal government is normally reviewed by the **Institutional Review Board (IRB)** of the institution with which the researcher is affiliated.

STUDY SUGGESTIONS

Chapter 5 of the accompanying *Study Guide to Accompany Essentials of Nursing Research*, 4th edition offers various exercises and study suggestions for reinforcing the concepts presented in this chapter.

Suggested Readings

References on Research Ethics

American Nurses' Association. (1975). *Human rights guidelines for nurses in clinical and other research.* Kansas City, MO: ANA.

American Nurses' Association. (1985). *Code for nurses with interpretive statements.* Kansas City, MO: ANA.

American Psychological Association. (1982). *Ethical principles in the conduct of research with human participants.* Washington, DC: APA.

American Sociological Association. (1984). *Code of ethics.* Washington, DC: ASA.

Code of Federal Regulations. (1983). *Protection of human subjects: 45CFR46* (revised as of March 8, 1983). Washington, DC: Department of Health and Human Services.

Davis, A. J. (1989). Informed consent process in research protocols: Dilemmas for clinical nurses. *Western Journal of Nursing Research, 11,* 448–457.

Munhall, P. L. (1988). Ethical considerations in qualitative research. *Western Journal of Nursing Research, 10,* 150–162.

National Commission for the Protection of Human Subjects of Biomedical and Behavioral Research. (1978). *Belmont Report: Ethical principles and guidelines for research involving human subjects.* Washington, DC: U. S. Government Printing Office.

Substantive References

Caruso, C. C., Hadley, B. J., Shukla, R., Frame, P., & Khoury, J. (1992). Cooling effects and comfort of four cooling blanket temperatures in humans with fever. *Nursing Research, 41,* 68–72.

Holdcraft, C., & Williamson, C. (1991). Assessment of hope in psychiatric and chemically dependent patients. *Applied Nursing Research, 4,* 129–133.

Kearney, M. H., Murphy, S., Irwin, K., & Rosenbaum, M. (1995). Salvaging self: A grounded theory of pregnancy on crack cocaine. *Nursing Research, 44,* 208–213.

Larson, D. E. (1994). Resuscitation discussion experiences of patients hospitalized in a coronary care unit. *Heart & Lung, 23,* 53–58.

Powell-Cope, G. M. (1995). The experiences of gay couples affected by HIV infection. *Qualitative Health Research, 5,* 36–62.

Williams, J. K. (1994). Behavioral characteristics of children with Turner syndrome and children with learning disabilities. *Western Journal of Nursing Research, 16,* 26–35.

Designs
for Nursing Research

PART III

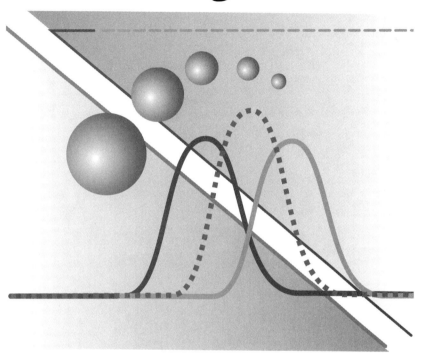

6

Research Design for Quantitative Studies

Student Objectives

On completion of this chapter, the student will be able to:

- describe the various types of decisions that are specified in a research design for a quantitative study
- describe the characteristics of experimental, quasi-experimental, preexperimental, and nonexperimental designs
- discuss the strengths and weaknesses of true experiments, quasi-experiments, preexperiments, and nonexperiments
- identify several specific designs (*e.g.,* factorial design, repeated measures design, randomized block design, nonequivalent control group design, retrospective design) and describe some of their advantages and disadvantages
- distinguish between and evaluate cross-sectional and longitudinal designs
- identify the purposes and some of the distinguishing features of surveys, evaluations, needs assessments, methodologic studies, and meta-analyses
- describe various aspects of research control
- identify and evaluate alternative methods of controlling external and intrinsic extraneous variables
- describe various threats to the internal and external validity of quantitative studies
- identify the type of research design (*e.g.,* experimental, cross-sectional) used in a study as described in a research report
- evaluate a quantitative study in terms of its overall research design and methods of controlling extraneous variables, including the resulting internal and external validity of the design
- define new terms in the chapter

New Terms

After-only design
Analysis of covariance
Attrition
Baseline data
Before–after design
Between-subjects design
Blocking variable
Case-control design
Cell
Clinical trial
Comparison group
Constancy of conditions
Control group

Correlational research
Cost–benefit analysis
Crossover design
Cross-sectional study
Descriptive correlational study
Descriptive research
Double-blind experiment
Evaluations
Ex post facto research
Experiment
Experimental group
External validity
Extraneous variable

Factor
Factorial design
Follow-up study
Hawthorne effect
History threat
Homogeneity
Impact analysis
Implementation analysis
Interaction effects
Internal validity
Intervention
Key informant
Level
Longitudinal study
Main effects
Manipulation
Matching
Maturation threat
Mediating variable
Meta-analysis
Methodologic research
Mortality threat
Needs assessment
Net effects
Nonequivalent control-group design
Nonexperimental research
Outcome analysis
Panel study

Posttest data
Posttest-only design
Preexperimental design
Pretest data
Pretest–posttest design
Process analysis
Prospective study
Protocol
Quasi-experimental design
Random assignment
Randomization
Randomized block design
Repeated measures design
Research control
Research design
Retrospective study
Rival hypothesis
Selection threat
Self-report
Self-selection
Survey
Systematic bias
Table of random numbers
Threats to internal validity
Time series design
Treatment
Trend study
Within-subjects design

 **PURPOSES AND DIMENSIONS
OF RESEARCH DESIGN
IN QUANTITATIVE STUDIES**

Research design refers to the researcher's overall plan for obtaining answers to
the research questions or for testing the research hypotheses. In a quantitative
study, the research design spells out in advance the strategies the researcher plans
to adopt to develop information that is accurate and interpretable. Typically, the
research design for a quantitative study involves decisions with regard to the following aspects of the study:

  • *Will there be an intervention?* In some situations, nurse researchers want
    to study the effects of a specific intervention (*e.g.,* an innovative program to

promote breast self-examination); in others, researchers gather information about phenomena as they currently exist. This is a distinction between two basic types of research design: experimental and nonexperimental. When there is an intervention, the research design specifies the full nature of that intervention and how it is to be implemented.

- *What types of comparison will be made?* Researchers usually develop some type of comparison within their studies so their results will be interpretable. For instance, in an example presented in Chapter 2 (Box 2–4), the researchers studied the emotional consequences of having an abortion. To do this, they compared the emotional status of women who had an abortion with that of women from the same health clinic who delivered a baby. If they had not used a comparison group, it would have been difficult for the researchers to know whether the emotional status of the abortion group members was unusual. Sometimes, researchers use a before–after comparison (*e.g.,* preoperative and postoperative), and sometimes several comparisons are used to more fully understand the phenomena of interest.

- *What procedures will be used to control extraneous variables?* The complexity of relationships among variables characterizing humans may make it difficult to unambiguously test hypotheses unless efforts are made to isolate the independent variables and dependent variables and control other factors extraneous to the research question (that is, to control **extraneous variables**). This chapter discusses techniques for achieving control in quantitative investigations.

- *When and how many times will data be collected from study participants?* In many studies, data are collected from participants at a single point in time. For example, patients might be asked to complete a questionnaire about their nutritional practices. Some studies, however, involve multiple contacts with participants, to determine how things have changed over time, to determine the stability of some phenomenon, or to establish a baseline against which the effect of some intervention can later be compared. The research design designates how often and also when, relative to other events, the data will be collected (*e.g.,* 1 day after operation, in the 13th week of gestation).

- *In what setting will the study take place?* Sometimes, data for quantitative studies are collected in real-world settings, such as in clinics, hospitals, or people's homes. Other studies are conducted in laboratory settings (*i.e.,* in highly controlled environments established for research purposes).

- *What information will be communicated to study participants?* The researcher must decide how much information will be provided to participants. As discussed in Chapter 5, full disclosure to subjects before obtaining their consent to participate is highly desirable ethically, but may in some cases undermine the value of the research. The researcher must consider the costs and benefits of alternative communication strategies.

The research design incorporates some of the most important methodologic decisions the researcher makes in conducting a quantitative study. Other aspects of the study—the data collection plan, the sampling plan, and the analysis plan— also involve important decisions, but the research design stipulates the fundamental form the research will take. For this reason, it is critical for consumers to understand the implications of researchers' design decisions.

There is, unfortunately, no single, easy-to-describe typology of research designs for quantitative studies. Research designs vary along a number of dimensions. Table 6–1 lays out some of the major dimensions of research designs. The dimensions involve whether the researcher has control over the independent variable; what type of comparison is made; how many times data are collected; whether the researcher looks forward or backward in time for the occurrence of the independent and dependent variables; and what type of setting is used for the collection of research data. Each dimension is, with a few exceptions, totally independent of the others. For example, an experimental design can be a between-subjects or within-subjects design; experiments can also be cross-sectional or longitudinal, and so on (these terms are discussed below). Moreover, within any one category, there are a

Table 6–1. Dimensions of Quantitative Research Designs

Dimension	Design	Major Features
Control over independent variable	• Experimental	Manipulation of independent variable, control group, randomization
	• Quasi-experimental	Manipulation of independent variable but no randomization or no control group
	• Nonexperimental	No manipulation of independent variable
Type of group comparisons	• Between-subjects	Participants in groups being compared are different people
	• Within-subjects	Participants in groups being compared are the same people
Number of data collection points	• Cross-sectional	Data collected at one point in time
	• Longitudinal	Data collected at multiple points in time over extended period
Occurrence of independent and dependent variable	• Retrospective	Study begins with dependent variable and looks backward for cause or influence
	• Prospective	Study begins with independent variable and looks forward for the effect
Setting	• Naturalistic	Data collected in a real-world setting
	• Laboratory	Data collected in artificial, contrived setting

number of variants; for example, there are several alternative experimental designs. The sections that follow elaborate on different types of design for quantitative nursing research. Qualitative research design is discussed in Chapter 7.

◻ TYPES OF QUANTITATIVE RESEARCH DESIGN: EXPERIMENTAL, QUASI-EXPERIMENTAL, AND NONEXPERIMENTAL RESEARCH

This section reviews various designs that differ with regard to the amount of control the researcher has over the independent variable. We begin with a discussion of research designs that offer the greatest amount of control: experimental studies.

Experimental Research

Experiments differ from nonexperiments in one important respect: The researcher is an active agent in experimental work rather than a passive observer. Early physical scientists found that, although observation of natural phenomena is valuable and instructive, the complexity of the events occurring in the natural state often obscures the understanding of important relationships. This problem was handled by isolating the phenomenon of interest in a laboratory setting and controlling the conditions under which it occurred. The procedures developed by physical scientists were profitably adopted by biologists during the 19th century, resulting in many achievements in physiology and medicine. The 20th century has witnessed the use of experimental methods by scholars and researchers interested in human behavior and psychological states.

Characteristics of True Experiments

Contrary to a popular misconception, experiments are not necessarily performed in laboratories. Experiments can be conducted in any setting. To qualify as an experiment, a research design need only possess the following three properties:

1. *Manipulation.* The experimenter does something to at least some of the participants in the study.
2. *Control.* The experimenter introduces one or more controls over the experimental situation, including the use of a control group.
3. *Randomization.* The experimenter assigns participants to a control or experimental group on a random basis.

In experimental research, the investigator manipulates the independent variable by administering an experimental **treatment** (or experimental **intervention**) to some subjects while withholding it from others (or administering some alternative treatment, such as a placebo). The experimenter, in other words, has control over and consciously varies the independent variable and then observes its effect on the dependent variable of interest. Let us illustrate the concept of **manipulation** with an example.

Suppose we were interested in investigating the effect on heart rate of physical restraint with a Posey belt. We might choose to begin our experimentation with a nonhuman species, such as the rat. One possible experimental design for addressing the research problem is a **before–after design** (also known as a **pretest–posttest design**). This scheme involves the observation of the dependent variable (heart rate) at two points in time: before and after the administration of the experimental treatment. Each of the rats in the experimental group is restrained with a Posey belt, whereas those in the control group are not. This scheme permits us to examine what changes in heart rate were produced as a result of being physically restrained, because only some of the rats were exposed to restraint by the Posey belt. In this example, we met the first criterion of a true experiment by manipulating physical restraint of the rats, the independent variable.

This example also meets the second requirement for experimental research, the use of a control group. Campbell and Stanley (1963), in a classic monograph on research design, observed that obtaining scientific evidence requires making at least one comparison. But not all comparisons provide equally persuasive evidence. Let us look at an example. If we were to supplement the diet of a group of premature neonates with a particular combination of vitamins and other nutrients every day for 2 weeks, the weight of these infants at the end of the 2-week period would give us absolutely no information about the effectiveness of the treatment. At a bare minimum, we would need to compare their posttreatment weight with their pretreatment weight to determine if, at least, their weights had increased. But let us assume for the moment that we find an average weight gain of half a pound. Does this finding support the conclusion that there is a causative relationship between the nutritional supplements (the independent variable) and weight gain (the dependent variable)? No, it does not. Infants normally gain weight as they mature. Without a control group—a group that does not receive the special supplements—it is impossible to separate the effects of maturation from those of the treatment. The term **control group** refers to a group of participants whose performance on a dependent variable is used as a basis for evaluating the performance of the **experimental group** (the group that receives the treatment of interest to the researcher) on the same dependent variable.

An experimental intervention and a control group are not in themselves sufficient conditions for a true experiment. To qualify as an experiment, the design must also involve the assignment of subjects to groups on a random basis. Through such **randomization** (or **random assignment**), every participant has an equal chance of being included in any group. If people are assigned to groups randomly, there is no **systematic bias** in the groups with respect to attributes that may affect the dependent variable under investigation. Random assignment of subjects to one group or the other is designed to perform an equalization function. Participants who are randomly assigned to groups are expected to be comparable, on average, with respect to a wide range of human characteristics, such as age, gender, race, education, physical condition, and psychological adjustment. Through randomization, groups tend to be equivalent with respect to an infinite number of biologic, psychological, and social traits at the outset of the study. Any differences that emerge after random assignment can therefore be attributed to the experimental treatment.

Random assignment can be accomplished by flipping a coin or pulling names from a hat. Researchers typically either use computers to perform the randomization or rely on a **table of random numbers** (a table displaying hundreds of digits arranged in a random order).

Alternative Experimental Designs

Basic Designs. The most basic experimental design involves the random assignment of subjects to two groups and the subsequent collection of data. This design is sometimes called an **after-only** (or **posttest-only**) **design**. A more refined design, discussed above, is the pretest–posttest or before–after design, which involves the collection of **pretest data** (also known as **baseline data**) before the experimental manipulation and **posttest data** after it.

Factorial Designs. Researchers sometimes manipulate two or more variables simultaneously. Suppose, for example, that we were interested in comparing two therapeutic strategies for premature infants: one method involving tactile stimulation and another approach involving auditory stimulation. Suppose we were also interested in learning if the daily amount of stimulation is related to the progress of the infant. The dependent variables for this study might be various measures of infant development, such as weight gain and cardiac responsiveness. Figure 6–1 illustrates the structure of this experiment.

This type of study, which is an experiment with a **factorial design,** permits the testing of three hypotheses in a single experiment. In the present example, the three research questions being addressed are the following:

1. Does auditory stimulation have a more beneficial effect on the development of premature infants than tactile stimulation?
2. Is the amount of stimulation (independent of modality) related to infant development?
3. Is auditory stimulation most effective when linked to a certain dose and tactile stimulation most effective when coupled with a different dose?

The third question demonstrates a major strength of factorial designs: they permit us to evaluate not only **main effects** (effects resulting from the manipulated variables, as exemplified in questions 1 and 2) but also **interaction effects** (effects resulting from combining the treatment methods). Our results may, for example, indicate that 15 minutes of tactile stimulation and 45 minutes of auditory stimulation are the most beneficial treatments. We could not have learned this by conducting

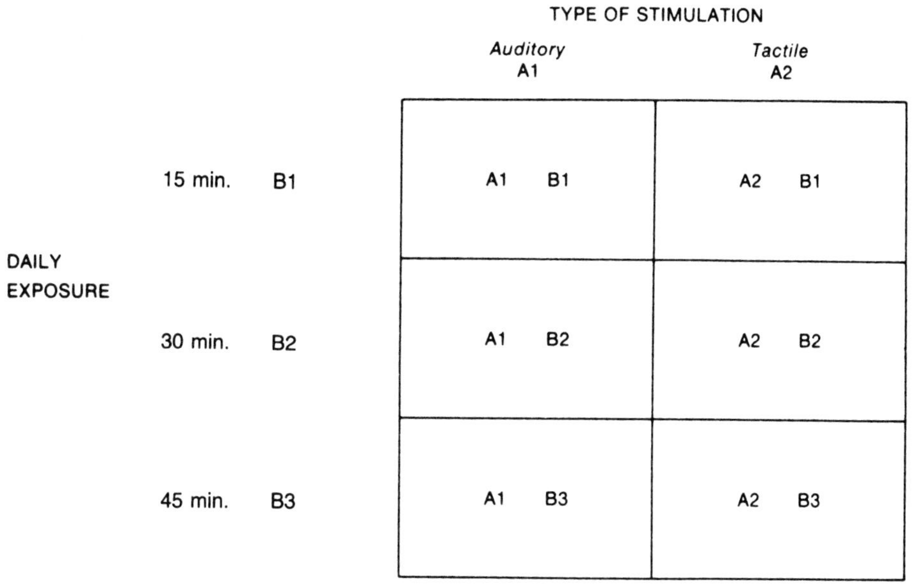

TYPE OF STIMULATION

Figure 6–1. Schematic diagram of a factorial experiment.

two separate experiments that manipulated one independent variable at a time and held the second one constant.

In factorial experiments, subjects are assigned at random to some combination of treatments. In the example that Figure 6–1 illustrates, the premature infants would be assigned randomly to one of the six cells. The term **cell** is used in experimental research to refer to a treatment condition; it is represented in a schematic diagram as a box in the design.

Figure 6–1 can also be used to define some design terminology encountered in the research literature. The two independent variables in a factorial design are referred to as the **factors.** The type-of-stimulation variable is factor A and the amount-of-daily-exposure variable is factor B. Each factor must have two or more **levels.** (If there were only one level, the factor would not be a variable.) Level one of factor A is *auditory* and level two of factor A is *tactile*. When describing the dimensions of the design, researchers refer to the number of levels. The design in Figure 6–1 would be described as a 2×3 design: two levels in factor A times three levels in factor B.

Factorial experiments can be performed with three or more independent variables (factors). Designs with more than three factors are rare, primarily because the number of subjects required becomes prohibitive.

Repeated Measures Design. Thus far, we have described experimental studies in which the subjects who are randomly assigned to different treatments are different people. For instance, in the previous example, infants exposed to 15 minutes of auditory stimulation were not the same infants as those exposed to the other five possible treatment conditions. This broad class of designs is sometimes referred to as **between-subjects designs** because the comparisons being made are between different people. When the *same* subjects are compared, the general class of designs is known as **within-subjects designs.**

A **repeated measures design** (sometimes called a **crossover design**) involves the exposure of the same study participants to more than one experimental treatment. Such studies are true experiments only if the participants are randomly assigned to different orderings of treatment. For example, if a repeated measures design were used to compare the effects of auditory and tactile stimulation on the development of premature infants, some infants would be randomly assigned to receive auditory stimulation first, whereas others would be randomly assigned to receive tactile stimulation first. In such a study, the three conditions for an experiment have been met: there is manipulation, randomization, and control—with subjects serving as their own control group.

A repeated measures design has the advantage of ensuring the highest possible equivalence among subjects exposed to different conditions. However, although repeated measures designs are extremely powerful, they are inappropriate for certain research questions because of the problems of carry-over effects. When subjects are exposed to two different treatments or conditions, they may be influenced in the second condition by their experience in the first condition. As one example, drug studies rarely use a repeated measures design because drug B administered after drug A is not the same treatment as drug B alone. Similarly, drug A administered after a placebo is not the same treatment as a placebo administered after drug A.

Clinical Trials. Medical researchers and epidemiologists often evaluate an innovative treatment through the use of a randomized clinical trial. **Clinical trials** involve the testing of a clinical treatment; random assignment of subjects to experimental and control conditions; the collection of information on outcomes of the treatment from subjects in all groups, sometimes after a long period has elapsed; and, generally, the use of a large and heterogeneous sample of subjects, frequently selected from multiple, geographically dispersed sites to ensure the findings are not unique to a single setting. Clinical trials typically use a before–after or after-only design and are thus not so much a specific design type as a distinctive application of experimental design.

Advantages and Disadvantages of True Experiments

True experiments represent the most powerful method available to scientists for testing hypotheses of cause-and-effect relationships between variables. Because of its special controlling properties, an experiment offers greater corroboration than any other research approach that the independent variable (*e.g.,* diet, drug dosage, teaching approach) has an effect on the dependent variable (*e.g.,* weight loss, recovery of health, learning). The great strength of experiments, then, lies in the confidence with which causal relationships can be inferred.

Lazarsfeld (1955) identified three criteria for causality. First, a cause must precede an effect in time. If we were testing the hypothesis that saccharin causes bladder cancer, it would be necessary to demonstrate that the subjects had not developed cancer before exposure to saccharin. Second, there must be an empirical relationship between the presumed cause and the presumed effect. In the saccharin and cancer example, the researchers would have to demonstrate an association between the ingestion of saccharin and the presence of a carcinoma (*i.e.,* that people who used saccharin experienced a higher incidence of cancer than those who did not). The final criterion for causality is that the relationship cannot be explained as being due to the influence of a third variable. Suppose, for instance, that people who use saccharin tend also to drink more coffee than nonusers. Thus, an empirical relationship between saccharin use and bladder cancer in humans may reflect an underlying causal relationship between a substance in coffee and bladder cancer. It is particularly because of this third criterion that the experimental approach is so strong. Through the controls imposed by manipulation, control groups, and randomization, alternative explanations to a causal interpretation can often be ruled out or discredited.

Despite the advantages of experimental research, this approach has several limitations. First, a number of interesting variables simply are not amenable to experimental manipulation. A large number of human characteristics, such as health problems, gender, or health habits, cannot be randomly conferred on people.

A second limitation is that there are many variables that could technically be manipulated, but ethical considerations prohibit their manipulation. For example, to date, there have not been any experiments using humans to study the effect of cigarette smoking on lung cancer. Such an experiment would require us to randomly assign people to a smoking group (people forced to smoke) or nonsmoking group (people prohibited from smoking). Experimentation with humans, therefore, is subject to a number of ethical constraints.

In many situations, experimentation may not be feasible simply because it is impractical. This often is the case in hospital settings. It may, for instance, be impossible to secure the necessary cooperation from administrators or other key people to conduct an experiment.

Another problem with experiments is the **Hawthorne effect,** which is a kind of placebo effect. The term is derived from a series of experiments conducted at the Hawthorne plant of the Western Electric Corporation in which various environmental conditions, such as light and working hours, were varied to determine their effect on worker productivity. Regardless of what change was introduced (*i.e.,* whether the light was made better or worse), productivity increased. Thus, it seems that the knowledge of being included in a study may be sufficient to cause people to change their behavior, thereby obscuring the effect of the variable of interest.

In a hospital situation, the researcher might have to contend with a double Hawthorne effect. For example, if an experiment investigating the effect of a new postoperative patient routine were conducted, nurses and hospital staff, as well as patients, might be aware of their participation in a study, and both groups could alter their actions accordingly. It is precisely for this reason that **double-blind experiments,** in which neither the subjects nor those who administer the treatment know who is in the experimental or control group, are so powerful. Unfortunately, the double-blind approach is not feasible for some kinds of nursing research because nursing interventions are harder to disguise than medications.

In summary, experimental designs are subject to a number of limitations that make them difficult to apply to many real-world problems; nevertheless, experiments have a clearcut superiority for testing causal hypotheses. Table 6–2 summarizes some recent examples of experimental studies conducted by nurse researchers.

Quasi-Experimental Research

Research that uses a **quasi-experimental design** looks much like an experiment because quasi-experiments also involve the manipulation of an independent variable (*i.e.,* the institution of a treatment). Quasi-experiments, however, lack either the randomization or control-group feature that characterizes true experiments—a fact that weakens the researcher's ability to make causal inferences.

Quasi-Experimental Designs

There are several quasi-experimental designs, but only the two most commonly found in the nursing research literature are discussed here.

Nonequivalent Control Group Design. The most frequently used quasi-experimental design is the **nonequivalent control-group design,** which involves an experimental treatment and two or more groups of subjects. Let us consider an example. Suppose we wished to study the effect of introducing primary nursing as the method of delivering nursing care on nursing staff morale. The system is to be implemented in a 600-bed hospital in a large metropolitan area. Because the new system of nursing care delivery is being implemented throughout the hospital, randomization is not possible. Therefore, we decide to collect comparison data from nurses in another similar hospital that is not instituting primary nursing. We decide to gather data on staff morale in both hospitals before implementing the new nursing care delivery system (the pretest) and again after the system is installed in the first hospital (the posttest).

This quasi-experimental research design is identical to the before–after experimental design discussed in the previous section, *except* subjects were not randomly assigned to the groups. The quasi-experimental design is substantially weaker because, without randomization, *it can no longer be assumed that the experimental and comparison groups are equal at the start of the study.* The design is, nevertheless, a strong one because the collection of pretest data allows us to determine whether the groups were initially similar in terms of their morale. If the comparison

Table 6–2. Examples of Studies Using Experimental Designs

Research Question	Manipulated Variable	Subjects
Design: After-Only		
Does a dextrose-saline solution containing low-dose heparin prolong the use of infusion sites in children? (Wright, Hecker, & McDonald, 1995)	Presence versus absence of low-dose heparin in intravenous infusion	36 children in low-dose heparin group; 44 children in control group
Design: Before–After		
What are the physiological and psychological effects of a back rub in the institutionalized elderly? (Corley, Ferriter, Zeh, & Gifford, 1995)	Back rub versus undisturbed rest	12 patients in backrub group; 7 patients in control group
Design: Factorial		
What is the effect of informational interventions on mothers' and children's ability to cope with an unplanned childhood hospitalization? (Melnyk, 1994)	Receipt of child behavioral information versus nonreceipt; receipt of parental role information versus nonreceipt	26 in child behavioral information group; 22 in parental role information group; 23 in group with neither; 27 in group with both
Design: Repeated Measures		
What is the effect of boomerang pillows on the respiratory capacity of hospitalized patients? (Roberts, Brittin, Cook, & deClifford, 1994)	Placement of patients on boomerang pillows versus straight pillows	42 patients exposed to both types of pillow in random order

and experimental groups responded similarly, on the average, on their pretest questionnaire, we could be relatively confident that any posttest difference in self-reported morale was the result of introducing the experimental treatment. (Note that in quasi-experiments, the term **comparison group** is generally used in lieu of *control group* to refer to the group against which outcomes in the treatment group are evaluated.)

Let us pursue this example a bit further. Suppose we had been unable to collect pretest data before the new method of nursing care delivery was introduced (*i.e.,* only posttest data were collected). This design has a flaw that is difficult to remedy. We have no basis on which to judge the initial equivalence of the two nursing staffs. If we found the morale of the experimental hospital staff was higher than that of the control hospital staff, could we conclude that the new method of delivering care caused an improvement in staff morale? There could be several alternative explanations for the posttest differences. Campbell and Stanley (1963), in fact, would call such a design **preexperimental** rather than quasi-experimental because of its weakness in permitting the desired inferences. Thus, even though quasi-experiments lack some of the controlling properties inherent in true experiments, the hallmark of the quasi-experimental approach is the effort to introduce other controls to compensate for the absence of either the randomization or control-group component.

Time Series Designs. In the above designs, a control group was used, but randomization was not. The design we examine next has neither a control group nor randomization. Let us suppose that a hospital decides to adopt a requirement that all its nurses accrue a certain number of continuing education units before being considered for a promotion or raise. The nurse administrators want to assess some of the positive and negative consequences of this mandate. Some of the dependent variables they might examine include turnover rate, absentee rate, and number of raises and promotions awarded. For the purposes of this example, let us assume there is no other hospital that can serve as a reasonable comparison for this study. In such a case, the only kind of comparison that can be made is a before–after contrast. If the requirement were inaugurated in January, one could compare the turnover rate, for example, for the 3-month period before the new rule with the turnover rate for the subsequent 3-month period.

Although this design seems logical and straightforward, there are actually a number of problems with it. What if one of the 3-month periods is atypical, apart from any regulation? What about the effects of any other hospital rules inaugurated during the same period? What about the effects of external factors, such as changes in the economy? The design in question offers no way of controlling any of these factors. This design again falls into the group called preexperimental by Campbell and Stanley because it fails to control so many possible extraneous factors.

The inability to obtain a meaningful control group, however, does not eliminate the possibility of conducting research with integrity. The previous design could be modified in such a way that at least some of the alternative explanations for any change in the turnover rate of nurses could be ruled out. A design that comes to our assistance in this case is known as the **time series design.** The basic notion underlying the time series design involves the collection of information over an extended time period and the introduction of an experimental treatment during the course of the data collection period. In the present example, the study could be designed with four observations before the new continuing education rule and four observations after it. For example, the first observation might be the number of nurses who resigned between January and March in the year before the new continuing education rule, the second observation might be the number of resignations between April and June, and so forth. After the rule is implemented, data on turnover similarly would be collected for four consecutive 3-month periods, giving us observations 5 through 8.

Although the time series design does not eliminate all the problems of interpreting changes in turnover rate, the extended time perspective immensely strengthens our ability to attribute any change to our experimental manipulation. This is because the time series design permits us to rule out the possibility that changes in resignations merely reflect a random fluctuation of turnover measured at only two points in time.

Advantages and Disadvantages of Quasi-Experiments

The great strength of quasi-experiments lies in their practicality, feasibility, and, to a certain extent, generalizability. It is sometimes impractical to conduct true experiments. Much of the research of interest to nurses occurs in natural settings, where it is often difficult to deliver an innovative treatment to some members of a group at random. Quasi-experimental designs introduce some research control when full experimental rigor is lacking.

The major disadvantage of quasi-experiments is that the kinds of cause-and-effect inferences that researchers often seek cannot be made as easily as with true experiments. With quasi-experiments, there are normally several alternative explanations for observed results. Take as an example the case in which we administer certain medications to a group of infants whose mothers are heroin addicts. Suppose we are interested in determining whether this treatment will result in a weight gain in these typically low-weight infants. If we use no comparison group or if we use a nonequivalent control group and then observe a weight gain, we must ask the following questions: Is it plausible that some other external factor caused or influenced the gain? Is it plausible that pretreatment group differences resulted in differential posttreatment weight gains? Is it plausible that the changes would have occurred in the absence of any intervention? If we answer yes to any of these **rival hypotheses,** then the inferences we can make about the effect of the experimental treatment are weakened considerably. With quasi-experiments, there is almost always at least one plausible rival explanation. We hasten to add, however, that the quality of a study is not necessarily a function of its design. There are many excellent quasi-experimental investigations as well as many weak experiments. Table 6–3 briefly summarizes several quasi-experimental and preexperimental studies conducted by nurse researchers.

Nonexperimental Research

Many research problems do not lend themselves to an experimental or quasi-experimental design. Let us say, for example, that we are interested in studying the effect of widowhood on physical and psychological functioning. Our independent variable here is widowhood versus nonwidowhood. Clearly, we would be unable to manipulate widowhood. Spouses become widows or widowers by a process that is neither random nor subject to research control. Thus, we would have to proceed by taking the two groups as they naturally occur (widows and nonwidows) and comparing them in terms of psychological and physical well-being.

As noted in the section on experimental studies, there are various reasons for doing nonexperimental research, including situations in which the independent variable is inherently nonmanipulable or in which it would be unethical to manipulate the independent variable. There are also many research questions for which an experimental design is not at all appropriate, such as studies whose main purpose is description.

Types of Nonexperimental Research

There are two broad classes of nonexperimental research. One is referred to as **ex post facto research** (or **correlational research**). The literal translation of the Latin term *ex post facto* is "from after the fact." This expression indicates that the research in question has been conducted after the variations in the independent variable have occurred in the natural course of events.

The basic purpose of ex post facto research is essentially the same as that of experimental research: to determine the relationships among variables. The most important distinction between the two is the difficulty of inferring causal relationships in ex post facto studies because of the lack of manipulative control of the independent variables. In experiments, the investigator makes a prediction that a deliberate variation in X, the independent variable, will result in changes to Y, the dependent variable. In ex post facto research, on the other hand, the investigator does not have control of the independent variable—the presumed causative factor—because it has already occurred. Therefore, attempts to draw any cause-and-effect conclusions may be totally unwarranted. There is a famous research dictum that is relevant here: *correlation does not prove causation* (that is, the mere existence of a relationship—even a strong one—between variables is not enough to warrant the conclusion that one variable has caused the other).

Ex post facto research that does attempt to elucidate causal relationships is sometimes described as either retrospective or prospective. **Retrospective studies** are ex post facto investigations in which the manifestation of some phenomenon in the present is linked to other phenomena occurring in the past. That is, the investigator is interested in some outcome and attempts to shed light on the antecedent

Table 6–3. Examples of Studies Using Quasi-experimental and Preexperimental Designs

Research Question	Manipulated Variable	Subjects
Design: One Group, Before–After (Preexperimental)		
Is a special educational program for nurses concerning causes of noise effective in decreasing noise levels in an intensive care unit for infants? (Elander & Hellstrom, 1995)	Nurses' participation in the special program	52 nurses
Design: Nonequivalent Control Group, After-Only (Preexperimental)		
How do four different methods of securing endotracheal tubes in orally intubated patients compare in terms of tube stability, facial skin integrity, and patient satisfaction? (Kaplow & Bookbinder, 1994)	Method of securing endotracheal tubes (Lillihei harness, Comfit, Dale, and SecureEasy)	120 intensive care unit patients (30 per method)
Design: Nonequivalent Control Group, Before–After (Quasi-Experimental)		
Does participation in the Cardiovascular Health Education Program (CHEP) improve adolescents' cardiovascular health knowledge? (MacDonald, 1995)	Participation versus nonparticipation in CHEP	22 adolescents in CHEP; 12 in control group
Design: Time Series (Quasi-Experimental)		
What is the effect of a dietary fiber and fluid intervention on the number of bowel movements and frequency of elimination among residents of a long-term care facility? (Rodrigues-Fisher, Bourguignon, and Good, 1993)	Participation in a dietary fiber and fluid program	15 laxative-dependent nursing home residents followed over a 6-month period

factors that have caused it. Many epidemiologic studies are retrospective in nature. For example, many lung cancer studies with humans have been retrospective in nature. In retrospective lung cancer research, the investigator begins with a sample of those who have already developed the disease and a sample of those who have not. Then the researcher looks for differences between the two groups in antecedent behaviors or conditions, such as smoking habits.

Prospective studies, by contrast, start with an examination of a presumed cause and then go forward in time to the presumed effect. For example, in prospective lung cancer studies, the investigators start with samples of smokers and nonsmokers and later compare the two groups in terms of lung cancer incidence. As a rule, prospective studies are more costly than retrospective studies but are considerably stronger. For one thing, any ambiguity concerning the temporal sequence of phenomena is resolved readily in prospective research (*i.e.,* the smoking preceded the lung cancer). In addition, samples are more likely to be representative of smokers and nonsmokers, and investigators may be in a position to impose controls to rule out competing explanations for observed effects.

However, researchers can sometimes strengthen a retrospective study by taking certain steps. For example, one type of retrospective design known as a **case-control design** involves the comparison of "cases" with a certain illness or condition (*e.g.,* breast cancer) with controls (women without breast cancer) who are carefully selected to be similar to the "cases" with regard to important background factors. To the degree that the researcher can demonstrate similarity between cases and controls with regard to extraneous traits, the inferences regarding the presumed cause of the disease are enhanced.

The second broad class of nonexperimental research is **descriptive research.** The purpose of descriptive studies is to observe, describe, and document aspects of a situation. For example, an investigator may wish to determine the percentage of teenaged mothers who receive inadequate prenatal care. Or a researcher might be interested in studying the average number of hours a woman with premenstrual symptoms experiences pain or discomfort. Because the intent in these cases is not to explain or to understand the underlying causes of the variables of interest, a nonexperimental design is appropriate.

Advantages and Disadvantages
of Nonexperimental Research

The major disadvantage of nonexperimental research is that, relative to experimental and quasi-experimental research, it is weak in its ability to reveal causal relationships. Ex post facto studies, which examine the relationships among variables, are, susceptible to faulty interpretation. This situation stems in large part from the fact that, in ex post facto studies, the researcher works with preexisting groups that have not formed by a random process but rather by what might be termed a self-selecting process. Kerlinger (1986) has offered the following description of **self-selection:**

Self-selection occurs when the members of the groups being studied are in the groups, in part, because they differentially possess traits or characteristics extraneous to the research problem, characteristics that possibly influence or are otherwise related to the variables of the research problem. (p. 349)

In other words, preexisting differences may be a plausible alternative explanation for any observed differences on the dependent variable of interest.

An example may help to make the problems of interpreting ex post facto results more clear. Let us suppose we were interested in studying differences in the level of depression of cancer patients who do or do not have adequate social support (*i.e.,* adequate assistance and emotional sustenance through a social network). Our independent variable in this hypothetical study is social support adequacy, and our dependent variable is level of depression. Let us say that we find that the patients without social support are significantly more depressed than the patients whose social support is adequate. We could interpret this finding to mean that people's emotional state is influenced by the adequacy of their social supports. This relationship is diagrammed in Figure 6–2A. There are, however, alternative explanations for the findings. Perhaps there is a third variable that influences *both* social support and depression, such as the patients' family configuration (*e.g.,* whether they are married, have children, and so forth). It may be that the availability or quantity of significant others is a powerful influence on how depressed cancer patients feel *and* on the quality of their social

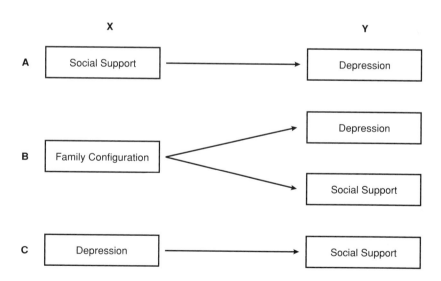

Note: Arrows show direction of causation or influence; variable *X* is presumed to cause variable *Y*

Figure 6–2. Alternative explanations for relationship between depression and social support in cancer patients.

support. This set of relationships is diagrammed in Figure 6–2B. A third possibility may be reversed causality, as shown in Figure 6–2C. Depressed cancer patients may find it more difficult to elicit needed social support from others than patients who are more cheerful or sociable. In this interpretation, it is the person's depression that causes the amount of received social support, and not the other way around. Undoubtedly, you will be able to invent other alternatives. The point is that interpretations of most ex post facto results should be considered tentative, particularly if the research has no theoretical basis.

Despite the interpretive problems associated with ex post facto studies, they continue to play a crucial role in nursing because many of the interesting problems to be solved are not amenable to experimentation. Correlational research is often an efficient and effective means of collecting a large amount of data about a problem area. For example, it would be possible to collect extensive information about the health histories and eating habits of a large number of people. Researchers could then examine which health problems correlate with which diets. By doing this, a large number of interrelationships could be discovered in a relatively short time. By contrast, an experimenter looks at only a few variables at a time. For example, one experiment might be devoted to manipulating foods with different cholesterol levels to observe the effects on certain medical symptoms, while another experiment could manipulate protein consumption, and so forth.

One final advantage is that nonexperimental research tends to be high in realism. Correlational and descriptive research can seldom be criticized for their artificiality and may, in fact, go far in advancing our understanding of what the world around us is like. Table 6–4 presents several examples of nonexperimental nursing studies.

◻ TYPES OF QUANTITATIVE RESEARCH DESIGN: THE TIME DIMENSION

As mentioned in the first section of this chapter, the research design generally specifies when and how often data will be collected in a study. In many nursing studies, data are collected at a single point in time; other studies involve data collection several times. Indeed, several designs involving multiple measurements have already been discussed, such as the pretest–posttest experimental design, the time series design, and the prospective design.

There are four situations in which it might be appropriate to design a study with multiple points of data collection:

1. *Time-related processes.* Certain research problems are concerned with phenomena that evolve over time. Examples include such phenomena as healing, learning, growth, recidivism, and physical development.
2. *Time-sequenced phenomena.* It is sometimes important to ascertain correctly the temporal sequencing of phenomena. For example, if it is hypothe-

Table 6–4. Examples of Nonexperimental Studies

Research Question	Study Participants
Design: Correlational, Retrospective	
What hospital workload factors are predictive of nurse medication errors? (Roseman & Booker, 1995)	Patient records over a 5-year period in an acute care medical center
Design: Correlational, Prospective	
What factors best predict functional status after percutaneous transluminal coronary angioplasty (PTCA)? (Fitzgerald, Zlotnick, & Kolodner, 1996)	135 adults who underwent PTCA, followed-up 12 months after the PTCA procedure
Design: Case-Control	
Can assaultive patients be distinguished from nonassaultive patients on the basis of behavioral asessments or sociodemographic variables? (Lanza, Kayne, Pattison, Hicks, & Islam, 1996)	36 patients who were assaultive (cases) and 36 patients randomly selected from ones who were not assaultive (controls)
Design: Descriptive	
What factors do intensive care unit resident physicians and nurses perceive as influential in making decisions about level of aggressiveness of patient care? (Baggs & Schmitt, 1995)	33 ICU resident physicians and 57 ICU nurses

sized that infertility contributes to depression, then it would be important to determine that depression did not precede the fertility problem.

3. *Comparative purposes.* Sometimes, a time dimension is useful for placing findings in a broader context to determine if changes have occurred over time. For example, a study might be concerned with documenting trends in the incidence of child abuse over a 10-year period. Another example is a study using a time series design, in which the intent is to see if changes over time can reasonably be attributed to some intervention.

4. *Enhancement of research control.* Some research designs collect data at multiple points to enhance the interpretability of the results. For example, in nonequivalent control-group designs, the collection of preintervention data allows the researcher to detect and control for any initial differences between groups.

Because of the importance of the time dimension in designing research, studies are often categorized in terms of how they deal with time. The major distinction is between cross-sectional and longitudinal designs.

Cross-Sectional Designs

Cross-sectional studies involve the collection of data at one point in time. The phenomena under investigation are captured, as they manifest themselves, during one period of data collection. Cross-sectional designs are especially appropriate for describing the status of phenomena or relationships among phenomena at a fixed point in time. For example, a researcher might be interested in determining whether psychological symptoms in menopausal women are correlated contemporaneously with physiologic symptoms. Retrospective studies are almost always cross-sectional. Data with regard to the independent and dependent variables are collected concurrently (*e.g.,* the lung cancer status of respondents and their smoking habits), but the independent variable usually captures events or behaviors occurring in the past.

Cross-sectional designs are sometimes used for time-related purposes such as the four described previously, and, in such instances, these designs are generally weaker than longitudinal designs. Suppose, for example, we were interested in studying the changes in nursing students' attitudes toward nursing research as they progress through a 4-year baccalaureate program. One way to investigate this issue would be to survey students when they are freshmen and resurvey them every year until they graduate. On the other hand, we could use a cross-sectional design by surveying members of the four classes at one point in time and then comparing the responses of the four groups. If seniors manifested more positive attitudes toward research than freshmen, it might be inferred that nursing students become increasingly socialized professionally by their educational experiences. To make this kind of inference, the researcher must assume that the senior students would have responded as the freshmen responded had they been questioned 3 years earlier, or, conversely, that freshmen students would demonstrate increased favorability toward research if they were surveyed 3 years later.

The main advantage of cross-sectional designs is that they are practical. They are relatively economical and easy to manage. There are, however, a number of problems in inferring changes and trends over time using a cross-sectional design. The overwhelming amount of social and technologic change that characterizes our society makes it questionable to assume in many instances that differences in the behaviors, attitudes, or characteristics of different age groups are the result of the passage through time rather than cohort or generational differences. In the previous example, seniors and freshmen may have different attitudes toward nursing research independent of any experiences they had during their 4 years of education. In cross-sectional studies, there are frequently several alternative explanations for any observed differences.

Longitudinal Designs

Research projects designed to collect data over an extended time period are referred to as **longitudinal studies.** The main value of longitudinal designs lies in their ability to demonstrate clearly (1) trends or changes over time and (2) the temporal sequencing of phenomena, which is an essential criterion for establishing causality.

Three types of longitudinal studies deserve special mention: trend, panel, and follow-up studies. **Trend studies** are investigations in which samples from a general population are studied over time with respect to some phenomenon. Different samples are selected at repeated intervals, but the samples are always drawn from the same population. Trend studies permit researchers to examine patterns and rates of change over time and to make predictions about future directions. For example, trend studies have been conducted to analyze the number of students entering nursing programs and to forecast future supplies of nursing personnel.

Panel studies differ from trend studies in that the same participants are used to supply the data at two or more points in time. The term *panel* refers to the sample of people involved in the study. Panel studies typically yield more information than trend studies because the investigator is in a better position to examine patterns of change and reasons for the changes. Because the same people are contacted at two or more points in time, the researcher can identify those who did and did not change and then isolate the characteristics of the subgroups in which changes occurred. As an example, a panel study could be designed to explore over time the coping mechanisms of caretakers of AIDS patients. Panel studies are intuitively appealing as an approach to studying change but are extremely difficult and expensive to manage. The most serious problem is the loss of participants at different points in the study. Subject **attrition** is problematic for the researcher because those who drop out of the study may differ in important respects from those who continue to participate; hence, the generalizability of the findings may be impaired.

Follow-up studies are undertaken to determine the subsequent development of subjects with a specified condition or who have received a specified intervention. For example, patients who have received a particular nursing intervention or clinical treatment may be followed up to ascertain the long-term effects of the treatment. To take a nonexperimental example, samples of premature and normal infants may be followed up to assess their later perceptual and motor development. Prospective studies generally fall in this category.

Longitudinal designs are useful for studying the dynamics of a variable or phenomenon over time. The number of data collection periods and the time intervals between the data collection points depend on the nature of the study. When change or development is rapid, numerous time points at relatively short intervals may be required to document the pattern and to make accurate forecasts. By convention, however, the term *longitudinal* implies multiple data collection points over an extended period of time. Our earlier example of a time series study, which involved the collection of data on nurse turnovers over a 2-year period, would be considered longitudinal. However, a time series design involving the collection of patient data on vital signs preoperatively and postoperatively at 2-hour intervals over a 3-day period would not be described as longitudinal.

Many nursing studies involve a time dimension. Table 6–5 presents a brief description of several nursing studies that have used different research designs to address time-related research questions.

Table 6–5. Examples of Studies with a Time Dimension

Research Question	Study Participants
Design: Cross-Sectional	
What is the pattern of development of nutritive sucking in very low birth weight (VLBW) infants of different gestational ages? (Medoff-Cooper, Verklan, & Carlson, 1993)	50 VLBW infants born at 27 to 32 weeks of gestational age
Design: Longitudinal (Trend Study)	
What are the trends in the academic achievement, values, and personal attributes of college freshmen aspiring to nursing careers from the 1960s to the 1980s? (Williams, 1988)	Samples of 500 college freshmen surveyed in 1966, 1972, 1982, 1983, 1984, and 1985
Design: Longitudinal (Panel Study)	
What is the relationship between preschool children's mental health and maternal depression measured 1 year earlier? (Gross, Conrad, Fogg, Willis, & Garvey, 1995)	Two panels of children, one followed from age 2 to 3 and the other followed from age 3 to 4
Design: Longitudinal (Follow-Up Study)	
What is the extent to which social support from the spouse and a health care provider is associated with long-term recovery outcomes in individuals after a cardiac illness? (Yates, 1995)	73 cardiac patients questioned 2 months and then 1 year after a cardiac event

ADDITIONAL TYPES OF QUANTITATIVE RESEARCH

The previous sections discussed different types of quantitative research based on several dimensions of research design. This section is devoted to a brief description of some additional types of quantitative research that vary according to the study's purpose rather than the dimensions outlined in Table 6–1.

Surveys

A **survey** is designed to obtain information regarding the prevalence, distribution, and interrelationships of variables within a population. Political opinion polls, such as those conducted by Gallup or Harris, are examples of surveys. Surveys obtain information from a sample of people by means of **self-report** (*i.e.,* the people in the sample respond to a series of questions posed by the investigator). Surveys collect information on people's actions, knowledge, intentions, opinions, attitudes, and values. Survey data can be collected in a number of ways. The three most common methods are personal, face-to-face interviews; interviews by telephone; and self-administered questionnaires distributed through the mail. The greatest advantages of survey research are its flexibility and broadness of scope. It can be applied to many populations, it can focus on a wide range of topics, and its information can be used for many purposes. The information obtained in most surveys, however, tends to be relatively superficial. Survey research is better suited to extensive rather than intensive analysis. Although surveys can be performed within the context of large-scale experiments, surveys are usually done as part of a nonexperimental study.

Evaluations

The purpose of **evaluations** is to find out how well a program, treatment, practice, or policy is working. In clinical nursing, nursing administration, and nursing education, there is often a need to sit back and pose such questions as the following: How are we doing? Are we accomplishing our goals? Is there a more effective way to do things? In this era of accountability, evaluations of the effectiveness of nursing actions are becoming increasingly common. In evaluation research, the purpose of the research is to answer pressing questions of people who must make decisions: Should the practice be continued? Do current policies need to be modified, or should they be abandoned altogether? Evaluations can employ experimental, quasi-experimental, or nonexperimental designs and can either be cross-sectional or longitudinal.

Evaluations are undertaken to address a variety of questions. A **process analysis** (sometimes called an **implementation analysis**) is undertaken when there is a need for descriptive information about the process by which a program or procedure gets implemented, and how it functions in actual operation. An **outcome analysis** documents the extent to which the goals of a program are attained (*i.e.,* the extent to which positive outcomes occur). An **impact analysis** attempts to identify (usually using an experimental design) the impacts or **net effects** of an intervention (*i.e.,* the effects over and above what would have occurred in the absence of the intervention). Finally, evaluations sometimes include a **cost–benefit analysis** to determine whether the benefits of the program outweigh the monetary costs.

Needs Assessments

A **needs assessment** is a study in which a researcher collects data for estimating the needs of a group, community, or organization. Surveys can be used to assess needs. Through a survey approach, the researcher can obtain information on the needs and perceived needs of a broad spectrum of people, directly from those whose needs are being determined. For example, nursing staff in a mental health outreach clinic might wish to gather information about the treatment needs of the elderly in the community by surveying a sample of elderly community residents.

Another approach is to use **key informants,** wherein the needs of a group are determined on the basis of reports from authoritative people who are in a position to know those needs. Needs assessments are useful planning tools because resources are seldom limitless, and information that can help in establishing priorities is almost always valuable.

Methodologic Research

Methodologic research refers to investigations of the methods of obtaining, organizing, and analyzing data. Methodologic studies address the development, validation, and evaluation of research tools or techniques. The methodologic researcher may, for example, concentrate on the development of an instrument that accurately measures patients' satisfaction with nursing care. The researcher in such a case is not interested in the level of patient satisfaction nor in how that satisfaction relates to other factors. The goals of the researcher are to develop an accurate, serviceable, and trustworthy instrument that can be used by other researchers and to evaluate his or her success in doing so. Methodologic studies are indispensable in any scientific discipline, and perhaps especially so when a field is relatively new and deals with highly complex phenomena, such as human behavior or health, as is the case in nursing research.

Meta-analysis

Chapter 4 described the function of a literature review as a preliminary step in a research project. However, there is growing recognition of the fact that the careful integration of knowledge on a topic in itself constitutes an important scholarly endeavor that can contribute new knowledge. The procedure known as **meta-analysis** represents an application of statistical procedures to findings from research reports. In essence, meta-analysis treats the findings from one study as a single piece of data. The findings from multiple studies on the same topic can, therefore, be combined to yield a data set that can be analyzed in a manner similar to that obtained from individuals. Meta-analytic procedures provide a convenient and objective method of integrating a large body of findings and of observing patterns and relationships that might otherwise have gone undetected. Meta-analysis can thus serve as an important scholarly tool in theory development, as well as in research utilization.

Examples of a survey, evaluation, needs assessment, methodologic study, and meta-analysis are briefly summarized in Table 6–6.

▧ TECHNIQUES OF RESEARCH CONTROL

A major purpose of research design in quantitative studies is to maximize the amount of control that an investigator has over the research situation and variables. This section describes what is meant by research control and then discusses methods of achieving it.

Table 6–6. Examples of Various Types of Quantitative Nursing Studies

Research Question	Type of Study
How do nurses initially learn about the medical devices they use and the consequences of their use? (McConnell, 1995)	Survey
What is the effect of a dyadic remediation program on functional outcomes of older care recipients with dementia? (Quayhagen, Quayhagen, Corbeil, Roth, & Rodgers, 1995)	Evaluation
What are the psychosocial and physiological health care needs of persons with HIV/AIDS in hospital, outpatient, home care, and long-term care settings? (Berk, Baigis-Smith, & Nanda, 1995)	Needs assessment
What organizational and client-centered factors function as barriers to the recruitment, retention, and protocol compliance of subjects in community-based clinical trials? (Morse, Simon, Besch, & Walker, 1995)	Methodologic study
What are the effects of psychoeducational care on blood pressure, knowledge about hypertension, medication compliance, weight, compliance with health care appointments, and anxiety, based on existing research? (Devine & Reifschneider, 1995)	Meta-analysis

Research Control

Essentially, **research control** is concerned with holding constant possible influences on the dependent variable under investigation so that the true relationship between the independent and dependent variables can be understood. In other words, research control attempts to eliminate any contaminating factors that might otherwise obscure the relationship between the variables that are of central interest. A detailed example should clarify this point.

Let us suppose that a researcher is interested in studying whether teenaged women are at higher risk of having low-birth-weight infants than older mothers specifically because of their age. In other words, the researcher wants to test whether there is something about the physiologic development of women that causes differences in the birth weights of their infants. Existing studies have shown that, in fact, teenagers have a higher rate of low-birth-weight infants than women in their twenties. The question, however, is whether age itself causes this difference or whether there are other **mediating variables** that intervene in the relationship between maternal age and infant birth weight.

The researcher in this example would probably want to design the study in such a way that other possible mechanisms are controlled. But which variables should be controlled? To answer this, one must ask the following critical question: What variables could affect the dependent variable under study and at the same time be related to the independent variable?

In the present study, the dependent variable is infant birth weight and the independent variable is maternal age. Two variables that are candidates for concern (although there are several other possibilities) are the nutritional habits of the mother and the amount of prenatal care received. Teenagers are not always as careful as older women about their eating patterns during pregnancy and are also less likely to obtain adequate prenatal care. Both nutrition and the amount of care could, in turn, affect the baby's birth weight. Thus, if these two mediating factors are not controlled, then any observed relationship between the mother's age and her baby's weight at birth could be caused by the mother's age, by her diet, or by her prenatal care.

These three possible explanations are shown schematically.

1. Mother's age → infant birth weight
2. Mother's age → prenatal care → infant birth weight
3. Mother's age → nutrition → infant birth weight

The arrows symbolize a causal mechanism or an influence. The researcher's task is to design a study in which the true explanation is made clear. If the researcher is testing the first explanation, then both nutrition and prenatal care must be controlled.

How can the researcher impose this control? A number of ways are discussed later, but the general principle underlying each alternative is the same: the competing influences—referred to as extraneous variables—must be held constant. The extraneous variables must somehow be handled in such a way that, in the context of the study, they are not related to the independent variable or dependent variable.

Research control is viewed as essential in most quantitative studies because the world is extremely complex and many variables are interrelated in complicated ways. When studying a particular problem, it is difficult to examine this complexity directly. Researchers analyze a few relationships at one time and put the pieces together like a jigsaw puzzle. That is why even modest quantitative studies can make contributions to science. The extent of the contribution, however, is often related to how well a researcher is able to control contaminating influences. Consumers of research reports must consider whether the researcher has, in fact, appropriately controlled extraneous variables.

Controlling External Factors

In carefully controlled quantitative research, steps usually are taken to minimize situational contaminants (that is, to achieve **constancy of conditions** for the collection of data). Researchers often try to make the conditions under which the data are collected as similar as possible for every participant in the study so they can be confident that the conditions are not influencing the data.

The environment has been found to exert a powerful influence on people's emotions and behavior. In designing research, therefore, investigators often pay attention to the environmental context within which the study is being conducted.

Control over the environment is most easily achieved in laboratory experiments in which all subjects are brought into an environment that the experimenter is in a position to arrange. Researchers have much less freedom in controlling the environment in studies that occur in natural settings, but there are opportunities for control even in these settings. For example, in interview studies, researchers sometimes restrict data collection to a single type of setting (*e.g.,* the respondents' homes).

A second external factor that may need to be controlled is time. Depending on the topic of the study, the criterion variable may be influenced by the time of day or the time of year in which the data are collected, or both. In these cases, it probably would be important for the researcher to ensure that constancy of time is maintained. If an investigator were studying fatigue or perceptions of well-being, it would probably matter a great deal whether the data were gathered in the morning, afternoon, or evening or in the summer as opposed to the winter.

Another aspect of maintaining constancy of conditions concerns constancy in the communications to the subjects and in the treatment itself in the case of experiments or quasi-experiments. To ensure constancy of communication, formal scripts are often prepared for research personnel assisting in quantitative studies. In research involving the implementation of a treatment, formal research **protocols,** or specifications for the interventions, are developed. For example, in an experiment to test the effectiveness of a new drug to cure a medical problem, great care would have to be taken to ensure that the subjects in the experimental group received the same chemical substance and the same dosage, that the substance was administered in the same way, and so forth.

Controlling Intrinsic Factors

Characteristics of the study participants are the primary targets of research control in most studies. For example, suppose we were investigating the effects of a physical training program on the cardiovascular functioning of nursing home residents. In this study, such variables as age, gender, prior occupation of the participants, and smoking history might be considered extraneous variables. Each of these characteristics might be related to the outcome of interest (cardiovascular functioning) independent of the physical training program. In other words, the effects that these variables have on the dependent variable are extraneous to the research topic. In this section, we review methods of controlling extraneous participant characteristics.

Randomization. We have already discussed the most effective method of controlling subject characteristics: randomization. The primary function of randomization is to secure comparable groups (*i.e.,* to equalize the groups with respect to the extraneous variables). A distinct advantage of random assignment, compared with most other methods of controlling extraneous variables, is that randomization controls *all* possible sources of extraneous variation, without any conscious decision on the researcher's part about which variables need to be controlled. Randomization within a repeated measures context is especially powerful, unless carry-over effects from one condition to another threaten the integrity of the manipulated variable (*e.g.,* drug A followed 2 hours later by drug B is not necessarily the same as drug B followed by drug A). In a repeated measures design, participants serve as their own controls, thereby totally controlling all extraneous variables. In our example of the physical training intervention, random assignment of subjects to an experimental (intervention) group and control (no intervention) group would be possible, but a repeated measures design does not seem appropriate in this case.

Homogeneity. When randomization is not feasible, there are several other methods of controlling extraneous subject characteristics. The first alternative is **homogeneity** (*i.e.,* using only subjects who are homogeneous with respect to the variables that are considered extraneous). The extraneous variables, in this case, are not allowed to vary. In the example of the physical training program, if gender were considered to be an important confounding variable, the researcher might wish to use only men (or only women) as participants. If the researcher were concerned about the effects of the participants' ages on physical fitness, participation in the study could be limited to those within a specified age range. This method of using a homogeneous pool of participants is fairly easy and offers considerable control. The limitation of this approach lies in the fact that the research findings can only be generalized to the type of subjects who participated in the study. If the physical training program was found to have beneficial effects on the cardiovascular functioning of a sample of men aged 65 to 75 years, its usefulness for improving the cardiovascular status of women in their eighties would be strictly a matter of conjecture.

Blocking. Another approach to controlling extraneous variables is to include them in the design of a study as independent variables. To pursue our example of the physical training program, if gender were thought to be a confounding variable, it could be built into the study design, as shown in Figure 6–3. This procedure would allow us to make an assessment of the impact of the physical training program on physical fitness for both men and women.

The design in Figure 6–3 is known as a **randomized block design.** The variable gender, which cannot be manipulated by the researcher, is known as a **blocking variable.** In an experiment to test the effectiveness of the physical training program, the experimenter obviously cannot randomly assign subjects to one of four cells: the gender of the subjects is a given. But the experimenter can randomly assign men and women separately to the experimental and control conditions.

Matching. A fourth method of dealing with extraneous variables is known as **matching.** Matching involves using information about subject characteristics to form comparison groups. For example, suppose the researcher began with a sample of nursing home residents already participating in the physical training program. A

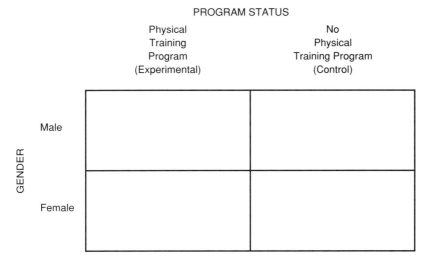

Figure 6–3. Schematic diagram of a randomized block design.

comparison group of nonparticipants could be created by matching subjects, one by one, on the basis of important extraneous variables (*e.g.,* age and gender). This procedure would result in two groups known to be comparable in terms of the extraneous variables of concern. Matching is the technique used to form comparable groups in case-control designs.

Matching has some drawbacks as a control technique. To match effectively, the researcher must know in advance what the relevant extraneous variables are. This information is not always available or may be imperfect. Second, after two or three variables, it often becomes impossible to match adequately. Let's say we are interested in controlling for the age, gender, race, and length of nursing home stays of the participants. Thus, if participant 1 in the physical training program is an African-American woman, aged 80 years, whose length of stay is 5 years, the researcher must seek another woman with these same or similar characteristics as a comparison group counterpart. With more than three variables, the matching procedure becomes extremely cumbersome, if not impossible. For these reasons, matching as a technique for controlling extraneous variables should, in general, be used only when more powerful procedures are not feasible.

Analysis of Covariance. Yet another method of controlling extraneous variables is through statistical analysis. We recognize that many readers are unfamiliar with basic statistical procedures, let alone sophisticated techniques such as those referred to here. Therefore, a detailed description of a powerful statistical control mechanism, known as **analysis of covariance,** will not be attempted. Consumers should recognize, however, that nurse researchers are increasingly using powerful statistical techniques to control extraneous variables. A brief description of analysis of covariance is presented in Chapter 11.

Evaluation of Control Methods

Overall, the random assignment of subjects to groups is the most effective approach to managing extraneous variables because randomization tends to cancel out individual variation on all possible extraneous variables. Repeated measures designs, although extremely useful in controlling all sources of extraneous variation, cannot be applied to all nursing research problems because of the possibility of strong carry-over effects. The four remaining alternatives described here have one disadvantage in common: the researcher must know or predict in advance the relevant extraneous variables. To select homogeneous samples, develop a blocking design, match, or perform an analysis of covariance, the researcher must make a decision about which variable or variables need to be controlled. This constraint may pose severe limitations on the degree of control that is possible, particularly because the researcher can seldom deal explicitly with more than two or three extraneous variables at a time.

Although we have repeatedly hailed randomization as the ideal mechanism for controlling extraneous subject characteristics, it is clear that randomization is not always possible. If the independent variable cannot be manipulated, then other techniques must be used. In our previous example concerning the effects of maternal age on infant birth weight, for example, it would not be possible to randomly assign women to different age groups. However, control methods such as matching, blocking, homogeneity, and statistical techniques could be used. All the control techniques discussed in this section have been profitably used by nurse researchers. Table 6–7 presents some research examples of these procedures.

INTERNAL AND EXTERNAL VALIDITY

Consumers evaluating the merits of a quantitative study need to pay careful attention to its research design. One framework for evaluating the adequacy of a research design in a quantitative study is to assess its internal and external validity.

Internal Validity

Campbell and Stanley (1963), in a classic monograph, use the term **internal validity** to refer to the extent to which it is possible to make an inference that the independent variable is truly influencing the dependent variable. True experiments possess a high degree of internal validity because the use of such procedures as control groups and randomization enables the researcher to control extraneous variables, thereby ruling out most alternative explanations for the results. With

Table 6–7. Examples of Studies Using Various Control Techniques

Research Question	Control Technique	Extraneous Variables Controlled
What is the effect of indwelling versus intermittent feeding tube placement on weight gain, apnea, and bradycardia in premature neonates? (Symington, Ballantyne, Pinelli, & Stevens, 1995)	Randomization	All
How effective are various comfort measures in alleviating nipple soreness in breastfeeding women? (Buchko, Pugh, Bishop, Cochran, Smith, & Lerew, 1994)	Homogeneity	Parity, riskiness of pregnancy, method of delivery, gestational age
Is massage an effective intervention for alleviating pain in cancer patients? (Weinrich & Weinrich, 1990)	Blocking Randomization	Patients' gender All other
What is the impact of the perceived quality of parental relationships on coping strategies, received support, and well-being in adolescents from separated/divorced versus married households? (Grossman & Rowat, 1995)	Matching	Adolescents' gender, age class, and parents' occupation
Do women who receive different treatments for breast cancer (mastectomy, mastectomy with delayed or immediate reconstruction, conservative surgery) differ with respect to body image? (Mock, 1993)	Analysis of covariance	Age

quasi-experiments and correlational studies, the investigator must always contend with competing explanations (rival hypotheses) for the obtained results. These competing explanations, referred to as **threats to internal validity,** have been grouped into several classes, a few of which are discussed here.

Threats to Internal Validity

History. The threat of **history** refers to the occurrence of events that take place concurrently with the independent variable that can affect the dependent variables. For example, suppose we were studying the effect of a hospital requirement for continuing education on nurses' turnover rate using a time series design. Now let us further suppose that, at about the same time the continuing education rule was put into effect, a nurse in the hospital was sued for malpractice. The lawsuit might bring to the nurses' attention a host of problems concerning their legal liability and the method used by the hospital in handling these problems. Our dependent variable in this case, turnover rate, is now subject to the influence of at least two forces, and it becomes impossible for us to disentangle the two effects. In a true experiment, history is rarely a threat to the internal validity of a study because external events are as likely to affect one group as another.

Selection. The threat of **selection** encompasses biases resulting from preexisting differences between groups. When people are not assigned randomly to groups, the possibility always exists that the groups are not equivalent. They may differ, in fact, in ways that are subtle and difficult to detect. If the groups are not equivalent, the researcher is faced with the possibility that any differences with respect to the dependent variable are due to differences in factors other than the independent variable. Selection biases are the most problematic threats to the internal validity of studies not using an experimental design.

Maturation. In a research context, **maturation** refers to processes occurring within the subjects during the course of the study as a result of time (*e.g.,* growth, fatigue) rather than as a result of the independent variable. For example, if we wanted to evaluate the effects of a special sensorimotor-development program for developmentally retarded children, we would have to take into account the fact that progress does take place in these children even without special assistance. Maturation is a relevant consideration in many areas of nursing research. Remember that the term here does not refer to aging or developmental changes exclusively but rather to any kind of change that occurs as a function of time. Thus, wound healing, postoperative recovery, and many other bodily changes that can occur with little or no nursing intervention must be considered as explanations for posttreatment results that rival an explanation based on the independent variable.

Mortality. **Mortality** refers to the threat that arises from differential attrition from the groups being compared. The loss of subjects during the course of a study may differ from one group to another because of initial differences in interest, motivation, and the like. For example, suppose we used a nonequivalent control-group design to assess the morale of the nursing personnel from two different hospitals, one of which was initiating primary nursing. The dependent variable, nursing staff satisfaction, is measured before and after the intervention. The comparison group, which may have no particular commitment to the study, may be reluctant to complete a posttest questionnaire. Those who do fill it out may be totally unrepresentative of the group as a whole; they may be highly enthusiastic about their work environment, for example. Thus, on the average, it may appear that the morale of nurses in the comparison hospital improved, but this improvement might only be an artifact of the mortality of a selective segment of this group.

Internal Validity and Research Design

Quasi-experimental, preexperimental, and correlational studies are especially susceptible to threats to internal validity. The four threats described above represent alternative explanations that compete with the independent variable as an influence on the dependent variable. The aim of a good research design is to rule out these competing explanations. The control mechanisms reviewed in the previous section are all strategies for improving the internal validity of studies.

Experimental designs normally minimize competing explanations, but this is not always the case. For example, if constancy of conditions is not maintained for experimental and control groups, then history might be a rival explanation for obtained results. Experimental mortality is, in particular, a salient threat in true experiments. Because the experimenter does different things with the experimental control groups, participants may drop out of the study differentially among these groups. This is particularly apt to happen if the experimental treatment is painful, inconvenient, or time-consuming or if the control condition is boring or considered a nuisance. When this happens, the participants remaining in the study may differ from those who left in important ways, thereby nullifying the initial equivalence of the groups.

Consumers should pay careful attention to the possibility of competing explanations for reported results, especially in nonexperimental studies. When the investigator does not have control over critical extraneous variables, caution in interpreting the results and drawing conclusions from them is appropriate. Consumers should also examine whether the researcher made any effort to detect and correct for biases such as selection and attrition.

External Validity

The term **external validity** refers to the generalizability of the research findings to other settings or samples. Quantitative studies are almost never conducted with the intention of discovering relationships among variables for one group of people at one point in time. For example, if a nursing intervention under study was found to be successful, others would want to adopt the procedure. Therefore, an important question is whether the intervention would work in another setting or with different patients.

One aspect of a study's external validity concerns the adequacy of the sampling design. If the characteristics of the sample are representative of those of the population, then the generalizability of the results is enhanced. Sampling designs are described at length in Chapter 8.

In addition to participant characteristics, various characteristics of the environment or research situation affect the study's external validity. For example, when a treatment is new (*e.g.,* a new curriculum for nursing students), subjects and researchers alike might alter their behaviors in a variety of ways. People may be either enthusiastic or skeptical about new methods of doing things. Thus, the results may reflect reactions to the novelty rather than to the intrinsic qualities of the treatment.

Sometimes the demands for internal and external validity conflict. If a researcher exercises tight control over a study to maximize internal validity, the setting may become too artificial to generalize to a more naturalistic environment. Therefore, a compromise must sometimes be reached. The need for replication of studies in different settings with new subjects cannot be overemphasized.

ASSISTANCE TO CONSUMERS OF NURSING RESEARCH

What to Expect in the Research Literature

To evaluate the utility of research findings from quantitative studies, consumers need to pay critical attention to the research design decisions that investigators make. Here are a few tips that should help you as you begin to think about the material in this chapter while reading research reports:

- Research reports typically present information about the research design used in the study early in the methods section, often in the first sentence. Complete information about the design is not always provided, however, and some researchers use terminology that is slightly different than that used in this book. (Occasionally, researchers even misidentify the study design.)
- Most nursing studies are nonexperimental, but there has been an increasing use of experimental designs in the past decade. Many studies using experimental (or quasi-experimental) designs are evaluations.
- Researchers using an experimental design generally report this explicitly, but they may also refer to the designs as randomized designs or as clinical trials. After-only, before–after, and repeated measures designs are the most commonly used experimental designs. The research report does not always identify which specific experimental design was used; this may have to be inferred from information about the data collection plan (in the case of after-only and

before–after designs) or from such statements as: The subjects were used as their own controls (in the case of a repeated measures design).

- Quasi- and preexperimental designs are less commonly found in the nursing research literature than true experimental designs. Researchers often do not identify their studies as quasi- or preexperimental. If a study involves the introduction of a treatment or intervention (*i.e.,* if the researcher has control over the independent variable) and if the report does not explicitly mention random assignment or the use of an experimental design, it is probably safe to conclude that the design is quasi- or preexperimental.

- Research reports sometimes say that a repeated measures design was used when the design is longitudinal or prospective (*i.e.,* in nonexperimental studies in which measures were obtained on repeated occasions). In such a study, the repeated measures do not necessarily serve to control intrinsic extraneous variables. A design is a true repeated measures design only when the researcher introduces two or more different treatment conditions and randomizes the order of presentation of those conditions to a *single* group of subjects.

- Most nursing studies using nonexperimental designs are correlational or ex post facto. Relatively few studies are purely descriptive. Sometimes a report refers to the design of a study as **descriptive correlational,** meaning that the researcher was interested primarily in describing relationships among variables, without necessarily seeking to establish a causal connection.

- Retrospective ex post facto studies are more common in nursing than prospective studies. Research reports, however, rarely point out that the design was retrospective. The reader has to determine whether the researcher measured the dependent variable in the present and then attempted to identify antecedent causes or determinants of that variable. By contrast, researchers almost always make explicit reference to the use of a prospective (or longitudinal) design.

- In nursing studies that are not experimental, statistical procedures such as analysis of covariance and similar sophisticated techniques are the most frequently used methods of controlling extraneous intrinsic variables. Matching, which was a commonly used control technique a few decades ago, has become much less prevalent since computers have become widely available for statistical analysis.

- The external validity of nursing studies is typically limited because most studies are done in a single local setting with relatively few subjects. Therefore, an important consideration is the extent to which a study's findings replicate those of other, similar studies.

Critiquing Research Designs

The overriding consideration in evaluating a research design is whether the design enables the researcher to answer the research question. This must be determined in terms of both substantive and methodologic issues.

Substantively, we must ask: What was the overall intent of the research project? If the researcher selected a design that does not match the overall aims of the research, then even sophisticated techniques will not advance knowledge. If the purpose of the research is primarily descriptive or exploratory, then clearly an experimental design is inappropriate. Furthermore, if the researcher is searching to understand the full nature of some phenomenon about which little is known, a design that is highly structured and allows little flexibility may only serve to block understanding. We have discussed techniques of research control as mechanisms for controlling bias, but there are situations in which too much control can introduce bias (*e.g.*, when the researcher tightly controls the ways in which the phenomena under study can be manifested, thereby obscuring the true nature of those variables). When the phenomena of interest are poorly understood or are ones whose dimensions have not been clarified, then a design that allows some flexibility may be best suited to the study aims (flexible designs are discussed in Chapter 7).

The main methodologic issues about the design of quantitative studies are whether the research design provides the most accurate, unbiased, interpretable answers possible to the research question and whether the design yields results that are replicable. Box 6–1 provides questions to assist consumers in evaluating the methodologic aspects of research design.

Research Examples

Below is a description of the research design used in three actual nursing studies. Use the guidelines in Box 6–1 to evaluate the research designs, referring to the full reports (cited at the end of the chapter), if necessary.

Research Example of a Longitudinal Experimental Evaluation

Koniak-Griffin, Ludington-Hoe, and Verzemnieks (1995) evaluated the effects of unimodal and multimodal stimulation on the mental, psychomotor, and behavioral development of healthy full-term infants using a posttest-only experimental design. A sample of 81 primiparous mothers and their newborns were randomly assigned to a control group or to one of three experimental conditions: daily administration of a stroking procedure, placement on a multisensory hammock during sleep periods, or a combination of the two treatments. The authors examined the success of randomization by comparing groups with respect to background characteristics; no group differences were found, thereby allowing the researchers to conclude that the groups were equivalent at the outset.

Follow-up data were collected at 4 months, 8 months, and 24 months after birth. At the 24-month follow-up, only 49 mother–child dyads were available to participate. The high rate of attrition resulted primarily from families moving out of the area. A comparison between the study dropouts and subjects who remained

---

Guidelines for Critiquing Research Designs in Quantitative Studies

Box 6-1

1. Given the nature of the research question, what type of design is most appropriate? How does this correspond to the type of design used?
2. Does the design used in the study involve an intervention? If yes, was a true experimental, quasi-experimental, or preexperimental design used—and was this the most appropriate design?
3. If the design is nonexperimental, why didn't the researcher manipulate the independent variable? Was the decision regarding manipulation appropriate?
4. Was the study longitudinal or cross-sectional? Was the number of points of data collection appropriate, given the research question?
5. What type of comparisons were called for in the research design (*e.g.,* was the study design within-subjects or between-subjects)? Are these comparisons the most appropriate for illuminating the relationship between the independent and dependent variables?
6. Can the study be described as a survey, evaluation, needs assessment, methodologic study or meta-analysis?
7. What procedures, if any, did the researcher use to control external (situational) factors and intrinsic (subject characteristic) factors? Were these procedures appropriate and adequate?
8. To what extent is the study internally valid? What types of alternative explanations must be considered (*i.e.,* what are the threats to the study's internal validity)? Does the research design enable the researcher to draw causal inferences about the relationship among study variables?
9. To what extent is the study externally valid? Can the design be criticized for its artificiality?
10. What are the major limitations of the design used? Are these limitations acknowledged by the researcher and taken into account in interpreting the results?

---

revealed few differences between these groups, suggesting no attrition bias.

At 24-months postbirth, data were collected in the study participants' homes on the children's mental and psychomotor development; the quality of mother–child interaction; and child behavior problems. All data were collected by pediatric nurses who were unaware of the subjects' experimental or control group status.

The results indicated that there were no significant group differences with respect to any of the dependent variables. The authors concluded that "These findings suggest that supplementary stimulation provided no benefits beyond those associated with natural caregiving and raise questions about the value of the interventions with nonrisk infants in middle-class families" (p. 27).

Research Example of a Quasi-Experimental Study

Pickler, Higgins and Crummette (1993) used a very strong quasi-experimental design to examine the effects of nonnutritive sucking on the physiologic and behavioral stress reactions of preterm infants at early bottle feedings. The sample consisted of 20 preterm infants, 10 of whom were provided nonnutritive sucking for 5 minutes before and 5 minutes after an early bottle feeding. The ten infants who served as a comparison group (and who received no nonnutritive sucking) were matched to the experimental group on the basis of gender, race, birthweight, and gestational age.

Physiologic stress was measured in terms of heart rate and oxygen saturation rate. For each, mean rates were computed for three periods: the 5 minutes before feeding, the first 5 minutes of bottle feeding, and the 5 minutes after total feeding. Behavioral stress was measured by observation of the infant's behavioral state at four points: immediately before the 5-minute prefeeding period, immediately after the initiation of bottle feeding, immediately after the conclusion of bottle feeding, and immediately after the conclusion of the 5-minute postfeeding period.

The results indicated that infants who received nonnutritive sucking before and after bottle feedings were more likely to be in a quiescent behavior state 5 minutes after feeding. However, there were no treatment, time, or time × treatment interaction effects for heart rate; oxygen saturation was unaffected by the treatment, but did change between different measurements in time.

Research Example of a Nonexperimental Survey

Pollow, Stoller, Forster, and Duniho (1994) conducted a survey of elderly people living in community settings and managing their own health, to examine their use of over-the-counter (OTC) medications and their consumption of alcohol. A major purpose of the study was to document drug-utilization patterns among community-dwelling elders and their risk of adverse drug reactions.

The sample for the study included 667 people living in community settings in northeastern New York, all of whom were 65 years of age or older. Of the people who were approached for the study, 79% agreed to participate.

Data were gathered through personal interviews in the respondents' homes. The interview covered a wide range of topics, including the respondents' health and disabilities, their use of prescription and OTC medications, consumption of alcohol, and other health-related behaviors (*e.g.,* smoking, exercise, eating patterns). Respondents who had difficulty remembering the names or therapeutic intent of any medications were asked to show the medicine to the interviewers, who recorded the names of the medications.

The findings indicated that almost two thirds of the respondents reported one or more drug–drug or drug–alcohol combinations associated with a possible adverse reaction. The potential for risk was highest among people taking psychoactive drugs, antidiabetics, anticoagulants, and ulcer medications. The results suggest the need for health-care practitioners to obtain more detailed drug histories when treating elderly clients who are taking certain categories of medications.

▧ SUMMARY

The **research design** is the researcher's overall plan for answering the research question. In quantitative studies, the design indicates whether there is an intervention; the type of intervention; the nature of any comparisons to be made; the methods to be used to control **extraneous variables** and enhance the study's interpretability; and the timing and location of data collection.

Research in which the researcher actively intervenes or introduces a **treatment** is referred to as an **experiment.** A true experimental design is characterized by **manipulation** (the researcher manipulates or varies the independent variable); control (including the use of a **control group**—a group whose performance on the dependent variables is used for assessing the performance of the experimental group); and **randomization** (whereby subjects are allocated to experimental and control groups at random so the groups have a strong likelihood of being comparable at the outset). Experiments are the most rigorous approach for studying cause-and-effect relationships.

Various experimental designs can be used. The **after-only design** involves collecting data only once, after random assignment and the introduction of the treatment. In the **before–after** (or **pretest–posttest) design,** data are collected both before and after the experimental manipulation. When a researcher manipulates more than one variable at a time, the design is known as a **factorial design,** which allows researchers to test both **main effects** (effects from the experimentally manipulated variables) and **interaction effects** (effects resulting from combining the treatments). These **between-subjects designs,** in which different groups of people are compared, contrast with **within-subjects designs** that involve comparisons of the same subjects. A **repeated measures design** (or **crossover design**) is used when the research subjects are exposed to more than one experimental condition and therefore serve as their own controls. When an experiment is used to test the efficacy of a clinical treatment in a large, heterogeneous population, the study is often referred to as a **clinical trial.**

Quasi-experimental designs involve a manipulative component but lack a comparison group or randomization. Quasi-experimental designs are designs in which efforts are made to introduce controls into the study to compensate for these missing components. By contrast, **preexperimental designs** have no such safeguards and are considerably weaker. The most frequently used quasi-experimental design is the **nonequivalent control-group design,** which involves the use of a **comparison group** that was not created through random assignment. Because the problem with the use of such a comparison group is the possibility that the groups are initially different in ways that will affect the research outcomes, the collection of pretreatment data becomes an important means of assessing their initial equivalence. In studies in which there is no comparison group, the **time series design** can be used, wherein information on the dependent variable is collected over a period of time before and after the treatment is instituted.

Nonexperimental research includes two broad categories: descriptive research and ex post facto or correlational research. **Descriptive research** is designed to summarize the status of some phenomena of interest as they currently exist. **Ex post facto** (or **correlational**) studies examine the relationships among variables but involve no manipulation of the independent variable. Because the researcher lacks control of the independent variable in ex post facto studies, it is difficult to draw cause-and-effect conclusions about relationships among variables. Nevertheless, researchers do use **retrospective** and **prospective** designs in attempts to infer causality. One of the major difficulties of ex post facto studies is that the findings are generally open to numerous interpretations. Nonexperimental research, however, plays an important role in nursing because not all variables of interest to nurses can be manipulated and because nonexperimental studies are often high in realism and can be particularly efficient.

Research design also stipulates the timing of data collection. **Cross-sectional designs** involve the collection of data at one point in time, whereas **longitudinal designs** involve data collection at two or more points in time over an extended time period. Research problems that involve trends, changes, or development over time are best addressed through longitudinal research. Three types of longitudinal studies are **trend studies, panel studies,** and **follow-up studies.**

Several types of research that vary according to the study purpose were discussed in this chapter. **Survey research** is research that examines the characteristics, attitudes, behaviors, and intentions of a group of people by asking individuals to answer questions either through interviews or self-administered questionnaires. **Evaluations** involve the collection and analysis of information relating to the effectiveness and functioning of a program or procedure. **Needs assessments** are investigations of the needs of a group or community for certain types of services or programs. In **methodologic research,** the researcher focuses on the development, assessment, and improvement of methodologic tools and strategies. **Meta-analysis** is an approach to integrating the findings of prior research using statistical procedures.

A major purpose of research design in quantitative studies is to enhance the interpretability of study results by exerting research control. **Research control** is used to control external factors that could affect the study outcomes (*e.g.,* the environment) and to control intrinsic subject characteristics extraneous to the research question. Several techniques can be used to control subject characteristics, including randomization; **homogeneity** (selecting a group such that variability on the extraneous variable is eliminated); **blocking** (building extraneous variables into the design of the study); **matching** (matching on a one-to-one basis subjects in different groups to make them comparable with regard to the extraneous variables); and statistical procedures, such as **analysis of covariance.** Randomization and repeated measures are the most effective control procedures because they control for all possible extraneous variables without the researcher having to identify or measure them.

Control mechanisms help to improve the **internal validity** of studies. Internal validity is concerned with whether the results of a study are attributable to the independent variable or to other extraneous factors. A number of plausible rival explanations, known as **threats to internal validity,** were discussed. These threats include **history, selection, maturation,** and **mortality** (caused by subject **attrition**). These threats are least likely to emerge in experimental studies. **External validity** refers to the generalizability of study findings to other samples and settings.

STUDY SUGGESTIONS

Chapter 6 of the accompanying *Study Guide to Accompany Essentials of Nursing Research,* 4th edition offers various exercises and study suggestions for reinforcing the concepts presented in this chapter.

Suggested Readings

Methodologic References

Campbell, D. T., & Stanley, J. C. (1963). *Experimental and quasi-experimental designs for research.* Chicago: Rand McNally.

Cook, T. D., & Campbell, D. T. (1979). *Quasi-experimental design and analysis issues for field settings.* Chicago: Rand McNally.

Kerlinger, F. N. (1986). *Foundations of behavioral research* (3rd ed.). New York: Holt, Rinehart and Winston.

Lazarsfeld, P. (1955). Foreword. In H. Hyman (Ed.), *Survey design and analysis.* New York: The Free Press.

Substantive References

Baggs, J. G., & Schmitt, M. H. (1995). Intensive care decisions about level of aggressiveness of care. *Research in Nursing and Health, 18,* 345–355.

Berk, R. A., Baigis-Smith, J., & Nanda, J. P. (1995). Health care needs of persons with HIV/AIDS in various settings. *Western Journal of Nursing Research, 17,* 647–671.

Buchko, B. L., Pugh, L. C., Bishop, B. A., Cochran, J. F., Smith, L. R., & Lerew, D. J. (1994). Comfort measures in breastfeeding, primiparous women. *Journal of Obstetric, Gynecologic & Neonatal Nursing, 23,* 46–52.

Corley, M. C., Ferriter, J., Zeh, J., & Gifford, C. (1995). Physiological and psychological effects of back rubs. *Applied Nursing Research, 8,* 39–43.

Devine, E. C., & Reifschneider, E. (1995). A meta-analysis of the effects of psychoeducational care in adults with hypertension. *Nursing Research, 44,* 237–243.

Elander, G., & Hellstrom, G. (1995). Reduction of noise levels in intensive care units for infants: Evaluation of an intervention program. *Heart and Lung, 24,* 376–379.

Fitzgerald, S. T., Zlotnick, C., & Kolodner, K. B. (1996). Factors related to functional status after percutaneous transluminal coronary angioplasty. *Heart and Lung, 25,* 24–30.

Gross, D., Conrad, B., Fogg, L., Willis, L., & Garvey, C. (1995). A longitudinal study of maternal depression and preschool children's mental health. *Nursing Research, 44,* 96–101.

Grossman, M., & Rowat, K. M. (1995). Parental relationships, coping strategies, received support, and well-being in adolescents of separated or divorced and married parents. *Research in Nursing and Health, 18,* 249–261.

Kaplow, R., & Bookbinder, M. (1994). A comparison of four endotracheal tube holders. *Heart and Lung, 23,* 59–66.

Koniak-Griffin, D., Ludington-Hoe, S., Verzemnieks, I. (1995). Longitudinal effects of unimodal and multimodal stimulation on development and interaction of healthy infants. *Research in Nursing and Health, 18,* 27–38.

Lanza, M. L., Kayne, H. L., Pattison, I., Hicks, C., & Islam, S. (1996). The relationship of behavioral cues to assaultive behavior. *Clinical Nursing Research, 5,* 6–27.

MacDonald, S. A. (1995). An assessment of the Cardiovascular Health Education Program in primary health care. *Applied Nursing Research, 8,* 114–117.

McConnell, E. A. (1995). How and what staff nurses learn about the medical devices they use in direct patient care. *Research in Nursing and Health, 18,* 165–172.

Medoff-Cooper, B., Verklan, T., & Carlson, S. (1993). The development of sucking patterns and physiologic correlates in very-low-birthweight infants. *Nursing Research, 42,* 100-105.

Melnyk, B. M. (1994). Coping with unplanned childhood hospitalization: Effects of informational interventions on mothers and children. *Nursing Research, 43,* 50–55.

Mock, V. (1993). Body image in women treated for breast cancer. *Nursing Research, 42,* 153–157.

Morse, E. V., Simon, P. M., Besch, C. L., & Walker, J. (1995). Issues of recruitment, retention, and compliance in community-based clinical trials with traditionally underserved populations. *Applied Nursing Research, 8,* 8–14.

Pickler, R. H., Higgins, K. E., & Crummette, B. D. (1993). The effect of nonnutritive sucking on bottle-feeding stress in preterm infants. *Journal of Obstetric, Gynecologic, and Neonatal Nursing, 22,* 230–234.

Pollow, R. L., Stoller, E. P., Forster, L. E., & Duniho, T. S. (1994). Drug combinations and potential for risk of adverse drug reaction among community-dwelling elderly. *Nursing Research, 43,* 44–49.

Quayhagen, M. P., Quayhagen, M., Corbeil, R. R., Roth, P. A., & Rodgers, J. A. (1995). A dyadic remediation program for care recipients with dementia. *Nursing Research, 44,* 153–159.

Roberts, K. L., Brittin, M., Cook, M. A., & deClifford, J. (1994). Boomerang pillows and respiratory capacity. *Clinical Nursing Research, 3,* 157–165.

Rodrigues-Fisher, L., Bourguignon, C., & Good, B. V. (1993). Dietary fiber nursing intervention: Prevention of constipation in older adults. *Clinical Nursing Research, 2,* 464–453.

Roseman, C., & Booker, J. M. (1995). Workload and environmental factors in hospital medication errors. *Nursing Research, 44,* 226–230.

Symington, A., Ballantyne, M., Pinelli, J., & Stevens, B. (1995). Indwelling versus intermittent feeding tubes in premature neonates. *Journal of Obstetric, Gynecologic, and Neonatal Nursing, 24,* 321–326.

Weinrich, S. P., & Weinrich, M. C. (1990). The effect of massage on pain in cancer patients. *Applied Nursing Research, 3,* 140–145.

Williams, R. P. (1988). College freshmen aspiring to nursing careers: Trends from the 1960s to the 1980s. *Western Journal of Nursing Research, 10,* 94–97.

Wright, A., Hecker, J., & McDonald, G. (1995). Effects of low-dose heparin on failure of intravenous infusions in children. *Heart and Lung, 24,* 79–82.

Yates, B. C. (1995). The relationships among social support and short- and long-term recovery outcomes in men with coronary heart disease. *Research in Nursing and Health, 18,* 193–203.

Qualitative Research Design and Approaches

Student Objectives

On completion of this chapter, the student will be able to:

- describe the features of and rationale for an emergent design in qualitative research
- identify areas in which a qualitative researcher can plan for broad design contingencies
- describe the three major phases typical in the design of a qualitative study
- identify the major research traditions for qualitative research and describe the domain of inquiry of each
- describe the basic characteristics of ethnographic, phenomenologic, and grounded theory studies
- identify several advantages of an integrated qualitative and quantitative design
- describe several specific applications of an integrated design
- define new terms in the chapter

New Terms

Being-in-the-world
Black box
Bracketing
Cognitive anthropology
Constant comparison
Corporeality
Discourse analysis
Ecological psychology
Embodiment
Emergent design
Emic perspective
Ethnography
Ethnomethodology
Ethnonursing research
Ethnoscience
Ethology
Etic perspective
Grounded theory
Hermeneutics

Historical research
Integration of qualitative and
    quantitative data
Intuiting
Lived body
Lived human relation
Lived space
Lived time
Macro ethnography
Micro ethnography
Multimethod research
Phenomenology
Relationality
Researcher as instrument
Semiotics
Spatiality
Symbolic interaction
Tacit knowledge
Temporality

◣ THE DESIGN OF QUALITATIVE STUDIES

As we have seen, quantitative researchers carefully specify a research design before collecting even one piece of data, and rarely depart from that design once the study is underway. In qualitative research, by contrast, the study design typically evolves over the course of the project. Decisions about how best to obtain data, from whom to obtain data, how to schedule data collection, and how long each data collection session should last are made in the field, as the study unfolds. The design for a qualitative study is often referred to as an **emergent design**—a design that emerges as the researcher makes ongoing decisions reflecting what has already been learned. As noted by Lincoln and Guba (1985), an emergent design in qualitative studies is not the result of sloppiness or laziness on the part of the researcher, but rather a reflection of the researcher's desire to have the inquiry based on the realities and viewpoints of those under study—realities and viewpoints that are not known or understood at the outset of the study.

Qualitative Design and Planning

Although design decisions are not specified in advance, the qualitative researcher typically does considerable advance planning that can support an emergent design. In the total absence of planning, flexibility in the design might actually be constrained. For example, the researcher initially might project a 6-month period for data collection, but must be prepared (financially and emotionally) to spend even longer periods of time in the field to pursue data collection opportunities that could not be foreseen. In other words, the qualitative researcher plans for broad contingencies that may be expected to pose decision opportunities once the study has begun. Example of the areas where advance planning is especially useful include the following:

- Selection of the site where the study will take place, and identification of the types of settings within the site that are likely to be especially fruitful for the collection of meaningful data
- Identification of the names and roles of key "gatekeepers" who can provide (or deny) access to important sources of data; arrangement of mechanisms for gaining entrée
- Determination of the maximum amount of time available for the study, given costs and other constraints
- Identification of all foreseeable types of equipment that could aid in the collection and analysis of data in the field (*e.g.*, audio and video recording equipment, laptop computers, and so forth)
- Determination of the number and type of assistants needed (if any) to complete the project

Thus, a qualitative researcher needs to plan for a variety of potential circumstances, but decisions about how he or she will deal with them must be resolved when the social context of time, place, and human interactions is better understood.

Qualitative Design Features

Some of the design features described in connection with quantitative studies (Chapter 6) also apply to qualitative ones. However, qualitative design features are often post hoc characterizations of what happened in the field rather than features specifically planned in advance. As a further means of contrasting qualitative and quantitative research design, we refer to the design elements identified in Table 6–1.

- *Control over independent variable.* Qualitative researchers do not normally conceptualize their studies as having independent and dependent variables, and they rarely control or manipulate any aspect of the setting under study. Qualitative research is almost always nonexperimental—although, as we discuss later in this chapter, a qualitative study sometimes can be embedded within an experimental project.
- *Type of group comparisons.* Qualitative researchers typically do not plan in advance to focus on group comparisons. Nevertheless, patterns emerging in the data sometimes suggest that certain comparisons are relevant and illuminating. For example, Astrom, Furaker, and Norberg (1995) studied nurses' skills in managing ethically difficult care situation with cancer patients. Their analysis revealed that interesting patterns emerged when nurses with limited experience in managing ethically difficult care situations were compared to nurses with extensive experience.
- *Number of data collection points.* Qualitative research, like quantitative research, can be either cross-sectional (one data collection point per study participant) or longitudinal (multiple data collection points over an extended time period, to observe the evolution of some phenomenon). Sometimes a qualitative researcher plans in advance for multiple sessions, but, in other cases, the decision to study a phenomenon longitudinally may be made in the field after preliminary data have been collected and analyzed.
- *Occurrence of independent and dependent variables.* Qualitative researchers typically would not apply the terms *retrospective* or *prospective* to their studies. Nevertheless, in trying to elucidate the full nature of some phenomenon, they may look back retrospectively (with the assistance of study participants) for antecedent factors leading up to the occurrence of some phenomenon. For example, Kerr (1994) studied adult women's perceptions of how the death of a parent, which had occurred years earlier, resulted in changes in their lifestyle. Qualitative researchers may also study the evolution of development of some phenomenon prospectively. For example, Dellasega and Mastrian (1995) studied the decision-making process

of family members who placed an elder in a long-term care facility, and then examined the immediate consequences of that decision.

- *Setting.* Qualitative researchers almost always collect their data in real-world, naturalistic settings. And, whereas a quantitative researcher usually strives to collect data in one type of setting to maintain constancy of conditions (*e.g.,* conducting all interviews with study participants in their homes), qualitative researchers may deliberately strive to study their phenomena in a variety of natural contexts. For example, Hatton (1994) conducted an in-depth study of health perceptions among older urbanized American Indians. The investigator made a conscious effort to conduct the study in numerous settings, including sessions in the study participants' homes, on fishing trips, at senior citizen lunches, and on outings to outlying reservations.

Phases in a Qualitative Inquiry

Although the exact form of a qualitative study cannot be known and specified in advance, Lincoln and Guba (1985) noted that a naturalistic inquiry typically progresses through three broad phases while the researcher is in the field:

- *Orientation and overview.* Quantitative researchers generally believe they know what they do not know (*i.e.,* they know exactly what type of knowledge they expect to obtain by doing a study and then strive to obtain it). A qualitative researcher, by contrast, enters the study "not knowing what is not known" (*i.e.,* not knowing what it is about the phenomenon that will drive the inquiry forward). Therefore, the first phase of many qualitative studies is to get a handle on what *is* salient about the phenomenon of interest.
- *Focused exploration.* The second phase of the study is a more focused scrutiny and in-depth exploration of those aspects of the phenomenon that are judged to be salient. The questions asked and the types of people invited to participate in the study are shaped by the understandings developed in the first phase.
- *Confirmation and closure.* In the final phase, qualitative researchers undertake efforts to establish that their findings are trustworthy, often by going back and discussing their understanding with study participants. Phase 3 activities are described at greater length in Chapter 10.

The three phases are not discrete events. Rather, they overlap to a greater or lesser degree in different projects. For example, even the first few interviews or observations are typically used as a basis for selecting subsequent informants, even though the researcher is still striving to understand the full scope of the phenomenon and to identify its major dimensions. The various phases might take only a few days to complete—or may take many months.

▧ QUALITATIVE RESEARCH TRADITIONS

Although qualitative studies cannot be characterized by their research designs in the same way that quantitative ones can, there are many different types of qualitative studies. Unfortunately, there is no readily agreed-upon classification system or taxonomy for the various approaches. Some authors have categorized qualitative studies in terms of analysis styles; others have classified studies according to their broad focus. We believe the most useful system is to describe various types of qualitative research according to disciplinary traditions. These traditions vary in their conceptualization of what types of questions are important to ask in understanding the world in which we live. The next section provides an overview of several qualitative research traditions, and subsequent sections describe in greater detail three traditions that have been especially useful for nurse researchers.

Overview of Qualitative Research Traditions

The research traditions that have provided a theoretical underpinning for qualitative studies come primarily from the disciplines of anthropology, psychology, and sociology.[1] As shown in Table 7–1, each discipline has tended to focus on one or two broad domains of inquiry.

The discipline of anthropology is concerned with human cultures. **Ethnography** is the primary research tradition within anthropology and provides a framework for studying the meanings, patterns, and experiences of a defined cultural group in a holistic fashion. Ethnographic research is described at greater length in the next section. **Ethnoscience** (sometimes referred to as **cognitive anthropology**) focuses on the cognitive world of a culture, with particular emphasis on the semantic rules and the shared meanings that shape behavior. Ethnoscience often relies on quantitative as well as qualitative data.

Phenomenology, which has its disciplinary roots in both philosophy and psychology, is concerned with the lived experiences of humans. Because many nursing studies have adopted a phenomenologic approach, this research tradition is described more fully in a subsequent section. A closely related research tradition is **hermeneutics,** which uses the lived experiences of people as a tool for better understanding the social, cultural, political, and/or historical context in which those experiences occur. Hermeneutic inquiry often focuses on *meaning*—how socially and historically conditioned individuals interpret the world within their given context.

The discipline of psychology has several other qualitative research traditions that focus on human *behavior.* Human **ethology,** which is sometimes described

[1]**Historical research**—the systematic collection and critical evaluation of data relating to past occurrences—is also a tradition that relies primarily on qualitative data and that has relevance for nursing.

Table 7–1. Overview of Qualitative Research Traditions

Discipline	Research Tradition	Domain of Inquiry
Anthropology		Culture
	Ethnography	Holistic view of a culture
	Ethnoscience (cognitive anthropology)	Mapping of the cognitive world of a culture; a culture's shared meanings, semantic rules
Psychology/ Philosophy		Lived Experience
	Phenomenology	Experiences of individuals within their lifeworld
	Hermeneutics	Experiences of individuals as access to sociocultural context
Psychology		Behavior and Events
	Ethology	Behavior observed over time in natural context
	Ecologic psychology	Behavior as influenced by the environment
Sociology		Social Settings
	Grounded theory	Social structural processes within a social setting
	Ethnomethodology	Manner by which shared agreement is achieved in social settings
	Symbolic interaction (semiotics)	Manner by which people make sense of social interactions
Sociolinguistics		Human Communication
	Discourse analysis	Forms and rules of conversation

as the biology of human behavior, studies human behavior as it evolves in its natural context. Human ethologists use primarily observational methods in an attempt to discover universal behavioral structures. **Ecological psychology** focuses more specifically on the influence of the environment on human behavior and attempts to identify principles that explain the interdependence of humans and their environmental context.

Sociologists study the social world in which we live and have developed several research traditions of importance to qualitative researchers. The **grounded theory** tradition (described briefly in Chapter 4 and elaborated on in a later section of this chapter) seeks to describe and understand the key social psychological and structural processes that occur in a social setting. **Ethnomethodology** seeks to discover how people make sense of their everyday activities and interpret their social worlds so as to behave in socially acceptable ways. Within this tradition, researchers attempt to understand a social group's norms and assumptions that are so deeply ingrained that the members no longer think about the underlying reasons for their behaviors. **Symbolic interaction** focuses on the manner in which people make sense of social interactions and the interpretations they attach to social symbols, such as language. Symbolic interactionists sometimes use **semiotics,** which refers to the study of signs and their meanings.

Finally, the domain of inquiry for sociolinguists is human communication. The tradition often referred to as **discourse analysis** seeks to understand the rules, mechanisms, and structure of conversations. The data for discourse analysis typically are transcripts from naturally occurring conversations, such as those between nurses and their patients.

Researchers in each of these traditions have developed methodologic guidelines for the design and conduct of relevant studies. Thus, once a researcher has identified what aspect of the human experience is of greatest interest, there is typically a wealth of advice available with regard to methods likely to be productive.

Ethnography

Ethnography, as noted above, focuses on the culture of a group of people. Ethnographic researchers can study both broadly defined cultures (*e.g.,* a Samoan village culture), in what is sometimes referred to as a **macro ethnography,** and more narrowly defined ones (*e.g.,* the culture of homeless shelters) in a **micro ethnography.** An underlying assumption of the ethnographer is that every human group eventually evolves a culture that guides the members' view of the world and the way they structure their experiences.

The aim of the ethnographer is to learn from (rather than to study) members of a cultural group—to understand their world view as they define it. Ethnographic researchers sometimes refer to emic and etic perspectives. An **emic perspective** refers to the way the members of the culture envision their world—it is the insiders' view. The **etic perspective,** by contrast, is the outsiders' interpretation of the experiences of that culture. Ethnographers strive to acquire an emic perspective of a culture under study. Moreover, they strive to reveal what has been referred to as **tacit knowledge,** information about the culture that is so deeply embedded in cultural experiences that members do not talk about it or may not even be consciously aware of it.

Ethnographers almost invariably undertake extensive field work to learn about the cultural group in which they are interested. Ethnographic research typically is a labor-intensive endeavor that requires long periods of time in the field—months and even years of fieldwork may be required. In most cases, the researcher strives to actively participate in cultural events and activities. The study of a culture requires a certain level of intimacy with members of the cultural group, and such intimacy can only be developed over time and by working directly with those members as an active participant. The concept of **researcher as instrument** is frequently used by anthropologists to describe the significant role the ethnographer plays in analyzing and interpreting a culture.

Three broad types of information are usually sought by ethnographers: cultural behavior (what members of the culture do); cultural artifacts (what members of the culture make and use); and cultural speech (what people say). This implies that the ethnographer relies on a wide variety of data sources, including observations, in-depth interviews, records, charts, and other types of physical evidence (photographs, diaries, letters, and so forth). Ethnographers typically conduct in-depth interviews with about 25 to 50 informants.

The product of ethnographic research usually includes very rich and holistic descriptions of the culture under study. Ethnographers also make interpretations of the culture, describing normative behavioral and social patterns. Among health-care researchers, ethnography provides access to the health beliefs and health practices of a culture or subculture. Ethnographic inquiry can thus help to facilitate understanding of behaviors affecting health and illness. Many nurse researchers have undertaken ethnographic studies. Indeed, Madeleine Leininger has coined the phrase **ethnonursing research,** which she defines as "the study and analysis of the local or indigenous people's viewpoints, beliefs, and practices about nursing care behavior and processes of designated cultures" (1985, p. 38).

Phenomenology

Phenomenology, rooted in a philosophical tradition developed by Husserl and Heidegger, is an approach to thinking about what the life experiences of people are like. The phenomenologic researcher asks the question: What is the *essence* of this phenomenon as experienced by these people? The phenomenologist assumes there is an essence that can be understood, in much the same way that the ethnographer assumes that cultures exist. The phenomenologist investigates subjective phenomena in the belief that essential truths about reality are grounded in people's lived experiences.

The focus of phenomenologic inquiry, then, is what people experience in regard to some phenomenon and how they interpret those experiences. The phenomenologist believes that lived experience gives meaning to each person's perception of a particular phenomenon. The goal of phenomenologic inquiry is to fully describe lived experience and the perceptions to which it gives rise. Four aspects of lived experience that are of interest to phenomenologists are **lived space** or **spatiality; lived body** or **corporeality; lived time** or **temporality;** and **lived human relation** or **relationality.**

Phenomenologists assume that human existence is meaningful and interesting because of people's consciousness of that existence. The phrase **being-in-the-world** (or **embodiment**) is a concept that acknowledges that people have physical ties to their world—they think, see, hear, feel, and are conscious through their bodies' interaction with the world.

In a phenomenologic inquiry, the main source of data typically is in-depth conversations in which the researcher and the informant are full coparticipants. The researcher helps the informant to describe lived experiences without leading the discussion. Through in-depth conversations, the researcher strives to gain entrance into the informants' world, to have full access to their experiences as lived. Sometimes two separate interviews or conversations may be needed. Typically, phenomenologic studies involve a small number of study participants—often five or fewer. For some phenomenologic researchers, the inquiry includes not only learning about the experience by gathering information from those people under study but also efforts to experience the phenomenon in the same way, typically through participation, observation, and introspective reflection.

There have been a number of methodologic interpretations of phenomenology, and hence different authors suggest different steps in the conduct of a phenomenologic inquiry. However, a phenomenologic study often involves the following four steps: bracketing, intuiting, analyzing, and describing. **Bracketing** refers to the process of identifying and holding in abeyance any preconceived beliefs and opinions one might have about the phenomenon under investigation. The researcher brackets out the world and any presuppositions in an effort to confront the data in pure form. **Intuiting** occurs when the researcher remains open to the meanings attributed to the phenomenon by those who have experienced it. Phenomenologic researchers then proceed to the analysis phase (*i.e.,* coding, categorizing, and making sense of the essential meanings of the phenomenon). Finally, the descriptive phase occurs when the researcher comes to understand and define the phenomenon.

The phenomenologic approach is especially useful when a phenomenon of interest has been poorly defined or conceptualized. The topics appropriate to phenomenology are ones that are fundamental to the life experiences of humans; for health researchers, these include such topics as the meaning of stress, the experience of bereavement, and the quality of life with a chronic illness.

Grounded Theory

Grounded theory has become a strong research tradition that began more as a systematic method of qualitative research than as a philosophy. Grounded theory was developed in the 1960s by two sociologists, Glaser and Strauss, whose own theoretical links were in symbolic interactionism.

Grounded theory is an approach to the study of social processes and social structures. The focus of most grounded theory studies is the development and evolution of a social experience—the social and psychological stages and phases that characterize a particular event or episode. As noted in Chapter 4, the primary purpose of the grounded theory approach is to generate comprehensive explanations of phenomena that are grounded in reality.

Grounded theory methods constitute an entire approach to the conduct of field research. For example, a study that truly follows Glaser and Strauss' precepts does not begin with a highly focused research question; the question emerges from the data. One of the fundamental features of the grounded theory approach is that data collection, data analysis, and sampling of study participants occur simultaneously. A procedure referred to as **constant comparison** is used to develop and refine theoretically relevant categories. The categories elicited from the data are constantly compared with data obtained earlier in the data collection so commonalities and variations can be determined. As data collection proceeds, the inquiry becomes increasingly focused on emerging theoretical concerns. Data analysis within a grounded theory framework is described in greater depth in Chapter 12.

Data for a grounded theory study may come from many sources. In-depth interviews are the most common data source, but observational methods and existing documents may also be used. Typically, a grounded theory study involves interviews with a sample of about 25 to 50 informants.

Grounded theory has become an important research method for the study of nursing phenomena and has contributed to the development of many middle-range theories of phenomena relevant to nurses. The majority of qualitative nursing studies that identify a research tradition claim grounded theory as the tradition to which they are linked.

 # INTEGRATION OF QUALITATIVE AND QUANTITATIVE APPROACHES

An emerging trend, and one that we believe will gain momentum in the years to come, is the **integration of qualitative and quantitative data** within single studies or coordinated clusters of studies. This section discusses the reasons for such integration and a few applications of it.

Rationale for Integrated Designs

The dichotomy between quantitative and qualitative data represents the key epistemologic and methodologic distinction within the social and behavioral sciences. Some argue, and are likely to continue to argue, that the paradigms that underpin qualitative and quantitative research are fundamentally incompatible. Others, however, believe that many areas of inquiry can be enriched through the judicious blending of qualitative and quantitative data—that is, by undertaking **multimethod research**. There are many noteworthy advantages of designing a study that combines various types of data in a single investigation:

- *Complementarity.* One argument in support of multimethod research is that qualitative and quantitative data are complementary, representing words and numbers, the two fundamental languages of human communication. As we have noted previously, researchers address their problems with methods and measures that are invariably fallible. By integrating different research methods, the weaknesses of a single approach may be diminished or overcome. Researchers who engage in multimethod research have noted that the strengths and weaknesses of quantitative and qualitative data are complementary. Combined judiciously in a single study, qualitative and quantitative data can "mutually supply each other's lack," which is one definition of complementarity. By using multiple methods, the researcher can allow each method to do what it does best, with the possibility of avoiding the limitations of a single approach.

- *Enhanced Theoretical Insights.* The world in which we live is complex and multidimensional, as are most of the theories we have developed to make sense of it. Qualitative and quantitative research constitute alternative ways of viewing and interpreting the world. These alternatives are not necessarily correct or incorrect; rather, they reflect and reveal different aspects of reality. To be maximally useful, nursing research should strive to understand these multiple aspects.

- *Incrementality.* It is sometimes argued that qualitative methods are well suited to exploratory or hypothesis-generating research early in the development of a research problem area, and quantitative methods are needed as the problem area matures for the purposes of verification. Although this argument has some merit, the fact remains that the evolution of a theory or problem area is rarely linear and unidirectional. The need for exploration and in-depth insights is rarely confined to the beginning of an inquiry in an area, and subjective impressions may need to be checked for accuracy and transferability early and continuously. Thus, progress in a developing area tends to be incremental and to rely on multiple feedback loops. It could be productive to build a loop into the design of a single study, thereby potentially speeding the progress toward understanding.

- *Enhanced Validity.* When a researcher's hypothesis or model is supported by multiple and complementary types of data, the researcher can be much more confident about the validity of the results. Scientists are basically skeptics, constantly seeking evidence to validate their theories and models. Evidence derived from different approaches can be especially persuasive. In Chapter 6, we discussed various types of validity problems in quantitative studies, such as rival hypotheses to explain the data and difficulties of generalizing beyond the study circumstances. The use of a single approach often leaves the study vulnerable to several of these problems. The integration of qualitative and quantitative data can provide better opportunities for testing alternative interpretations of the data and for examining the extent to which the context helped to shape the results.

- *Creating New Frontiers.* Inevitably, researchers sometimes find that qualitative and quantitative data are inconsistent with each other. This lack of congruity—when it happens in the context of a single investigation—can actually lead to insights that can push a line of inquiry further than would otherwise have been possible. When separate investigations yield inconsistent results, the differences are difficult to reconcile and interpret because they may reflect differences in study participants and circumstances rather than theoretically meaningful distinctions that merit further study. In a single study, any discrepancies that emerge can be tackled head on. The incongruent findings, in other words, can be used as a springboard for the investigation of the reasons for the discrepancies and for a thoughtful analysis of both the methodologic and theoretical underpinnings of the study.

Applications of Integrated Designs

Researchers make decisions about study design and procedures based on the specific objectives of their investigations. In this section, we illustrate how the integration of qualitative and quantitative data can be used in addressing a variety of research goals.

Instrumentation

One of the most frequent uses of an integrated approach in nursing research involves the development and validation of formal, structured instruments designed for research or clinical purposes, such as quantitative measures of anxiety, social support, or coping. When a researcher becomes aware of the need for a new measuring tool, where do the questions that comprise the tool come from, and how can the researcher be assured that he or she has adequately captured the construct? The questions are sometimes generated by the researcher based on theory, his or her clinical experience, readings in the field, or prior research. When a construct is new, however, these mechanisms may be inadequate to capture its full complexity and dimensionality. No matter how rich the researcher's experience or knowledge base, the fact remains that this base is highly personal and inevitably biased by the researcher's values and world view. In recognition of this situation, many nurse researchers have begun to use data obtained from qualitative inquiries as the basis for generating questions for quantitative instruments that are subsequently subjected to rigorous testing. For example, Gulick (1991) developed the Work Assessment Scale to evaluate situations that impede or enhance the work capabilities of people with multiple sclerosis. The questions for her formal instrument were developed on the basis of conversational responses to questions regarding the conditions and situations that make the performance of tasks easy or difficult.

Illustration

Qualitative data are sometimes combined with quantitative data to illustrate the meaning of descriptions or relationships. Such illustrations help to clarify important concepts and further serve as a method of corroborating the understandings gleaned from the statistical analysis. In this sense, these illustrations help to illuminate the analysis and give guidance to the interpretation of results.

As an example, Hough and her colleagues (Hough, Lewis & Woods, 1991; Lewis, Woods, Hough & Bensley, 1989) conducted a study on family coping and adaptation to a mother's chronic illness. Using data from structured questionnaires, the researchers performed a sophisticated statistical analysis to test a theoretical model of family functioning under stress. The quantitative analyses suggested that the mother's illness had an impact on the spouse and on the quality of his relationship with his wife. Qualitative data were also gathered in the course of the same study through observations and unstructured interviews. The following excerpt illustrating a family that adjusted poorly after the mother's diagnosis of breast cancer adds a perspective that the quantitative results alone could not provide:

> It was a tremendous surprise how I felt about myself after losing part of my body. The fact that this is a life-threatening disease and you could die is quite sobering. The relationships within the family have been difficult. My husband's a denier—he can't understand why I can't forget about it. He left the house when he knew I was going to get a call regarding the lab results. The denial and the sexuality change is a strain on our relationship. (Hough et al., 1991, p. 577)

Qualitative materials can be used to illustrate specific statistical findings or can also be used to provide more global and dynamic views of the phenomena under study, often in the form of illustrative case studies.

Understanding Relationships and Causal Processes

Quantitative methods often demonstrate that variables are systematically related to one another, but they may fail to provide insights about *why* the variables are related. This situation is especially likely to occur with ex post facto research.

Typically, the discussion section of research reports is devoted to an interpretation of the findings. In quantitatively oriented studies, the interpretations are often speculative, representing the researcher's best guess (a guess that may, of course, be built on solid theory or prior research) about what the findings mean. In essence, the interpretations represent a new set of hypotheses that could be tested in another study. When a study integrates both qualitative and quantitative data, however, the researcher may be in a much stronger position to derive meaning immediately from the statistical findings.

A collaborative study by a group of researchers (Meleis, Norbeck & Laffrey, 1989; Hall, Stevens & Meleis, 1992) provides a good illustration of this application of multimethod research. These researchers examined how married, low-income, working women from different cultural backgrounds integrate their multiple roles on a daily basis. The data were collected by means of lengthy interviews that included both structured questions and in-depth, probing questions that focused on role integration. In the quantitative analysis, these researchers learned that role integration was important in predicting health outcomes—but not *why* this was so. By means of an analysis of the qualitative data, the researchers developed a theoretical understanding of the construct of role integration that provided insights into how it could affect health.

Quantitative analyses can also help to clarify and give shape to findings obtained in qualitative analyses. For example, Lipson (1992) conducted an in-depth field study to investigate the health and adjustment of Iranians who had immigrated to the United States. The primary data were qualitative, gathered by means of observation and in-depth interviews. After a dozen interviews, Lipson noticed that many of the immigrants reported numerous stress-related physical symptoms.

Thereafter, interview respondents were also asked to complete the Health Opinion Survey, a structured instrument that measured in a more systematic fashion the symptoms that are common reactions to stress.

Theory Building, Testing, and Refinement

The most ambitious application of an integrated approach is in the area of theory development. As we have pointed out, a theory is never proven nor confirmed, but rather is supported to a greater or lesser extent. A theory gains acceptance as it escapes disconfirmation. The use of multiple methods provides greater opportunity for potential disconfirmation of the theory. If the theory can survive these assaults, then it can provide a substantially stronger context for the organization of our clinical and intellectual work.

As an example, Salazar and Carter (1993) conducted a study that promotes the development of theory in the area of decision making. These researchers sought to identify the factors that influence the decision of working women to practice breast self-examination (BSE). The first phase of the study involved in-depth interviews with 19 women, selected on the basis of how frequently the women said they practiced BSE. The transcribed interviews were qualitatively analyzed and led to the development of a hierarchical scheme of factors influencing the BSE decision. In the next phase of the research, the researchers used the hierarchy as the basis for developing a survey questionnaire, which was administered to 52 women. BSE performers and nonperformers were compared, and a complex statistical analysis was used to identify factors in the decision hierarchy that best distinguished the two groups.

Integration Strategies

The ways in which a researcher might choose to integrate qualitative and quantitative methods in a single study are almost limitless—or rather, are limited only by the ingenuity of the investigator. Therefore, it is impossible to develop a catalog of integration strategies. However, some of the following scenarios are apt to be especially common.

Embedding Qualitative Approaches Within a Survey

By far the most common data collection method used by nurse researchers is structured interviews and questionnaires, as in a survey situation. Once the researcher has gained the cooperation of the sample for the structured portion of a study, he or she is in an ideal position to move into a second in-depth stage with a subset of the initial respondents. From a practical point of view, it is efficient to have the two forms of data collection occurring simultaneously. However, a two-stage approach has two distinct advantages. If the second stage data collection can be postponed until after the quantitative data have been collected and analyzed, then the researcher will have greater opportunity to probe deeply into the reasons for any obtained results. This is especially likely to be beneficial if the quantitative analyses did not confirm the researcher's hypotheses or if there were any inconsistencies in the results. The second-stage respondents, in other words, can be used as informants to help the researcher interpret the outcomes.

Murphy's longitudinal study of the consequences and processes relating to a natural disaster (the eruption of Mount St. Helens in southwestern Washington state in 1980) provides an example of multimethod research in which qualitative interviews were embedded within a larger survey (Murphy, 1989). In the study, the bulk of the data were collected by way of structured questionnaires administered to three groups of individuals: (1) a bereaved group (individuals who experienced the loss of a family member or close friend); (2) a property loss group (individuals who experienced serious damage or destruction to their homes); and (3) a matched "no disaster loss" group for comparison purposes. Complex analyses of the quantitative data were undertaken to test alternative theories regarding disaster-related effects. In addition, in-depth interviews were conducted with subsets of the study group participants to obtain richer information regarding disaster-induced stress, coping strategies, and processes of recovery.

Embedding Quantitative Measures Into Field Work

Although qualitative data prevail in field studies, field researchers can, in some cases, profit from the collection of more structured information from a larger or more representative sample than is possible in collecting the qualitative data. For instance, the quantitative portion of the study could be used to gather descriptive information about the characteristics of the community or group, so the qualitative findings could be understood in a broader context. Having already gained entrée into the community and the trust and cooperation of its members, the field researcher may be in an ideal position to pursue a survey or a record-extraction activity. For example, if the researcher's in-depth field work focused on family violence, police and hospital records could be used to gather systematic data amenable to statistical analysis.

A study by Grau and Wellin (1992) provides an example of a field study that included the use of structured, quantitative data. Their ethnographic study focused on the question of how nursing homes cope with the demands of government regulation for state licensure and Medicaid/Medicare certification. Two skilled care nursing facilities were studied in depth over a 6-month period. The researchers provided a context for interpreting the qualitative data by administering structured interviews to nurses and others working in the two facilities; these interviews obtained information on the employees' daily work routines, knowledge of regulatory strategies, and experience with regulatory surveys.

Qualitative and Quantitative Data in Experimental Research

Because experimental research involves highly controlled designs and the testing of causal hypotheses, it is easy to get the impression that only quantitative data are appropriate. However, qualitative data can greatly enrich studies that use an experimental or quasi-experimental design. Through in-depth, unstructured approaches, the researcher can better understand qualitative differences between groups, including differences in the reactions of subjects to the experimental conditions, and experiences and processes underlying experimental effects.

Qualitative data collection methods may be especially useful when the researcher is evaluating complex interventions. When an experimental treatment is simple and straightforward (*e.g.,* a new drug), it might be relatively easy to interpret the results. Any posttreatment group differences (assuming that sufficient controls have been instituted) can be attributed to the intervention. However, many nursing interventions are not so straightforward. They may involve new ways of interacting with patients or new approaches to organizing the delivery of care. Sometimes the intervention is multidimensional, involving several different components. At the end of the experiment, even when hypothesized results are obtained, people may ask, What *was* it that really caused the group differences? (If there were no group differences, then the important question would be, *Why* was the intervention unsuccessful?) In-depth qualitative interviews with participants could help to address these questions. In other words, qualitative data may help researchers to address the **black box** question—understanding what it is about the complex intervention that is driving any observed effects. This knowledge can be helpful for theoretical purposes and can also help to streamline an intervention and make it more efficient and cost-effective.

A study in which one of the authors was a coinvestigator (Quint, Polit, Bos & Cave, 1994; Quint & Musick, 1994) provides an example of using both qualitative and quantitative data collection/analysis in an experimental study. The study was a multifaceted evaluation of a comprehensive program for poor teenage mothers, implemented in 16 sites nationwide. The intervention included educational, health, employment, parenting, and social services for participating young mothers and their children. Data were collected over a 4-year period from a sample of over 2000 young mothers. The quantitative data, obtained primarily through structured interviews with the young mothers, suggested relatively modest beneficial treatment effects. In-depth ethnographic interviews with a small sample of the mothers provided insights into the personal problems that undermined program success.

ASSISTANCE TO CONSUMERS OF NURSING RESEARCH

What to Expect in the Research Literature

Qualitative research is increasingly common in the nursing literature, and we can expect this trend to continue in the years to come. In this section, we present some information designed to help consumers in approaching qualitative and integrated studies.

- A decade ago, the *Western Journal of Nursing Research* was the major publication outlet for qualitative nurse researchers. However, every major nursing journal that includes research reports, including specialty journals, now includes qualitative studies. A relatively new journal, *Qualitative Health Research,* specializes in qualitative studies.
- Design decisions for a qualitative study are usually summarized in the method section of a report (*e.g.,* a decision to interview a subset of study participants a second time), but the decision-making process for design decisions is rarely described.
- Some qualitative research reports do not specifically identify a research tradition (*e.g.,* ethnography or phenomenology) but simply describe themselves as qualitative. A research tradition may need to be inferred from information about the types of questions that were asked and the methods used to collect and analyze data. The research tradition most likely to be cited in a nursing research report is grounded theory.
- Sometimes a research report will identify more than one tradition as having provided the framework for a qualitative inquiry. For example, Mayo (1992) studied patterns of physical activity and processes of managing physical activity among African-American women. She described her investigation as an ethnographic study that used a grounded theory method.
- Integrated studies rarely combine qualitative and quantitative findings in a single report. Typically, the quantitative findings are reported in one journal article, and the qualitative findings appear in a separate article in a different journal. However, the authors often summarize the results of the other component of the study in the introduction or discussion section of the report.

Critiquing Qualitative and Integrated Designs

Evaluating a qualitative design is difficult. Qualitative researchers do not always document design decisions and are even less likely to describe the process by which such decisions were made. However, readers should carefully consider whether the design could have been enhanced in some way (*e.g.,* by drawing certain comparisons that might have been supported by the data).

Researchers often do, however, indicate whether the research was conducted within a specific qualitative tradition. This information can be used to come to some conclusions about the study design. For example, if a report indicated that the researcher conducted 1 month of field work for an ethnographic study, there would be reason to suspect that insufficient time had been spent in the field to obtain a true emic perspective of the culture under study.

Most qualitative studies—quite appropriately—do not collect any quantitative data. However, it might be useful to consider how and in what way the addition of quantitative data might have improved the study design. Conversely, not all integrated studies are well suited to a multimethod approach, so integrated studies should be carefully evaluated in terms of the incremental value of having both types of data in a single study.

The guidelines in Box 7–1 are designed to assist you in critiquing the designs of qualitative and integrated studies.

RESEARCH EXAMPLES

Nurse researchers have conducted studies within all of the qualitative research traditions described in this chapter. Table 7–2 provides several examples of research questions addressed within various traditions. Below we present more detailed descriptions of three nursing studies, including two multimethod investigations.

Example of an Ethnographic Study

Dreher and Hayes (1993) spent 6 years in the field studying marijuana use among pregnant Jamaican women and subsequent effects on the offspring. The researchers combined two types of investigations: an ethnographic study of perinatal use of

---

Guidelines for Critiquing Qualitative and Integrated Designs

Box 7–1

1. Is the research tradition within which the qualitative study was undertaken identified? What was that tradition? If no research tradition was identified, can one be inferred?
2. Does the research question appear to be congruent with the research tradition (*i.e.*, is the domain of inquiry for the study congruent with the domain encompassed by the tradition)? Do the data sources and general methodology of the study (*e.g.*, data sources) appear consistent with the tradition?
3. How well is the actual research design described? Does the design appear thoughtful and appropriate? What design elements might have strengthened the study (*e.g.*, would a longitudinal perspective have been preferable, although a cross-sectional design was used)?
4. Is the study exclusively qualitative, or were both qualitative and quantitative data collected? Could the study have been strengthened by the inclusion of some quantitative data?
5. If both qualitative and quantitative data were collected, were they used in a complementary fashion? How (if at all) did the inclusion of both types of data contribute to enhanced theoretical insights, enhanced validity, or movement toward new frontiers?

Table 7–2. Examples of Qualitative Studies Within Various Traditions

Research Tradition	Research Question
Ethnography	How does the culture of 12-step recovery programs empower individuals in making changes in their relationships and identity? (Eastland, 1995)
Phenomenology	What is the essential meaning of stressful life experiences in 9- to 11-year-old children? (Jacobson, 1994)
Hermeneutics	How do patients who have had a near-death experience (NDE) understand and experience the early aftermath of the NDE? (Orne, 1995)
Ethology	What are the interaction dynamics between nurses and patients at transitions from one type of nurse attending to another? (Bottorff & Varcoe, 1995)
Grounded theory	What are the social psychological processes in surviving and recovering from a serious traumatic injury? (Morse & O'Brien, 1995)
Ethnomethodology	What are the social dynamics of home visits by community psychiatric nurses? (Bowers, 1992)
Discourse analysis	What are some of the major ways in which a cancer patient and her oncologist claim power in a medical encounter? (Ainsworth-Vaughn, 1995)

marijuana in rural Jamaican communities, and a quantitative clinical study of a sample of women (including both users and nonusers of marijuana) and their children. The field researchers lived in a rural parish for most of the 6-year period and had regular contact with each of the families in the study.

The ethnographic portion of the study involved in-depth observations and interviews related to perinatal use of marijuana (called *ganja* in Jamaica). The researchers found that most female users prepared and consumed ganja for themselves and their families in the form of teas and tonics for medicinal or health-rendering purposes. Ganja smoking was less common among Jamaican women than Jamaican men, although the researchers found that smoking increased among women over the course of the field work. Women who smoked ganja often smoked throughout pregnancy, during labor, and into the breastfeeding period.

In the clinical portion of the study, the researchers compared the offspring of 30 ganja users and 30 nonusers using standardized measures of development (*e.g.,* the Bayley Scales of Infant Development). The ethnographic work proved to be critical in suggesting adaptations that made these instruments appropriate for a different culture.

Example of an Integrated Study

Reed (1991) studied the link between developmental resources on the one hand and mental health on the other among the oldest-old (those over 80 years of age). Specifically, she was interested in a resource that she labeled "self-transcendence"—the expansion of one's conceptual boundaries inwardly through introspective activities, outwardly through concerns about the welfare of others, and temporally by integrating perceptions of one's past and future.

Reed collected a variety of both quantitative and qualitative data from a sample of 55 older adults living independently. Several structured instruments that yielded quantitative data were administered, including the Center for Epidemiological Studies Depression Scale and the Self-Transcendence Scale, which the author herself developed. Additionally, because the construct of self-transcendence had not been widely studied previously, Reed used an in-depth interview designed to elicit the respondents' own descriptions of self-transcendence perspectives and respondents' perspectives about their past, present, and future and about the bodily changes they were experiencing.

Reed used a highly systematic, iterative process to analyze the qualitative data. A conceptually clustered matrix was constructed to answer questions about patterns of variables across respondents. This analysis revealed four conceptual clusters that the researcher labeled *generativity, introjectivity, temporal integration,* and *body-transcendence.* Table 7–3 presents Reed's clusters and categories for the qualitative data. The relationship between self-transcendence and depression was examined by juxtaposing the qualitatively generated self-transcendence patterns and quantitative depression scores for each respondent. Reed found a relationship between self-transcendence and positive mental health among the very elderly.

Example of a Phenomenologic Study

Building on Reed's concepts and framework, Coward (1995) used a phenomenologic approach to studying the lived experience of self-transcendence in women with AIDS. Coward defined self-transcendence as reaching out beyond the boundaries of the self—either outward beyond personal concern or inward toward increased understanding—to achieve broader perspectives and behaviors that facilitate the discovery of meaning.

Coward obtained her data primarily through unstructured interviews with 10 women with class IV HIV infection (AIDS) recruited through support groups and a family clinic. The women were asked to fully describe situations in which they experienced self-transcendence, including all their thoughts, feelings, and perceptions.

The audiotaped interviews were transcribed verbatim, and phenomenologic analysis techniques were used to organize and synthesize the descriptions. The analysis revealed eight central themes: experiencing fear and aloneness; experiencing uncertainty; using others as role models; finding inner strength; reaching out to give and to receive; making a difference/having purpose; viewing AIDS as opportunity; and having hope. Here is an excerpt that contributed to the theme of "making a difference":

Table 7–3. Reed's Clusters and Categories of Self-Transcendence

Clusters, Categories	Sample Responses
I. Generativity	
(1)* Helping others	Visit the sick; volunteer work; teaching; church work
(1) Family involvement	Visiting siblings, helping children
II. Introjectivity	
(1) Interiority	Hobbies; travel; housework
(1) Lifelong learning	Reading; taking formal courses; spiritual or self-reflection
III. Temporal Integration	
Past	
(2) Active acceptance	Sense of pride in past; feelings of joy about past
(1) Passive acceptance	The past is gone; I have no regrets
(0) Negative acceptance	It saddens me; I regret it
Present	
(2) Active positive	I make the best of it; I am happy; one must change to grow
(1) Passive positive	Take one day at a time; you have to roll with the punches
(0) Negative	I am existing, not living; it is worrisome; discouraging
Future	
(2) Active anticipation	I look forward to it; I am at peace; I have hope
(1) Passive anticipation	Que sera sera; I don't think about it
(0) Negative anticipation	I worry about my health then; I have fears about it
IV. Body-Transcendence	
(2) Flexibility	Learn how to live with it; have to accept it; don't dwell on it
(1) Maybe or unsure	Never thought about it; I think I'm able to accept the changes
(0) Negative	I get disgusted; I feel trapped by my body; I hate my body

From Reed, 1991.
* Indicates weighting used to code the score for each cluster.

I've not always been a strong person. As a matter of fact, I was a follower more than a leader. But now that I have this AIDS, it's like, I'm not going to follow no more. I want people to know—teenagers especially—that AIDS is out there and no one can hide from it.

SUMMARY

Qualitative research typically involves an **emergent design**—a design that emerges in the field once the study is underway. Nevertheless, the qualitative researcher can plan for broad contingencies that can be expected to pose decision opportunities about the design of the study in the field. Although the exact form of a qualitative study is not known in advance, a naturalistic inquiry typically progresses through three broad phases in the field: an orientation and overview phase to determine what it is about the phenomenon under investigation that is salient; a focused exploration phase that closely examines important aspects of the phenomenon; and a confirmation and closure phase to confirm findings.

A variety of research traditions stemming from several disciplines fall within the broad umbrella of qualitative research. These traditions have their roots in anthropology (*e.g.,* **ethnography** and **ethnoscience**); philosophy (**phenomenology** and **hermeneutics**); psychology (**ethology, ecological psychology**); sociology (**grounded theory, ethnomethodology, symbolic interaction**); and sociolinguistics (**discourse analysis**). The various research traditions vary in their conceptualization of what types of questions are important to ask about humans and our social contexts.

Ethnography, which has been used by many nurse researchers, focuses on the culture of a group of people and relies on extensive field work. The ethnographer strives to acquire an **emic,** or insider's, perspective of the culture under study; the outsider's perspective is known as **etic.** The concept of **researcher as instrument** is frequently used by ethnographers to describe the significant role the researcher plays in analyzing and interpreting a culture. Nurses doing ethnographic work sometimes refer to their studies as **ethnonursing research.**

Phenomenology strives to discover the *essence* of a phenomenon as it is experienced by some people. Four aspects of lived experience that are of interest to phenomenologists are **lived space** or **spatiality; lived body** or **corporeality; lived time** or **temporality;** and **lived human relation** or **relationality.** The phenomenologic researcher strives to **bracket** out any preconceived views so the data can be confronted in pure form and to **intuit** the essence of the phenomenon by remaining open to the meanings attributed to it by those who have experienced it.

Grounded theory is a research tradition that began as a systematic method of conducting qualitative research. Grounded theory is an approach to studying social psychological processes and social structures. The aim of grounded theory studies is to discover theoretical precepts grounded in the data. This approach makes use of a technique called **constant comparison:** categories elicited from the data are constantly compared with data obtained earlier so that shared themes and variations can be determined.

In some studies, the judicious integration of qualitative and quantitative data in a single investigation can offer many advantages. The most obvious advantage to a **multimethod research** design is that the qualitative and quantitative data have complementary strengths and weaknesses and offer the possibility of "mutually supplying each other's lack." The potential for confirmation of the study hypotheses through multiple and complementary types of data can strengthen the researcher's confidence in the validity of the findings. An integrated approach can also lead to theoretical and substantive insights into the multidimensional nature of reality that might otherwise be unattainable. Moreover, integration can provide feedback loops that augment the incremental gains in knowledge that a single-method study can achieve.

The integration of qualitative and quantitative data can be used in many applications. In nursing, one of the most frequent uses of multimethod research has been in the area of instrument development. Qualitative data are also used in some studies to illustrate the meaning of quantified descriptions or relationships. Integrated analyses are also used in efforts to interpret and give shape to relationships and causal processes. Finally, the most ambitious application of an integrated approach is in the area of theory development.

◩ STUDY SUGGESTIONS

Chapter 7 of the accompanying *Study Guide to Accompany Essentials of Nursing Research*, 4th edition offers various exercises and study suggestions for reinforcing the concepts presented in this chapter.

Suggested Readings

Methodologic References

Brewer, J., & Hunter, A. (1989). *Multimethod research: A synthesis of styles.* Newbury Park, CA: Sage Publications.

Chenitz, W. C., & Swanson, J. (Eds.). (1985). *Qualitative research in nursing: From practice to grounded theory.* Menlo-Park, CA: Addison-Wesley.

Glaser, B. G., & Strauss, A. L. (1967). *The discovery of grounded theory: Strategies for qualitative research.* Chicago: Aldine.

Leininger, M. M. (Ed.). (1985). *Qualitative research methods in nursing.* New York: Grune & Stratton.

Lincoln, Y. S., & Guba, E. G. (1985). *Naturalistic inquiry.* Newbury Park, CA: Sage Publications.

Morse, J. M. (1991). *Qualitative nursing research: A contemporary dialogue.* Newbury Park, CA: Sage Publications.

Morse, J. M., & Field, P. A. (1995). *Qualitative research methods for health professionals* (2nd ed.). Thousand Oaks, CA: Sage Publications.

Streubert, H. J., & Carpenter, D. R. (1995). *Qualitative research in nursing: Advancing the humanistic imperative.* Philadelphia: J. B. Lippincott.

Substantive References

Ainsworth-Vaughn, N. (1995). Claiming power in the medical encounter: The whirlpool discourse. *Qualitative Health Research, 5,* 270–291.

Astrom, G., Furaker, C., & Norberg, A. (1995). Nurses' skills in managing ethically difficult care situations: Interpretations of nurses' narratives. *Journal of Advanced Nursing, 21,* 1073–1080.

Bottorff, J. L., & Varcoe, C. (1995). Transitions in nurse-patient interactions: A qualitative ethology. *Qualitative Health Research, 5,* 315–331.

Bowers, L. (1992). Ethnomethodology II: A study of the community psychiatric nurse in the patient's home, part 2. *International Journal of Nursing Studies, 29,* 69–79.

Coward, D. D. (1995). The lived experience of self-transcendence in women with AIDS. *Journal of Obstetric, Gynecologic, and Neonatal Nursing, 24,* 314–318.

Dellasega, C., & Mastrian, K. (1995). The process and consequences of institutionalizing an elder. *Western Journal of Nursing Research, 17,* 123–140.

Dreher, M. C., & Hayes, J. S. (1993). Triangulation in cross-cultural research of child development in Jamaica. *Western Journal of Nursing Research, 15,* 216–229.

Eastland, L. S. (1995). Recovery as an interactive process: Explanation and empowerment in 12-step programs. *Qualitative Health Research, 5,* 292–314.

Grau, L., & Wellin, E. (1992). The organizational cultures of nursing homes: Influences on responses to external regulatory controls. *Qualitative Health Research, 2,* 42–60.

Gulick, E. E. (1991). Reliability and validity of the Work Assessment Scale for persons with multiple sclerosis. *Nursing Research, 40,* 107–112.

Hall, J. M., Stevens, P. E., & Meleis, A. I. (1992). Developing the construct of role integration: A narrative analysis of women clerical workers' daily lives. *Research in Nursing and Health, 15,* 447–457.

Hatton, D. C. (1994). Health perceptions among older urban American Indians. *Western Journal of Nursing Research, 16,* 392–403.

Hough, E. E., Lewis, F. M., & Woods, N. F. (1991). Family response to mother's chronic illness: Case studies of well- and poorly-adjusted families. *Western Journal of Nursing Research, 13,* 568–596.

Jacobson, G. (1994). The meaning of stressful life experiences in nine- to eleven-year-old children: A phenomenological study. *Nursing Research, 43,* 95–99.

Kerr, R. B. (1994). Meanings adult daughters attach to a parent's death. *Western Journal of Nursing Research, 16,* 347–365.

Lewis, F. M., Woods, N. F., Hough, E. E., & Bensley, L. (1989). The family's functioning with chronic illness in the mother. *Social Science and Medicine, 29,* 1261–1269.

Lipson, J. G. (1992). The health and adjustment of Iranian immigrants. *Western Journal of Nursing Research, 14,* 10–24.

Mayo, K. (1992). Physical activity practices among American black working women. *Qualitative Health Research, 4,* 51–71.

Meleis, A. I., Norbeck, J. S., Laffrey, S. (1989). Role integration and health among female clerical workers. *Research in Nursing and Health, 12,* 355–364.

Morse, J. M., & O'Brien, B. (1995). Preserving self: From victim, to patient, to disabled person. *Journal of Advanced Nursing, 21,* 886–896.

Murphy, S. A. (1989). An explanatory model of recovery from disaster loss. *Research in Nursing and Health, 12,* 67–76.

Orne, R. M. (1995). The meaning of survival: The early aftermath of a near-death experience. *Research in Nursing and Health, 18,* 239–247.

Quint, J. C., & Musick, S. J. (1994). *Lives of promise, lives of pain: Young mothers after New Chance.* New York, NY: Manpower Demonstration Research Corporation.

Quint, J. C., Polit, D. F., Bos, H., & Cave, G. (1994). *New Chance: Interim findings on a comprehensive program for disadvantaged young mothers and their children.* New York, NY: Manpower Demonstration Research Corporation.

Reed, P. G. (1991). Self-transcendence and mental health in oldest-old adults. *Nursing Research, 40,* 5–11.

Salazar, M. K., & Carter, W. B. (1993). Evaluation of breast self-examination beliefs using a decision model. *Western Journal of Nursing Research, 15,* 403–418.

8

Sampling Designs

Student Objectives

On completion of this chapter, the student will be able to:

- describe the rationale for sampling in research studies
- distinguish between nonprobability and probability samples
- compare the advantages and disadvantages of probability and nonprobability samples in quantitative studies
- identify several types of nonprobability and probability samples and describe their main characteristics
- identify differences in the logic and evaluation criteria used in sampling approaches for quantitative versus qualitative studies
- identify several approaches to theoretical/purposive sampling in qualitative studies
- identify the type of sampling method used in a research study as documented in a research report
- evaluate the sampling approach and sample size in a research study
- define new terms in the chapter

New Terms

Accessible population
Accidental sampling
Cluster sampling
Convenience sampling
Data saturation
Disproportionate sample
Elements
Eligibility criteria
Extreme/deviant case sampling
Homogenous sampling
Intensity sampling
Judgmental sampling
Maximum variation sampling
Multistage sampling
Network sampling
Nonprobability sampling
Nonresponse bias
Population
Power analysis
Probability sampling
Proportionate sample
Purposive (purposeful) sampling

Quota sampling
Random selection
Response rate
Sample
Sample size
Sampling
Sampling bias
Sampling error
Sampling frame
Sampling interval
Simple random sampling
Snowball sampling
Strata
Stratified random sampling
Systematic sampling
Target population
Theoretical sampling
Theory-based sampling
Typical case sampling
Volunteer sample
Weighting

Sampling is a process familiar to all of us. In the course of our daily activities, we gather information, make decisions, and formulate predictions through sampling. A nursing student may decide on an elective course for a semester by sampling two or three different classes on the first day of the semester. Patients may generalize about the quality of nursing care in a hospital as a result of their exposure to a sample of nurses during a 1-week hospital stay. We all come to conclusions about phenomena on the basis of contact with a limited portion of those phenomena.

Researchers, too, must derive knowledge from samples. In testing the efficacy of a nursing intervention for patients with Alzheimer's disease, a nurse researcher must reach a conclusion without testing the intervention with every victim of the disease. However, researchers cannot afford to draw conclusions about the effectiveness of nursing interventions based on a sample of only three or four subjects. The consequences of making erroneous decisions are much more momentous in disciplined inquiries than in private decision making.

Quantitative and qualitative researchers have very different approaches to the issue of sampling. Quantitative researchers seek to select samples that will allow them to generalize their results to much broader groups. They are, therefore, careful in developing plans that specify in advance how study participants are to be selected and how many to include. Qualitative researchers are not concerned with issues of generalizability but rather with an in-depth, holistic understanding of the phenomenon of interest. They allow sampling decisions to emerge during the course of data collection based on informational and theoretical needs, and typically do not develop a formal sampling plan in advance.

Because formal sampling designs are more relevant to quantitative than to qualitative research, most of this chapter is devoted to sampling plans for quantitative studies. However, a section of the chapter is devoted to sampling issues for qualitative research.

◫ BASIC SAMPLING CONCEPTS IN QUANTITATIVE RESEARCH

Sampling is an important step in the research process for quantitative studies. Let us first consider some terms associated with sampling—terms that are used primarily (but not exclusively) in connection with quantitative studies.

Populations

A **population** is the entire aggregation of cases that meets a designated set of criteria. For instance, if a nurse researcher were studying American nurses with doctoral degrees, the population could be defined as all U. S. citizens who are RNs and who have acquired a PhD, DScN, DEd, or other doctoral-level degree. Other possible populations might be (1) all the male patients who had undergone cardiac surgery in Memorial Hospital during the year 1996, (2) all women over 60 years of age who are under psychiatric care, or (3) all the children in Atlanta with cystic fibrosis. As this list illustrates, a population may be broadly defined, involving millions of people, or narrowly specified to include only several hundred people.

Populations are not restricted to human subjects. A population might consist of all the hospital records on file in the Belleview Hospital, or all the blood samples taken from clients of a health maintenance organization, or all the U. S. high schools with a school-based clinic that dispenses contraceptives. Whatever the basic unit, the population always comprises an aggregate of elements in which the researcher is interested.

Quantitative research reports should identify the **eligibility criteria** for inclusion in the study. These criteria are the characteristics that delimit the population of interest. For example, consider a population defined as American nursing students. Would this population include students in all three types of basic programs? Would part-time students be included? How about RNs returning to school for a bachelor's degree? Would foreign students enrolled in American nursing programs qualify? The researcher needs to establish these criteria before sample selection to make decisions about whether a person would be classified as a member of the population in question. A reader of a research report needs to know the eligibility criteria to understand the population to which the findings can be generalized. The eligibility criteria specified in one nursing study are presented in Table 8–1.

It is sometimes useful to make a distinction between target and accessible populations. The **target population** is the entire population in which the researcher is interested. The **accessible population** refers to those cases that conform to the eligibility criteria and that are accessible to the researcher as a pool of subjects for the study. For example, the researcher's target population might consist of all diabetics in the United States, but, in reality, the population that is accessible to a researcher might consist of all diabetics who are members of a particular health plan. Researchers sample from an accessible population, often in the hope of generalizing to a target population.

Samples and Sampling

Sampling refers to the process of selecting a portion of the population to represent the entire population. A **sample,** then, consists of a subset of the entities that make up the population. The entities that make up the samples and populations are

Table 8–1. Eligibility Criteria Specified in a Quantitative Nursing Study

Research Question	Eligibility Criteria
What is the degree to which hospital patients ready for discharge and with identifiable levels of need for service were referred for home health care? (Prescott, Soeken & Griggs, 1995)	To be eligible for the study, the patient must: • be hospitalized for a minimum of 48 hours with a medical or surgical condition • have a planned discharge to home • be age 18 or over • be English speaking • be able to participate in a discharge interview

sometimes referred to as **elements.** The element is the most basic unit about which information is collected. In nursing research, the elements are usually humans.

Samples and sampling plans vary in their adequacy. *The overriding consideration in assessing a sample in a quantitative study is its representativeness* (*i.e.,* the extent to which the sample behaves like or has characteristics similar to the population). Unfortunately, there is no method for ensuring absolutely that a sample is representative without obtaining the information from the entire population. Certain sampling procedures are less likely to result in samples that are biased than others, but there is never any guarantee of a representative sample. This may sound somewhat discouraging, but it must be remembered that researchers always operate under conditions in which error is possible. An important role of the researcher is to minimize or control those errors, or at least to estimate the magnitude of their effects.

Sampling plans can be grouped into two categories: **probability sampling** and **nonprobability sampling.** Probability samples use some form of random selection in choosing the sample units. The hallmark of a probability sample is that a researcher is in a position to specify the probability that each element of the population will be included in the sample. Probability samples are generally preferred because greater confidence can be placed in the representativeness of probability samples. In nonprobability samples, elements are selected by nonrandom methods. There is no way to estimate the probability that each element has of being included in a nonprobability sample, and every element usually does *not* have a chance for inclusion.

Strata

Sometimes it is useful to think of populations as consisting of two or more subpopulations, or **strata.** A stratum refers to a mutually exclusive segment of a population based on one or more characteristics. For instance, suppose our population consisted of all RNs currently employed in the United States. This population could be divided into two strata based on gender. Alternatively, we could specify three strata consisting of nurses younger than 30 years, nurses aged 30 to 45 years, and nurses aged 46 years or older. Strata are often identified and used in the sample selection process to enhance the representativeness of the sample.

Sampling Rationale

Researchers work with samples rather than with populations because it is more economical and efficient to do so. The typical researcher has neither the time nor the resources required to study all possible members of a population. Furthermore, it is unnecessary to gather information about some phenomenon from an entire population. It is almost always possible to obtain reasonably accurate information from a sample. Samples, thus, are practical and efficient means of collecting data.

Still, despite all the advantages of sampling, the data obtained from samples can lead to erroneous conclusions. Finding 50 willing subjects to participate in a research project seldom poses any difficulty, even to a novice researcher. It is considerably more problematic to select 50 subjects who adequately represent the population and who are not a biased subset of it. **Sampling bias** refers to the systematic overrepresentation or underrepresentation of some segment of the population in terms of a characteristic relevant to the research question.

Sampling bias is almost always unintentional. If a researcher studying students at Boston College systematically interviewed every tenth student who entered the library, the sample of students would be strongly biased in favor of students who use the library, even though the researcher may have exerted a conscientious effort to include every tenth entrant, irrespective of their appearance, gender, or other characteristic.

An important point to remember is that sampling bias is affected by the homogeneity of the population with respect to the critical variables. If the elements in a population were all identical on some critical attribute, then any sample would be as good as any other. Indeed, if the population were completely homogeneous (*i.e.*, exhibited no variability at all), then a single element would constitute a sufficient sample for drawing conclusions about the population. With regard to many physical or physiologic attributes, it may be safe to assume a reasonably high degree of homogeneity and to proceed in selecting a sample on the basis of this assumption. For example, the blood in a person's veins is relatively homogeneous. A single blood sample chosen haphazardly from a patient is usually adequate for clinical purposes. For many human attributes, however, homogeneity is the exception rather than the rule. Variables, after all, derive their name from the fact that traits vary from one person to the next. Age, blood pressure, occupation, stress level, and health habits are all attributes that reflect the heterogeneity of human beings. In assessing the risk of sampling bias, readers of quantitative research reports must consider the degree to which a population is heterogeneous with respect to key variables.

◪ NONPROBABILITY SAMPLING

As previously noted, nonprobability sampling involves selecting a sample through nonrandom methods. There are three primary methods of nonprobability sampling used in quantitative studies: convenience, quota, and purposive sampling.

Convenience Sampling

Convenience sampling (sometimes called **accidental sampling**) entails the use of the most conveniently available people as study participants. The nurse who distributes questionnaires about breastfeeding intentions to the first 100 available pregnant women is using a convenience sample. The problem with convenience sampling is that available subjects might be atypical of the population with regard to the critical variables being measured. Thus, the cost of convenience is the risk of bias and erroneous findings.

Convenience samples do not necessarily comprise people known to the researchers. Stopping people at the street corner to ask them to complete a question-naire is sampling by convenience. Sometimes a researcher seeking people with certain characteristics places an advertisement in a newspaper or places signs in clinics or community centers. Both these approaches may result in bias because people select themselves as pedestrians on certain streets or as volunteers in re-sponse to public notices. Self-selection generally leads to bias.

Another type of convenience sampling is known as **snowball sampling** or **network sampling.** With this approach, early sample members are asked to identify and refer other people who meet the eligibility criteria for the study. In quantitative studies, this method of sampling is most often used when the research population consists of people with specific traits who might be difficult to identify by ordinary means (*e.g.,* women who stopped breastfeeding their infants within 1 month of release from the hospital).

Convenience sampling is the least desirable form of sampling for quantitative studies. In cases in which the phenomena under investigation are fairly homoge-neous within the population, the risk of bias may be minimal. When the phenomena are heterogeneous, there is no other sampling approach in which the risk of bias is greater—and there is no way to evaluate the biases that may be operating. Caution should be exercised in interpreting findings from quantitative studies in which convenience samples were used.

Quota Sampling

Quota sampling is a form of nonprobability sampling in which the researcher uses knowledge about the population to build some representativeness into the sampling plan. The quota sample is one in which the researcher identifies strata of the population and specifies the proportions of elements needed from the various seg-ments of the population. By using information about the composition of the popula-tion, the investigator can ensure that diverse segments are represented in the sample. Quota sampling gets its name from the procedure of establishing quotas for the various strata from which data are to be collected.

Let us use as an example a researcher interested in studying the attitudes of undergraduate nursing students toward working on an AIDS unit. The accessible population for this study might be a school of nursing that has an undergraduate enrollment of 1000 students. A sample size of 200 students is desired. The easiest procedure would be to use a convenience sample by distributing questionnaires to students in classrooms or as they enter or leave the library. Suppose, however, that the researcher suspects that male students and female students, as well as members of the four classes, have different attitudes toward working with AIDS victims. A convenience sample could easily sample too many or too few students from these subgroups. Table 8–2 presents some fictitious data showing the numbers of students in each strata, both for the population and for a convenience sample. As this table shows, the convenience sample seriously overrepresents freshmen and women while underrepresenting men and members of the sophomore, junior, and senior classes. In anticipation of a problem of this type, the researcher can guide the selection of

Table 8–2. Numbers and Percentages of Students in Strata of a Population, Convenience Sample, and Quota Sample

	Freshmen	**Sophomores**	**Juniors**	**Seniors**	**Total**
Population					
Males	25 (2.5%)	25 (2.5%)	25 (2.5%)	25 (2.5%)	100 (10%)
Females	225 (22.5%)	225 (22.5%)	225 (22.5%)	225 (22.5%)	900 (90%)
TOTAL	250 (25%)	250 (25%)	250 (25%)	250 (25%)	1000 (100%)
Convenience Sample					
Males	2 (1%)	4 (2%)	3 (1.5%)	1 (0.5%)	10 (5%)
Females	98 (49%)	36 (18%)	37 (18.5%)	19 (9.5%)	190 (95%)
TOTAL	100 (50%)	40 (20%)	40 (20%)	20 (10%)	200 (100%)
Quota Sample					
Males	5 (2.5%)	5 (2.5%)	5 (2.5%)	5 (2.5%)	20 (10%)
Females	45 (22.5%)	45 (22.5%)	45 (22.5%)	45 (22.5%)	180 (90%)
TOTAL	50 (25%)	50 (25%)	50 (25%)	50 (25%)	200 (100%)

subjects so that the final sample includes an appropriate number of cases from each stratum. The bottom panel of Table 8–2 shows the number of cases that would be required for each stratum in a quota sample for this example.

If we pursue this example a bit further, you may better appreciate the dangers of inadequate representation of the various strata. Suppose that one of the key questions in this study was: Would you be willing to work on a unit that cared exclusively for AIDS patients? The percentage of students in the population who would respond "yes" to this inquiry is shown in the first column of Table 8–3. Of course, these values would not be known by the researcher; they are displayed to illustrate a point. Within the population, males and older students are more likely than females and younger students to express willingness to work on a unit with AIDS patients, yet these are the groups that were underrepresented in the convenience sample. As a result, there is a sizable discrepancy between the population and sample values: nearly twice as many students in the population are favorable toward working with AIDS victims (12.5%) than one would suspect based on the results obtained from the convenience sample (6.5%). The quota sample, on the other hand, does a reasonably good job of mirroring the viewpoint of the population.

Quota sampling is a relatively easy way to enhance the representativeness of a nonprobability sample. Researchers generally stratify on the basis of extraneous variables that, in their estimation, would reflect important differences in the dependent variable under investigation. Such variables as age, gender, ethnicity, socioeconomic status, educational attainment, and medical diagnosis are frequently used as stratifying variables in quantitative nursing studies.

Except for the identification of the key strata, quota sampling is procedurally

Table 8–3. Students Willing to Consider Working
with AIDS Patients

	Number in Population	Number in Convenience Sample	Number in Quota Sample
Freshmen males	2	0	0
Sophomore males	6	1	1
Junior males	8	1	2
Senior males	12	0	3
Freshmen females	6	2	1
Sophomore females	16	2	3
Junior females	30	4	7
Senior females	45	3	9
Number of willing students	125	13	26
Total number of students	1000	200	200
Percentage	12.5%	6.5%	13.0%

similar to convenience sampling. The subjects in any particular cell constitute, in essence, a convenience sample from that stratum of the population. Because of this fact, quota sampling shares many of the same weaknesses as convenience sampling. For instance, if the researcher were required by the quota sampling plan to interview 20 male nursing students, a trip to the college dormitories might be the most convenient method of obtaining those subjects. Yet this approach would fail to give any representation to any male commuter students, who may have distinctive views about working with AIDS patients. Despite its problems, however, quota sampling represents an important improvement over convenience sampling for quantitative studies.

Purposive Sampling

Purposive or **judgmental sampling** is based on the assumption that a researcher's knowledge about the population can be used to handpick the cases to be included in the sample. The researcher might decide purposely to select the widest possible variety of respondents or might choose subjects who are judged to be typical of the population in question or particularly knowledgeable about the issues under study. Sampling in this subjective manner, however, provides no external, objective method for assessing the typicalness of the selected subjects. Nevertheless, this method can be used to advantage in certain instances. For instance, newly developed instruments can be effectively pretested and evaluated with a purposive sample of divergent types of people. Purposive sampling is often used when the researcher wants a sample of experts, as in the case of a needs assessment using the key informant approach. Generalizing findings from a purposive sample to the broader population, however, is risky in most instances.

Evaluation of Nonprobability Sampling

Nonprobability samples are rarely representative of the researcher's target population. The difficulty stems from the fact that not every element in the population has a chance of being included in the sample. Therefore, it is likely that some segment of the population will be systematically underrepresented. If the population is homogeneous on the critical attributes, then biases will be small or nonexistent. Still, only a small fraction of the characteristics in which quantitative nurse researchers are interested are sufficiently homogeneous to render sampling bias an irrelevant consideration.

Why then are nonprobability samples used at all in quantitative research? Clearly, the advantage of these sampling designs lies in their convenience and economy. Probability sampling, which is discussed in the next section, requires resources and time. There is often no option but to use a nonprobability approach or to abandon the project altogether. Even hard-nosed research methodologists would hesitate to advocate a total abandonment of one's ideas in the absence of a random sample. The researcher using a nonprobability sample out of necessity must be cautious about the inferences and conclusions drawn from the data, and readers of the research report should be alert to the possibility of sampling bias.

▧ PROBABILITY SAMPLING

The hallmark of probability sampling is the random selection of elements from the population. Random selection should not be confused with random assignment, which was described in connection with experimental research in Chapter 6. Random assignment refers to the process of allocating subjects to different experimental conditions on a random basis. Random assignment has no bearing on how the subjects participating in an experiment were selected in the first place. A **random selection** process is one in which each element in the population has an equal, independent chance of being selected. The four most commonly used probability sampling designs are simple random, stratified random, cluster, and systematic sampling.

Simple Random Sampling

Simple random sampling is the most basic of the probability sampling designs. Because the more complex probability sampling designs incorporate the features of simple random sampling, the procedures are briefly described so consumers can appreciate what is involved.

Once the population has been defined, the researcher establishes what is known as a sampling frame. The term **sampling frame** is the technical name for the actual list of the population elements from which the sample will be chosen. If nursing students attending Wayne State University constituted the population, then a roster of those students would be the sampling frame. If the sampling unit consisted of 400-bed or larger general hospitals in the United States, then a list of all those hospitals would be the sampling frame. In actual practice, a population may be defined in terms of an existing sampling frame rather than starting with a population and then developing a list of the elements. For example, if a researcher wanted to use a telephone directory as a sampling frame, the population would have to be defined as the residents of a certain community who are clients of the telephone company *and* who have a listed number. Because not all members of a community have a telephone and others have unlisted numbers, it would be inappropriate to consider a telephone directory the sampling frame for the entire community population.

Once a listing of the population elements has been developed or located, the elements are numbered consecutively. A table of random numbers or a computer is then usually used to draw, at random, a sample of the desired size. (Another possibility is to draw names from a hat at random, but this is an unwieldy procedure if the sampling frame is large.)

It should be clear that the samples selected randomly in such a fashion are not subject to the biases of the researcher. There is no guarantee that the sample will be representative of the population. Random selection does, however, guarantee that differences in the attributes of the sample and the population are purely a function of chance. The probability of selecting a markedly deviant sample through random sampling is low, and this probability decreases as the size of the sample increases.

Simple random sampling tends to be an exceedingly laborious process. The development of the sampling frame, enumeration of all the elements, and selection of the sample elements are time-consuming chores, particularly if the population is large. Imagine enumerating all the telephone subscribers listed in the New York City telephone directory. Moreover, it is rarely possible to get a complete listing of every element in a population, so other methods are often used.

Stratified Random Sampling

Stratified random sampling is a variant of simple random sampling whereby the population is first divided into two or more strata or subgroups. As in the case of quota sampling, the aim of stratified sampling is to obtain a greater degree of representativeness. Stratified sampling designs subdivide the population into homogeneous subsets from which an appropriate number of elements can be selected at random.

The most common procedure for drawing a stratified random sample is to group together those elements that belong to a stratum and to select randomly the desired number of elements. The researcher may sample either proportionately (in relation to the relative size of the stratum) or disproportionately. For example, if an undergraduate population in a school of nursing consisted of 10% African Americans, 5% Hispanics, and 85% whites, then a **proportionate sample** of 100 students, with racial background as the stratifying variable, would consist of 10, 5, and 85 students from the respective subpopulations.

When the researcher is concerned with determining differences between the strata, then proportionate sampling may result in an insufficient base for making comparisons. In the previous example, would the researcher be justified in coming to conclusions about the characteristics of Hispanic nursing students based on only five cases? It would be extremely unwise to do so. Researchers often use a **disproportionate sample** whenever comparisons are sought between strata of greatly unequal membership size. In the example at hand, the sampling proportions might be altered to select 20 African Americans, 20 Hispanics, and 60 whites. This design would ensure a more adequate representation of the viewpoints of the two racial minorities. When disproportionate sampling is used, however, it is necessary to make a mathematical adjustment (known as **weighting**) to the data to arrive at the best estimate of overall population values.

Stratified random sampling offers the researcher the opportunity to sharpen the precision and representativeness of the final sample. When it is desirable to obtain reliable information about subpopulations whose membership is relatively small, stratification provides a means of including a sufficient number of cases in the sample by oversampling for that stratum. Stratified sampling may, however, be impossible if information on the stratifying variables is unavailable (*e.g.,* a sampling frame of students in a school of nursing might not include information on race and ethnicity). Furthermore, a stratified sample requires even more labor and effort than simple random sampling because the sample must be drawn from multiple enumerated listings.

Cluster Sampling

For many populations, it is simply not possible to obtain a listing of all the elements. The population consisting of all full-time nursing students in the United States would be extremely difficult to list and enumerate for the purpose of drawing a simple or stratified random sample. In addition, it would be prohibitively expensive to sample nursing students in this way because the resulting sample would consist of no more than one or two students per institution. Large-scale quantitative studies almost never use simple or stratified random sampling. The most common procedure for large-scale surveys is cluster sampling.

In **cluster sampling,** there is a successive random sampling of units. The first unit to be sampled is large groupings, or clusters. In drawing a sample of nursing students, the researcher might first draw a random sample of nursing schools. Or, if a sample of nursing supervisors is desired, a random sample of hospitals might first be obtained. The usual procedure for selecting a general sample of citizens is to sample such administrative units as states, cities, districts, blocks, and then households, successively. Because of the successive stages of sampling, this approach is often referred to as **multistage sampling.**

For a specified number of cases, cluster sampling tends to contain more sampling errors than simple or stratified random sampling. Despite this disadvantage, cluster sampling is considered more economical and practical than other types of probability sampling, particularly when the population is large and widely dispersed.

Systematic Sampling

Systematic sampling involves the selection of every kth case from some list or group, such as every 10th person on a patient list or every 100th person listed in a directory of American Nurses' Association members. Systematic sampling is sometimes used to sample every kth person who, for example, enters a bookstore or leaves a hospital. In these situations, unless the population is narrowly defined as consisting of all those people entering the bookstore, or leaving the hospital, the sampling is nonprobability in nature. If college students were sampled systematically on entering a bookstore, the resulting sample could not be called a random selection of students because not every student had a chance of being selected. Systematic sampling designs can, however, be applied in such a way that an essentially random sample is drawn. If the researcher used a list, or sampling frame, the size of the population (N) could be divided by the size of the desired sample (n) to obtain the sampling interval width (k). The **sampling interval** is the standard distance between the elements chosen for the sample. For instance, if we were seeking a sample of 150 from a population of 30,000, then our sampling interval would be as follows:

$$k = 30,000 \div 150 = 200$$

In other words, every 200th case on the list would be sampled. The first case would be selected randomly, using a table of random numbers. If the random number chosen is 73, then the people corresponding to numbers 73, 273, 473, 673, and so forth will be included in the sample.

Systematic sampling conducted in this manner is essentially identical to simple random sampling. Problems may arise if the list is arranged in such a way that a certain type of element is listed at intervals coinciding with the sampling interval. For instance, if every tenth nurse listed in a nursing personnel roster was a head nurse, and the sampling interval was ten, then head nurses would be included in the sample either always or never. Problems of this type are not common, fortunately. In most cases, systematic sampling is preferable to simple random sampling because the same results are obtained in a more convenient and efficient manner.

Evaluation of Probability Sampling

Probability sampling is the only reliable method of obtaining representative samples in quantitative studies. The superiority of probability sampling lies partially in its avoidance of conscious or unconscious biases. If all the elements in the population have an equal probability of being selected, then the likelihood is high that the resulting sample will do a good job of representing the population.

A further advantage is that probability sampling allows the researcher to estimate the magnitude of sampling error. **Sampling error** refers to the differences between population values (such as the average age of the population) and sample values (such as the average age of the sample). It is rare that a sample is perfectly representative of a population and contains no sampling error on any of the attributes under investigation. Probability sampling does, however, permit estimates of the degree of expected error.

The great drawbacks of probability sampling are its expense and inconvenience. Unless the population is narrowly defined, it is beyond the scope of most small-scale quantitative studies to sample using a probability design. A researcher adopting a nonprobability sampling design might well be able to argue that the homogeneity of the attribute under consideration makes an elaborate sampling scheme unnecessary. This justification, however, probably will not be acceptable if attributes of a psychological or social nature are being studied. In summary, probability sampling is the preferred and most respected method of obtaining sample elements in quantitative research, but it is often impractical or unnecessary.

◩ SAMPLE SIZE IN QUANTITATIVE STUDIES

A major issue in the conduct and evaluation of quantitative research is the **sample size,** or the number of subjects in a sample. Although there is no simple equation that can automatically answer the question of how large a sample is needed, quantitative researchers are generally advised to use the largest sample possible. The larger the sample, the more representative of the population it is likely to be. Every time a researcher calculates a percentage or an average based on sample data, the purpose is to estimate a population value. Smaller samples tend to produce less accurate estimates than larger samples. In other words, the larger the sample, the smaller the sampling error.

Let us illustrate this notion with the simple example of monthly aspirin consumption in a nursing home facility, as shown in Table 8–4. The population consists of 15 residents whose aspirin consumption averages 16 units per month. Two simple random samples with sample sizes of 2, 3, 5, and 10 were drawn from the population of 15 residents. Each sample average on the right represents an estimate of the population average, which we know is 16. (Under ordinary circumstances, the population value would be unknown to us, and we would draw only one sample.) With a sample size of two, our estimate might have been wrong by as many as eight aspirins in sample 1B. As the sample size increases, not only does the average get closer to the true population value, but also the differences in the estimates between samples A and B get smaller. As the sample size increases, the probability of getting a markedly deviant sample diminishes. Large samples provide the opportunity to counterbalance, in the long run, atypical values.

The advanced researcher can estimate how large the sample should be for an

Table 8–4. Comparison of Population and Sample Values and Averages in Nursing Home Aspirin Consumption Example

Number in Group	Group	Values (Monthly Number of Aspirins Consumed)	Average
15	Population	2, 4, 6, 8, 10, 12, 14, 16, 18, 20, 22, 24, 26, 28, 30	16.0
2	Sample 1A	6, 14	10.0
2	Sample 1B	20, 28	24.0
3	Sample 2A	16, 18, 8	14.0
3	Sample 2B	20, 14, 26	20.0
5	Sample 3A	26, 14, 18, 2, 28	17.6
5	Sample 3B	30, 2, 26, 10, 4	14.4
10	Sample 4A	18, 16, 24, 22, 8, 14, 28, 20, 2, 6	15.8
10	Sample 4B	14, 18, 12, 20, 6, 14, 28, 12, 24, 16	16.4

adequate test of the research hypotheses through a procedure known as **power analysis** (Cohen, 1977). It is beyond the scope of this introductory text to describe this technical topic in much detail, but a simple example can be used here to illustrate some basic principles. Suppose a researcher were testing a new intervention to help smokers quit smoking. Smokers would be randomly assigned to either an experimental or a control group. How many smokers should be used in the study? When using power analysis, the researcher must estimate how large a difference between the groups will be observed (*e.g.,* the difference in the mean number of cigarettes consumed in the week after the experimental treatment). This estimate might be based on previous research, on personal experience of the researcher, or on some other factors. When expected differences are large, it does not take a particularly large sample to ensure that the differences will actually be revealed in a statistical analysis; but when small differences are predicted, then large samples are needed. Cohen (1977) claims that, for most new areas of research, group differences are likely to be small. In our example, if a small group difference in postintervention smoking were expected, the sample size needed to test adequately the effectiveness of the new program would be in the vicinity of 800 smokers (400 per group), assuming standard statistical criteria. If a medium-sized difference were expected, the total sample size would still be several hundred smokers.

When samples are too small, quantitative researchers run a great risk of gathering data that will not confirm the study hypotheses—even when those hypotheses are correct. Large samples are no assurance of accuracy, however. When nonprobability sampling methods are used, even a large sample can harbor extensive bias. The famous example illustrating this point is the 1936 presidential poll conducted by the magazine *Literary Digest,* which predicted that Alfred M. Landon would defeat Franklin D. Roosevelt by a landslide. About 2.5 million people participated in this poll, which is a huge sample. Biases resulted from the fact that the sample was drawn from telephone directories and automobile registrations during a Depression year when only the well-to-do (who favored Landon) had a car or telephone.

A large sample cannot correct for a faulty sampling design; nevertheless, a large nonprobability sample is generally preferable to a small one. When critiquing quantitative studies, you must assess both the size of the sample and the method by which the sample was selected. An important point to remember is that the ultimate criterion for assessing a sample in quantitative research is its representativeness.

▧ SAMPLING IN QUALITATIVE RESEARCH

Qualitative studies almost always use small, nonrandom samples. This does not mean that qualitative researchers are unconcerned with the quality of their samples, but rather that they use different criteria for selecting study participants. This section examines considerations that apply to sampling in qualitative studies.

The Logic of Qualitative Sampling

Quantitative research is concerned with measuring attributes and relationships in a population, and therefore a representative sample is needed to ensure that the measurements accurately reflect and can be generalized to the population. The aim of most qualitative studies is to discover *meaning* and to uncover multiple realities, and so generalizability is not a guiding criterion.

The qualitative researcher begins a study with the following types of sampling question in mind: Who would be an information-rich data source for my study? Who should I talk to, or what should I observe first so as to maximize my understanding of the phenomenon? Clearly, with these types of question, a critical first step in qualitative sampling is the selection of a setting with high potential for "information-richness."

As the study progresses, new sampling questions emerge, such as the following: Whom can I talk to or observe to confirm my understandings? Challenge or modify my understandings? Enrich my understandings? Thus, as with the overall design in qualitative studies, sampling design is an emergent one that capitalizes on early learnings to guide subsequent direction.

Types of Qualitative Sampling

Qualitative researchers usually eschew probability samples. A random sample is not the best method of selecting people who will make good informants (*i.e.,* people who are knowledgeable, articulate, reflective, and willing to talk at length with the researcher).

Qualitative researchers may begin with a convenience sample (sometimes referred to in qualitative studies as a **volunteer sample**), especially if the researcher needs to have potential informants come forward to identify themselves (*e.g.,* by placing notices in newspapers for people with certain experiences). Qualitative researchers also use snowball sampling, asking early informants to make referrals for other study participants.

Although qualitative sampling may begin with volunteer informants and may be supplemented with new participants through snowballing, most qualitative studies eventually evolve to a purposive sampling strategy. (In qualitative research, purposive sampling is often referred to as **theoretical sampling** or **purposeful sampling.**) That is, regardless of how initial participants are selected, the researcher usually strives to purposefully select sample members based on the information needs emerging from the early findings. Whom to sample next depends on who has been sampled already.

Within purposive sampling, several alternative strategies have been identified (Patton, 1990), only a few of which will be mentioned here:

- **Maximum variation sampling**—involves purposefully selecting cases with a wide range of variation on dimensions of interest
- **Homogeneous sampling**—deliberately reduces variation and allows a more focused inquiry
- **Extreme/deviant case sampling**—provides opportunities for learning from the most unusual and extreme informants (*e.g.,* outstanding successes and notable failures)
- **Intensity sampling**—consists of information-rich cases that manifest the phenomenon of interest intensely, but not as extreme or potentially distorting manifestations
- **Typical case sampling**—involves selection of participants who will illustrate or highlight what is typical or average
- **Theory-based sampling**—involves selection of people or incidents on the basis of their potential representation of important theoretical constructs

Maximum variation sampling is often the sampling mode of choice in qualitative research because it is useful in documenting the scope of a phenomenon and in identifying important patterns that cut across variations. However, other strategies can also be used advantageously, depending on the nature of the research question.

Sample Size

There are no firmly established criteria or rules for sample size in qualitative research. Sample size is largely a function of the purpose of the inquiry, the quality of the informants, and the type of sampling strategy used. For example, a larger sample is likely to be needed with maximum variation sampling than with typical case sampling. Patton argues that purposive samples "be judged on the basis of the purpose and rationale of each study and the sampling strategy used to achieve the study's purpose. The sample, like all other aspects of qualitative inquiry, must be judged in context . . ." (p. 185).

In qualitative research, sample size should be determined on the basis of informational needs. Hence, a guiding principle in sampling is **data saturation** (*i.e.*, sampling to the point where no new information is obtained and redundancy is achieved). Redundancy can typically be achieved with a fairly small number of cases, if the information from each is of sufficient depth. With a fairly homogeneous sample, fewer than ten cases may suffice. However, when maximum variation is desired or when the researcher is interested in seeking potentially disconfirming evidence, a larger sample is usually required.

ASSISTANCE TO CONSUMERS OF NURSING RESEARCH

What to Expect in the Research Literature

Virtually all nursing studies involve the use of samples rather than entire populations. Here are a few suggestions to guide you as you read about sampling plans in the nursing literature:

- The sampling plan is almost always discussed in the methods section of a research report, sometimes in a separate subsection with the heading "Sample" or "Subjects" or "Study Participants." A description of the characteristics of the actual sample, however, is often postponed until the results section of the report.
- If the researcher has undertaken any analyses to detect sample biases in a quantitative study, these may be described in either the methods or results section (*e.g.*, the researcher might compare the characteristics of patients who were invited to participate in the study but who declined to do so with those of patients who actually became subjects).
- The research report is not always explicit about the type of sampling approach used. This is particularly apt to be true with nonprobability sampling plans. If the sampling design is not specified, it is probably safe to assume that a sample of convenience was used in a quantitative study and that some type of purposive sampling was used in a qualitative one.
- In some quantitative research reports, the researchers do not clearly identify the population under study. In others, the population is not clarified until the discussion section, when an effort is made to discuss the group to which the study findings can be generalized.
- The sampling plan is often one of the weakest aspects of quantitative nursing studies (this is also true of quantitative research in other disciplines). Most nursing studies use samples of convenience, and many are based on samples that are too small to provide an adequate test of the research hypotheses. Most quantitative studies are based on samples of under 200

subjects, and a great many studies have fewer than 100 subjects. Power analysis is not used by many nurse researchers. Typically, research reports offer no justification for the size of the study sample. Small samples run a high risk of leading researchers to erroneously reject their research hypotheses. Therefore, readers should be especially prepared to critique the sampling plan of studies that fail to support research hypotheses.

- The sample size adequacy of quantitative studies often can be determined by consumers after the fact through power analysis. However, sample size adequacy in a qualitative study is more difficult to judge on the basis of reading a research report because the main criterion is redundancy of information, which is difficult for consumers to judge. However, some qualitative reports explicitly state that data saturation was achieved.

Critiquing the Sampling Plan

The sampling plan of a research study—particularly a quantitative study—merits particular scrutiny because, if the sample is seriously biased or too small, the findings may be misleading or just plain wrong. In critiquing a description of a sampling plan, the consumer must consider two issues. The first and most basic issue is whether the researcher has adequately described the sampling plan that was used. Ideally, a research report includes a description of the following aspects of the sample:

- The type of sampling approach used (*e.g.,* convenience, snowball, purposive, simple random)
- The population under study and the eligibility criteria for sample selection in quantitative studies; the nature of the setting and study group in a qualitative one
- The method of recruiting study participants (*e.g.,* through direct invitation by the researcher, through notices placed on a bulletin board)
- The number of participants in the study and a rationale for the sample size
- A description of the main characteristics of the participants (*e.g.,* age, gender, medical condition, race, ethnicity, and so forth) and, in a quantitative study, of the population
- In quantitative studies, the number and characteristics of potential subjects who declined to participate in the study and of subjects who agreed to participate but who subsequently withdrew

If the description of the sample is inadequate, the reviewer may not be in a position to deal with the second and principal issue, which is whether the researcher made good sampling decisions.

Evaluating Quantitative Sampling Plans

We have stressed that the main criterion for assessing the adequacy of a sampling plan in quantitative research is whether the resulting sample is representative of the population. A research consumer never knows for sure, of course, but, if the sampling strategy is weak or if the sample size is small, then there is reason to suspect that the findings contain some degree of bias. The extent of this bias depends on several factors, including the homogeneity of the population with respect to the dependent variable. When the researcher has adopted a sampling plan in which the risk of bias is high, he or she should have taken steps to estimate the direction and degree of this bias so that the reader can draw some informed conclusions.

Even with a perfectly conceived and executed sampling plan, the resulting sample may contain some bias because not all people invited to participate in a research study actually agree to do so. If certain segments of the population systematically refuse to cooperate, then a biased sample can result, even when probability sampling is used. The research report ideally should provide information about **response rates** (*i.e.,* the number of people participating in a study relative to the number of people sampled) and some indication about possible **nonresponse bias**—differences between participants and those who refused to participate in the study.

In developing the sampling plan, the researcher makes decisions regarding the specification of the population as well as the selection of the sample. If the target population is defined too broadly, the researcher has missed opportunities to control extraneous variables and to delimit the heterogeneity of the dependent variables. Moreover, the gap between the accessible and the target population may be too great. Your job as reviewer is to come to some conclusion about the reasonableness of generalizing the findings from the researcher's sample to the accessible population and from the accessible population to a broader target population. If the sampling plan is seriously flawed, it may be risky to generalize the findings at all without further replication of the results with another sample.

Box 8–1 presents some guiding questions for critiquing the sampling plan of a quantitative research report.

Box 8–1

Guidelines for Critiquing Quantitative Sampling Designs

1. Is the target or accessible population identified and described? Are eligibility criteria specified? To whom can the study results be generalized?
2. Are the sample selection procedures clearly described? What type of sampling plan was used?
3. How adequate is the sampling plan in terms of yielding a representative sample?
4. Did some factor other than the sampling plan affect the representativeness of the sample (*e.g.,* a low response rate)?
5. Are possible sample biases identified?
6. Is the sample size sufficiently large? Was the sample size justified on the basis of a power analysis or is another rationale for the sample size offered?

Guidelines for Critiquing Qualitative
Sampling Designs

Box 8-2

1. Is the setting or study group adequately described? Is the setting appropriate for the research question?
2. Are the sample selection procedures described? What type of sampling strategy was used?
3. Given the information needs of the study, was the sampling approach appropriate? Were dimensions of the phenomenon under study adequately represented?
4. Is the sample size adequate? Did the researcher stipulate that information redundancy was achieved? Do the findings suggest a richly textured and comprehensive set of data without any apparent "holes" or thin areas?

Evaluating Qualitative Sampling Plans

In a qualitative study, the sampling plan can be evaluated in terms of its adequacy and appropriateness (Morse, 1991). Adequacy refers to the sufficiency and quality of the data the sample yielded. An adequate sample provides the researcher with data without any "thin" spots. When the researcher has truly obtained saturation with a sample, informational adequacy has been achieved, and the resulting description or theory is richly textured and complete.

Appropriateness concerns the methods used to select a sample. An appropriate sample is one resulting from the identification and use of study participants who can best supply information according to the conceptual requirements of the study. The researcher must use a strategy that will yield the fullest possible understanding of the phenomenon of interest. A sampling approach that excludes negative cases or that fails to include participants with unusual experiences may not meet the information needs of the study.

Further guidance to critiquing sampling in a qualitative study is presented in Box 8-2.

◰ RESEARCH EXAMPLES

Table 8-5 presents some examples of nursing studies with various sampling designs. Below, we describe at greater length the sampling plans of two nursing studies, one quantitative and the other qualitative. The guidelines in Boxes 8-1 and 8-2 can be used to evaluate the research samples.

Table 8–5. Examples of Sampling Designs Used in Nursing Studies

Research Question	Sample Description
Design: Convenience (Nonprobability)	
What is the relationship between perceived patient deviance and avoidance behaviors among nurses? (Carveth, 1995)	52 staff nurses providing direct patient care
Design: Quota (Nonprobability)	
To what extent can nursing home staff members accurately screen residents for competence? (Williams & Engle, 1995)	100 nursing home residents, 25 in each of four types of nursing home (for-profit home, not-for profit home, home for veterans, home for indigent county residents)
Design: Purposive/Theoretical (Nonprobability)	
What is the nature of the parenting process when a child has developmental delay including mental retardation? (Seideman & Kleine, 1995)	29 mothers and 13 fathers of children with developmental delay/ mental retardation
Design: Simple Random (Probability)	
What are the values influencing neonatal nurses' perceptions and choice of behavior in a clinical situation? (Raines, 1994)	331 neonatal nurses randomly sampled from members of the National Association of Neonatal Nurses
Design: Stratified Random (Probability)	
What level of confidence do nurse practitioners have regarding their practice skills and knowledge? (Thibodeau & Hawkins, 1994)	National sample of 900 nurses, stratified by specialty area
Design: Multistage (Probability)	
What are the work situation characteristics, levels of satisfaction, and individual characteristics of ICU and non-ICU nurses? (Boumans & Landeweerd, 1994)	Nurses in randomly selected ICU and non-ICU units from 16 randomly selected hospitals (Netherlands)
Design: Systematic (Probability)	
What is the extent to which nurses in a wide variety of practice settings discuss sexual concerns with their patients? (Matocha & Waterhouse, 1993)	Every 17th nurse listed by a state Board of Nursing in a south Atlantic state (500 nurses)

Research Example From
a Quantitative Study

Ferrans and Powers (1992) conducted a methodologic study to appraise a data collection instrument known as the Quality of Life Index (QLI). The QLI consists of 64 questions that measure satisfaction with various domains of life and the importance of those domains to people. Their study involved administering the QLI to a sample and analyzing the results to determine if the QLI is a good measure of a person's overall quality of life, so that the instrument could be used by other researchers interested in the quality-of-life construct.

The selected sample consisted of 800 respondents randomly selected from an accessible population of adult, in-unit hemodialysis patients from 93% of the counties in Illinois. A total of 2967 patients comprised the population. Patients undergoing treatment in Veterans Administration hospitals were not included in the population. Of the 800 sampled patients, 36 died or had a kidney transplantation. Of the 764 remaining subjects, 57% (434) returned a questionnaire. Eighty-five subjects were dropped from the study because they had left too many questions blank. The final sample consisted of 349 subjects, which represented a 46% response rate.

The representativeness of the research sample was evaluated by comparing the sample and the population in terms of a number of characteristics about which information was available: gender, number of months on dialysis, presence of diabetes mellitus, primary cause of renal failure, age, and race. The sample and population were comparable with respect to the first four characteristics, but the sample had a higher proportion of white patients and older patients than the population.

Research Example From
a Qualitative Study

Quinn (1993) conducted an in-depth study to examine how nurses explained their use of physical restraints with elderly patients and the extent to which the nurses perceived the restraint decision as a moral problem. A sample of nurses was recruited from the medical–surgical unit of a hospital. Nurses were eligible to participate in Quinn's study if they were female, were direct caregivers on the medical–surgical unit, and had cared for a restrained elderly patient (65 years old or older) within the previous 48 hours.

After the first few interviews were completed, theoretical sampling was used to guide the recruitment of subsequent respondents. For example, analysis of the early interviews revealed that nurses made a distinction between initiating physical restraint as opposed to continuing restraint that had been initiated by a previous caregiver. As a result, the researcher took care to include respondents with sufficient experience with both types of restraint. As another example, it was noted early in the study that respondents identified time of day as a factor in the use of restraint. Thereafter, Quinn made sure her sample included nurses who cared for restrained patients during all three tours of duty. The final sample consisted of 20 nurses ranging in age from 21 to 58 years, representing a wide range of nursing experience and educational preparation.

▧ SUMMARY

Sampling is the process of selecting a portion of the population to represent the entire population. Both qualitative and quantitative researchers use samples, but their approaches to sampling differ markedly.

Quantitative researchers use a sample to generalize about a **population,** which is the entire aggregate of cases that meet a designated set of criteria. In a sampling context, an **element** is the most basic unit about which information is collected. An element can be sampled from the population if it meets the researcher's **eligibility criteria.** Quantitative researchers usually sample from an **accessible population** rather than an entire **target population.** The overriding consideration in assessing the adequacy of a sample in a quantitative study is the degree to which it is representative of the population and avoids bias. **Sampling bias** refers to the systematic overrepresentation or underrepresentation of some segment of the population.

Sampling plans for quantitative research vary in their ability to reflect adequately the population from which the sample was drawn. In **nonprobability sampling,** elements are selected by nonrandom methods. Convenience, quota, and purposive sampling are the principal nonprobability methods. **Convenience sampling** (sometimes referred to as **accidental sampling**) consists of using the most readily available or most convenient group of people for the sample. **Snowball sampling** is a type of convenience sampling in which referrals for potential participants are made by those already in the sample. **Quota sampling** divides the population into homogeneous **strata** or subgroups to ensure representation of various subgroups in the sample. Within each stratum, the researcher selects participants by convenience sampling. In **purposive** (or **judgmental**) **sampling,** participants are handpicked to be included in the sample based on the researcher's knowledge about the population. Nonprobability sampling designs are convenient and economical; a major disadvantage is their potential for biases.

Probability sampling designs involve the random selection of elements from the population. **Simple random sampling** involves the selection on a random basis of elements from a **sampling frame** that enumerates all the elements. **Stratified random sampling** divides the population into homogeneous subgroups from which elements are selected at random. **Cluster sampling** (or **multistage sampling**) involves the successive selection of random samples from larger to smaller units by either simple random or stratified random methods. **Systematic sampling** is the selection of every kth case from some list or group. By dividing the population size by the desired sample size, the researcher is able to establish the **sampling interval,** which is the standard distance between the elements chosen for the systematic sample. Probability sampling designs are the preferred type of design for quantitative studies because they tend to result in more representative samples and because they permit the researcher to estimate the magnitude of sampling error. Probability samples, however, are time-consuming, expensive, inconvenient, and, in some cases, impossible to obtain.

There is no simple equation that can be used to determine how large a sample is needed for a particular quantitative study, but advanced researchers use a procedure known as **power analysis** to estimate **sample size** requirements. Large samples are usually preferable to small ones because, in general, the larger the sample, the more representative of the population it is likely to be. Even a large sample, however, does not guarantee representativeness.

In a qualitative study, sampling design is an emergent one that capitalizes on early learnings to guide subsequent direction. Qualitative researchers use the theoretical demands of the study as a framework for selecting articulate and reflective informants with certain types of experience. Qualitative researchers thus most often use purposive sampling—or **theoretical sampling** as it is often called—to guide them in using data sources that maximize the richness of the information obtained. Various strategies can be used to sample purposively, including such approaches as sampling to maximize variation, to select typical cases, and to learn from extreme cases. The criteria for evaluating qualitative sampling are informational adequacy and appropriateness.

STUDY SUGGESTIONS

Chapter 8 of the accompanying *Study Guide to Accompany Essentials of Nursing Research*, 4th edition offers various exercises and study suggestions for reinforcing the concepts presented in this chapter.

Suggested Readings

Methodologic References

Cohen, J. (1977). *Statistical power analysis for the behavioral sciences* (rev. ed.). New York: Academic Press.

Levey, P. S., & Lemeshow, S. (1980). *Sampling for health professionals.* New York: Lifetime Learning.

Morse, J. M. (1991). Strategies for sampling. In J. M. Morse (Ed.), *Qualitative nursing research: A contemporary dialogue.* Newbury Park, CA: Sage Publications.

Patton, M. Q. (1990). *Qualitative evaluation and research methods* (2nd ed.). Newbury Park, CA: Sage Publications.

Substantive References

Boumans, N. P. G., & Landeweerd, J. A. (1994). Working in an intensive or non-intensive care unit: Does it make a difference? *Heart & Lung, 23,* 71–79.

Carveth, J. A. (1995). Perceived patient deviance and avoidance by nurses. *Nursing Research, 44,* 173–178.

Ferrans, E. E., & Powers, M. J. (1992). Psychometric assessment of the Quality of Life Index. *Research in Nursing and Health, 15,* 29–38.

Matocha, L. K., and Waterhouse, J. K. (1993). Current nursing practice related to sexuality. *Research in Nursing and Health, 16,* 371–378.

Prescott, P. A., Soeken, K. L., & Griggs, M. (1995). Identification and referral of hospitalized patients in need of home care. *Research in Nursing and Health, 18,* 85–95.

Quinn, C. A. (1993). Nurses' perceptions about physical restraints. *Western Journal of Nursing Research, 15,* 148–158.

Raines, D. A. (1994). Values influencing neonatal nurses' perceptions and choices. *Western Journal of Nursing Research, 16,* 675–691.

Seideman, R. Y., & Kleine, P. F. (1995). A theory of transformed parenting: Parenting a child with development delay/ mental retardation. *Nursing Research, 44,* 38–44.

Thibodeau, J. A., & Hawkins, J. W. (1994). Moving toward a nursing model in advanced practice. *Western Journal of Nursing Research, 16,* 205–218.

Williams, J. S., & Engle, V. F. (1995). Staff evaluations of nursing home residents' competence. *Applied Nursing Research, 8,* 18–22.

Collection of
Research Data

PART IV

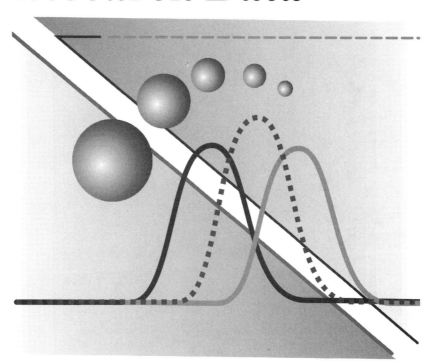

9

Methods of Data Collection

Student Objectives

On completion of this chapter, the student will be able to:

- evaluate a researcher's decision to use existing data versus collecting new data
- discuss the four dimensions along which data collection approaches vary
- critique a researcher's decisions regarding the data collection plan and its implementation
- define new terms in the chapter
- **Self-Reports**
    - distinguish between and evaluate structured and unstructured self-reports and open-ended and closed-ended questions
    - identify several types of unstructured self-report techniques
    - compare the advantages and disadvantages of interviews and questionnaires
    - describe and evaluate composite scales, vignettes, projective techniques, and Q sorts
    - evaluate a researcher's decision to use a self-report approach
    - evaluate a researcher's decision to use an interview versus questionnaire format and an unstructured versus structured approach
- **Observation**
    - identify several types of phenomena that lend themselves to observation
    - describe and evaluate unstructured observations
    - describe various methods of collecting structured observational data
    - identify several methods of sampling observations
    - evaluate a researcher's decision to use an observational data collection approach versus an alternative approach (*e.g.,* self-report)
    - evaluate a researcher's decision to use structured versus unstructured observation
- **Biophysiologic Measures**
    - distinguish in vitro and in vivo measures
    - describe the major features, advantages, and disadvantages of biophysiologic measures
    - evaluate a researcher's decision to use a biophysiologic measure as well as the choice of the specific measure

New Terms

Acquiescence response set bias	Checklist
Biophysiologic measure	Closed-ended question
Bipolar adjectives	Completely unstructured interviews
Category system	Counterbalancing

Critical incidents technique
Diary
Event sampling
Extreme response set bias
Field notes
Fixed-alternative question
Focus group interview
Focused interview
Grand tour question
Historical research
Instrument
Interview schedule
In vitro measures
In vivo measures
Item
Life history
Likert scale
Log
Methodologic notes
Mobile positioning
Moderator
Multiple positioning
Nay-sayer
Observation
Observational methods
Observational notes
Open-ended question
Participant observation

Personal notes
Pretest
Probing
Projective technique
Q sort
Questionnaire
Rating scale
Reactivity
Records
Response alternatives
Response set biases
Scale
Secondary analysis
Self-report
Semantic differential
Single positioning
Social desirability response set bias
Structured observation
Structured self-report
Summated rating scale
Theoretical notes
Time sampling
Topic guide
Unstructured observation
Unstructured self-report
Vignette
Visual analog scale
Yea-sayer

The phenomena in which a researcher is interested must ultimately be translated into concepts that can be measured, observed, or recorded. The task of selecting or developing appropriate methods for obtaining data are among the most challenging in the research process. Without high-quality data collection methods, the validity of research conclusions is easily challenged. Researchers generally choose from an array of alternatives in deciding how data are to be collected. This chapter discusses the characteristics of the major data collection approaches.

OVERVIEW OF DATA COLLECTION AND DATA SOURCES

Like research design, there are many alternative approaches to data collection, and these approaches vary along several dimensions. This introductory section provides an overview of some of the important dimensions.

Existing Data Versus New Data

One of the first decisions an investigator makes with regard to research data concerns the use of existing data versus the collection of new data generated specifically for the research project. Most of this chapter is devoted to methods researchers use to generate new data, but it is important to note that they often can take advantage of existing information. A meta-analysis (Chapter 6) is one example of a type of study that relies on available data (*i.e.,* research reports).

Historical research typically relies exclusively on available data. **Historical research** is the systematic collection and critical evaluation of data relating to past occurrences. Data for historical research are usually in the form of written records of the past: periodicals, diaries, letters, newspapers, minutes of meetings, legal documents, reports, and so forth. The historical researcher usually must evaluate the authenticity and accuracy of historical data before analyzing them. Nurses have used historical research methods to examine a wide range of phenomena. For example, Widerquist (1992) studied Florence Nightingale's spirituality and its influence on the development of modern nursing through an analysis of Nightingale's letters, diaries, essays, and journals.

Sometimes researchers perform what is referred to as a **secondary analysis,** which is the use of data gathered in a previous study (often by other researchers) to test new hypotheses or address new research questions. A secondary analysis can be performed with both quantitative and qualitative data. For example, Rajan (1994) did a secondary analysis of data from a large-scale quantitative study of pain relief during childbirth to study the effect of obstetric procedures on breastfeeding 6 weeks after delivery. Logan and Jenny (1990) did a secondary analysis of data from a grounded theory study of nurses' perceptions of weaning patients from mechanical ventilation; the secondary analysis yielded a new nursing diagnosis— dysfunctional ventilatory weaning response.

An important existing data source for nurse researchers is **records.** Hospital records, nursing charts, physicians' order sheets, and care plan statements all constitute rich data sources to which nurse researchers may have access. The use of information from records is advantageous to the researcher because records are an economical source of information. The collection of data is often the most time-consuming and costly step in the research process. Furthermore, the investigator does not have to be concerned with obtaining cooperation from participants. On the other hand, because the researcher has not been responsible for the collection and recording of information, he or she may be unaware of the limitations, biases, or incompleteness of the records. If the records available for use do not constitute the entire set of all of these records possible, the investigator often must deal with the question of the representativeness of the existing records. Existing records have been used in many nursing studies, including both qualitative and quantitative ones. For example, Micelli, Waxman, Cavalieri, and Lage (1994) used physician progress notes, medical records, physician order sheets, and nursing assessment records to examine whether falls among older nursing home residents predicted subsequent disease onset.

Key Dimensions of Data Collection Methods

If existing data are not available or suitable for the research question, the researcher must collect new data. In developing a plan for data collection, the investigator makes many important decisions. A primary decision concerns the basic form of data collection to use. Three types of approach have been used most frequently by nurse researchers: self-reports, observation, and biophysiologic measures. **Self-reports** are study participants' responses to questions posed by the researcher, such as in an interview. Direct **observation** of people's behaviors, characteristics, and circumstances is an alternative to self-reports for certain types of research questions. Nurses are increasingly using **biophysiologic measures** to assess important clinical variables. Sections of this chapter are devoted to these three major types of data collection.

Regardless of what specific approach is used, data collection methods vary along several important dimensions:

- *Structure.* Research data are often collected in a highly structured manner: exactly the same information is gathered from all participants in a comparable, prespecified way. Sometimes, however, it is more appropriate to be flexible and impose a minimum of structure and to provide participants with opportunities to reveal relevant information in a naturalistic way.
- *Quantifiability.* Data that will be subjected to statistical analysis must be gathered in such a way that they can be quantified. On the other hand, data that are to be analyzed qualitatively are collected in narrative form. Structured data collection approaches tend to yield data that are more easily quantified. It is sometimes possible and useful, however, to quantify unstructured information as well.
- *Obtrusiveness.* Data collection methods differ in terms of the degree to which participants are aware of their status as a study participant. If participants are fully aware of their role in a study, their behavior and responses might not be normal. When data are collected unobtrusively, however, ethical problems may emerge.
- *Objectivity.* Some data collection approaches require more subjective judgment than others. Quantitative researchers generally strive for methods that are as objective as possible. In qualitative research, however, the subjective judgment of the investigator is considered a valuable component of data collection.

Sometimes the nature of the research question dictates where on these four dimensions the method of data collection will lie. For example, questions that are best suited for a qualitative study normally use data collection methods that are low on structure, quantifiability, obtrusiveness, and objectivity, whereas research questions that call for a survey tend to use methods that are high on all four dimensions. However, the researcher often has considerable latitude in selecting or designing a suitable data collection plan.

◪ SELF-REPORT METHODS

In the human sciences, a good deal of information can be gathered by direct questioning of people (*i.e.,* by asking people to report on their own experiences). If, for example, we are interested in learning about patients' perceptions of hospital care, nursing home residents' fear of death, or women's knowledge about menopause, we are likely to try to find answers by posing questions to a group of relevant people. For some research variables, alternatives to direct questioning exist, but the unique ability of humans to communicate verbally on a sophisticated level makes it unlikely that self-reports will ever be eliminated from nurse researchers' repertoire of data collection techniques.

The self-report approach consists of a range of techniques that vary considerably in the degree of structure imposed on the data collection process. At one extreme are loosely structured methods that do not involve a formal written set of questions. At the other extreme are tightly structured methods involving the use of formal documents such as questionnaires. Some characteristics of different self-report approaches are discussed below.

Unstructured and Semistructured
Self-Report Techniques

Unstructured or loosely structured self-report methods offer the researcher flexibility in gathering information from research participants. When these methods are used, the researcher does not have a specific set of questions that must be asked in a specific order and worded in a given way. Instead, the researcher starts with some general questions or topics and allows the respondents to tell their stories in a naturalistic, narrative fashion. In other words, unstructured or semistructured self-reports, usually obtained in interviews, tend to be conversational in nature.

Investigations in almost all the qualitative research traditions use unstructured approaches to gathering self-report data. Unstructured interviews encourage respondents to define the important dimensions of a phenomenon and to elaborate on what is relevant to them, rather than being guided by the investigator's a priori notions of relevance. Unstructured interviews should be the mode of choice when the researcher does not have a clear idea of what it is he or she does not know.

Types of Unstructured Self-Reports

There are several different approaches to collecting self-report data in a loosely structured format:

- **Completely unstructured interviews** are used when the researcher proceeds with no preconceived view of the specific content or flow of information to be gathered. The aim of these interviews is to elucidate the respondents' perceptions of the world without imposing on them any of the researcher's views. Typically, the researcher begins by posing a broad question (sometimes referred to as a **grand tour question**), such as "What happened when you first learned that you had AIDS?" Subsequent questions are more focused and are guided by responses to the broad questions. Ethnographic and phenomenologic studies generally rely heavily on unstructured interviews.

- **Focused interviews** are used when a researcher has a list of topics that must be covered in an interview. The questions are of the type that encourage conversation rather than yes and no responses. The interviewer uses a **topic guide**—a list of broad questions—to ensure that all question areas are covered. The interviewer's function is to encourage participants to talk freely about all the topics on the list.
- **Focus group interviews** are interviews with groups of about 5 to 15 people whose opinions and experiences are solicited simultaneously. The interviewer (often called a **moderator**) guides the discussion according to a topic guide or written set of questions. The advantages of a group format are that it is efficient and can generate a lot of dialogue, but one disadvantage is that some people are uncomfortable expressing their views or describing their experiences in front of a group.
- **Life histories** are narrative self-disclosures about life experiences. With this approach, the researcher asks the respondents to provide, in chronologic sequence, their ideas and experiences regarding some theme, either orally or in writing. For example, some researchers have used this approach to obtain a total life health history.
- The **critical incidents technique** is a method of gathering data about people's behaviors by studying specific incidents relating to the behavior under investigation. The technique focuses on an observable and integral episode of human behavior; the word "critical" means that the incident must have a discernible impact on some outcome. The technique differs from other unstructured self-report approaches in that it focuses on something specific about which the respondent can be expected to testify as an expert witness.
- **Diaries** have been used by some researchers, who ask participants to maintain a daily log concerning some aspect of their lives over a specified period of time. Nurse researchers have used health diaries to collect information about how people prevent illness, maintain health, experience morbidity, or treat health problems.

Gathering Unstructured Self-Report Data

In most cases, the primary purpose of gathering unstructured self-report data is to enable the researcher to construct reality in ways that are consistent with the construction of the people being studied. This goal requires the researcher to take steps to overcome communication barriers and to enhance the flow of meaning. An important issue is that the researcher and the respondents should have a common vocabulary. For example, if the researcher is studying a different culture, or studying a subgroup that uses distinctive terms or slang, he or she should strive before going into the field to understand those terms and their nuances.

Although unstructured interviews are conversational in nature, this does not mean that researchers enter into them casually. The conversations are purposeful ones that require advance thought and preparation. For example, the wording of questions should make sense to the respondent and reflect his or her world view.

In addition to being good questioners, the researchers must be good listeners. Only by attending carefully to what the respondent is saying can the in-depth interviewer develop appropriate follow-up questions. Even when a topic guide is used, the interviewer must not let the flow of dialogue be bound by those questions; many questions that appear on a topic guide are answered spontaneously over the course of the interview, usually out of sequence.

Unstructured interviews are typically quite long—sometimes lasting up to several hours. Researchers often find that the respondents' construction of their experience only begins to emerge after lengthy, in-depth dialogues. The issue of how best to record such abundant information is a difficult one. Some researchers take sketchy notes as the interview progresses, filling in the details as soon as practical after the interview is completed. Many prefer tape recording the interviews for later transcription. Although some respondents balk or are overly self-conscious when their conversation is recorded, respondents typically forget about the presence of recording equipment after a few minutes.

Structured Self-Report Techniques

A structured approach to collecting self-report data is appropriate when the researcher knows in advance exactly what he or she needs to know and can, therefore, frame appropriate questions to obtain the needed information. Structured self-report data are usually collected in a quantitative study by means of a formal, written document referred to as an **instrument.** The instrument is known as the **interview schedule** when the questions are asked orally in either a face-to-face or telephone format and as the **questionnaire** when the respondents complete the instrument themselves in a paper-and-pencil format. Some features of structured self-report instruments are discussed below.

Question Form

In a totally structured or standardized instrument, the respondents are asked to respond to exactly the same questions in exactly the same order, and they are given the same set of options for their responses. **Closed-ended questions** (also referred to as **fixed-alternative questions**) are ones in which the **response alternatives** are designated by the researcher. The alternatives may range from a simple yes or no to rather complex expressions of opinion. The purpose of using questions with such a high degree of structure is to ensure comparability of responses and to facilitate analysis.

Many structured interviews, however, also include some **open-ended ques-**

tions, which allow participants to respond to questions in their own words. When open-ended questions are included in questionnaires, the respondent must write out his or her response. In interviews, the interviewer tries to write down the response verbatim or uses a tape recorder for later transcription. Some examples of open-ended and closed-ended questions are presented in Table 9–1.

Both open-ended and closed-ended questions have certain strengths and weaknesses that you should understand. Closed-ended questions are more difficult to construct than open-ended ones but easier to administer and, especially, to analyze. The analysis of open-ended questions is time consuming and difficult, and it is also more subjective. Furthermore, closed-ended questions are more efficient than open-ended questions in the sense that a respondent is normally able to complete more closed-ended questions than open-ended ones in a given amount of time. Also, in questionnaires, respondents may be unwilling to compose lengthy written responses to open-ended questions.

These various advantages of fixed-alternative questions are offset by some corresponding shortcomings. The major drawback of closed-ended questions lies in the possibility of the researcher neglecting or overlooking some potentially important responses. Another objection is that closed-ended questions are sometimes superficial. Open-ended questions allow for a richer and fuller perspective on the topic of interest if the respondents are verbally expressive and cooperative. Finally, some respondents object to being forced into choosing from among alternatives that do not reflect their opinions precisely.

Instrument Construction

The construction of a structured interview schedule or questionnaire is a time-consuming task requiring considerable attention to detail. The investigator must make many decisions, including whether to use an interview schedule or a self-administered questionnaire as well as how to balance open-ended and closed-ended questions.

Researchers generally work with an outline of the instrument if it is complex and encompasses a variety of topics. Questions for the relevant content areas are then drafted or, if possible, borrowed or adapted from other instruments. Researchers must carefully monitor the wording of each question for clarity, sensitivity to the respondent's psychological state, freedom from bias, and (in questionnaires) reading level. Questions must then be sequenced in a psychologically meaningful order and in a manner that encourages cooperation and candor.

When the instrument has been drafted, it should be critically reviewed by others who are knowledgeable about instrument construction and about the substantive area of the study. The instrument also should be pretested with a small sample of respondents and then revised if necessary. A **pretest** is a trial run to determine insofar as is possible whether the instrument is clearly worded and free from major biases and whether it solicits the type of information envisioned. In large studies, the development and pretesting of self-report instruments may take many months to complete.

Table 9–1. Examples of Question Types

Open-Ended

1. What led to your decision to stop using oral contraceptives?
2. What did you do when you discovered you had AIDS?

Closed-Ended

1. Dichotomous Question
   Have you ever been hospitalized?
   ( ) 1. Yes
   ( ) 2. No

2. Multiple-Choice Question
   How important is it to you to avoid a pregnancy at this time?
   ( ) 1. Extremely important
   ( ) 2. Very important
   ( ) 3. Somewhat important
   ( ) 4. Not at all important

3. "Cafeteria" Question
   People have different opinions about the use of estrogen-replacement therapy for women in menopause. Which of the following statements best represents your point of view?
   ( ) 1. Estrogen replacement is dangerous and should be totally banned.
   ( ) 2. Estrogen replacement may have some undesirable side effects that suggest the need for caution in its use.
   ( ) 3. I am undecided about my views on estrogen-replacement therapy.
   ( ) 4. Estrogen replacement has many beneficial effects that merit its promotion.
   ( ) 5. Estrogen replacement is a wonder cure that should be administered routinely to menopausal women.

4. Rank-Order Question
   People value different things about life. Below is a list of principles or ideals that are often cited when people are asked to name things they value most. Please indicate the order of importance of these values to you by placing a *1* beside the most important, *2* beside the next most important, and so forth.
   ( ) Achievement and success
   ( ) Family relationships
   ( ) Friendships and social interaction
   ( ) Health
   ( ) Money
   ( ) Religion

5. Forced-Choice Question
   Which statement most closely represents your point of view?
   ( ) 1. What happens to me is my own doing.
   ( ) 2. Sometimes, I feel I don't have enough control over my life.

6. Rating Question
   On a scale from 0 to 10, where 0 means extremely dissatisfied and 10 means extremely satisfied, how satisfied are you with the nursing care you received during your hospitalization?

   Extremely dissatisfied   Extremely satisfied
   0   1   2   3   4   5   6   7   8   9   10

Interviews Versus Questionnaires

An important decision that the researcher must make when using a structured self-report approach concerns the use of an interview versus a questionnaire. Interview schedules and questionnaires require different skills and considerations in their administration. Self-administered questionnaires can be distributed in a number of ways, such as through the mail or to self-contained groups (*e.g.,* a classroom of nursing students). The successful collection of interview data, in contrast to questionnaire data, is strongly dependent on interpersonal skills and the ability of the interviewer to probe in a neutral manner. **Probing** is the technique used by interviewers to elicit more useful or detailed information from a respondent than was volunteered in the initial reply. There are advantages and disadvantages to both the interview and questionnaire approaches. You should be aware of the limitations and strengths of these alternatives because the research findings may be affected by the researcher's decision.

Questionnaires, relative to interviews, have the following advantages:

- Questionnaires are much less costly and require less time and energy to administer.
- Questionnaires offer the possibility of complete anonymity, which may be crucial in obtaining information about illegal, immoral, or deviant behaviors or about embarrassing characteristics.
- The absence of an interviewer ensures that there will be no bias in the responses that reflect the respondent's reaction to the interviewer rather than to the questions themselves.

The strengths of interviews far outweigh those of questionnaires. These strengths include the following:

- The response rate tends to be high in face-to-face interviews. Respondents are generally more reluctant to refuse to talk to an interviewer than to ignore a questionnaire, especially a mailed questionnaire. Low response rates can lead to serious biases, because people who complete the questionnaire or interview are rarely a random subset of those whom the researcher intended for inclusion in the study.
- Many people simply cannot fill out a questionnaire; examples include young children, the blind, and the very elderly. Interviews are feasible with most people.
- Interviews are less prone to misinterpretation by the respondents because the interviewer is present to determine whether questions have been misunderstood.
- Interviewers can produce additional information through observation. The interviewer is in a position to observe or judge the respondent's level of understanding, degree of cooperativeness, lifestyle, and so on. These kinds of information can be useful in interpreting responses.

Many of the advantages of face-to-face interviews also apply to telephone interviews. Complicated or detailed schedules clearly are not well suited to tele-phone interviewing; but, for relatively brief instruments, the telephone interview combines the low cost and ease of administration of questionnaires with relatively high response rates.

Scales and Other Special Forms of Structured Self-Reports

Several special types of structured self-report are used by nurse researchers. These include composite social psychological scales, vignettes, projective techniques, and Q-sorts.

Composite Scales

The social–psychological scale is a special kind of self-report instrument that is used by many nurse researchers, often incorporated into a questionnaire or inter-view schedule. A composite **scale** is a device designed to assign a numeric score to participants to place them on a continuum with respect to attributes being measured, like a scale for measuring people's weight. The purpose of social–psycho-logical scales is to quantitatively discriminate among people with different attitudes, fears, motives, perceptions, personality traits, and needs.

Many sophisticated scaling techniques have been developed in connection with the measurement of attitudes. The most common technique is the **Likert scale,** named after the psychologist Rensis Likert. A Likert scale consists of several declarative state-ments (sometimes referred to as **items**) that express a viewpoint on a topic. Respondents are asked to indicate the degree to which they agree or disagree with the opinion expressed by the statement. Table 9–2 presents an illustrative, six-item Likert scale for measuring attitudes toward the mentally ill. After the scale is administered, the responses must be scored and combined. Typically, the responses are scored in such a way that agreement with positively worded statements and disagreement with negatively worded statements are assigned a higher score, as in Table 9–2. The first statement is positively phrased, so that agreement is indicative of a favorable attitude toward the mentally ill. The researcher would, therefore, assign a higher score to a person agreeing with this statement than to someone disagreeing with it. Because the item has five response alternatives, a score of 5 would be given to someone strongly agreeing, 4 to someone agreeing, and so forth. The responses of two hypothetical respondents are shown by a check or an X, and their scores for each item are shown in the right-hand columns of the table. Person 1, who agreed with the first statement, is given a score of 4, whereas person 2, who strongly disagreed, is given a score of 1. The second statement is negatively worded, and so the scoring is reversed—a 1 is assigned to those who strongly agree, and so forth. This reversal is necessary so that a high score will consistently reflect positive attitudes toward the mentally ill. When each item has been handled in this manner, a person's total score can be determined by adding together individual item scores. Because total scores are computed in this manner, these scales are sometimes

Table 9–2. Example of a Likert Scale to Measure Attitudes
Toward the Mentally Ill

Direction of Scoring*		Responses†					Score	
		SA	A	?	D	SD	Person 1 (✓)	Person 2 (X)
+	1. People who have had a mental illness can become normal, productive citizens after treatment.		✓			X	4	1
−	2. People who have been patients in mental hospitals should not be allowed to have children.			X		✓	5	3
−	3. The best way to handle patients in mental hospitals is to restrict their activity as much as possible.		X		✓		4	2
+	4. Many patients in mental hospitals develop normal, healthy relationships with staff members and other patients.			✓	X		3	2
+	5. There should be an expanded effort to get the mentally ill out of institutional settings and back into their communities.	✓				X	5	1
−	6. Because the mentally ill cannot be trusted, they should be kept under constant guard.		X			✓	5	2
	TOTAL SCORE						26	11

*Researchers would not indicate the direction of scoring on a Likert scale administered to subjects. The scoring direction is indicated in this table for illustrative purposes only.
†SA, strongly agree; A, agree: ?, uncertain; D, disagree; SD, strongly disagree.

called **summated rating scales.** The total scores of the two hypothetical respondents to the items in Table 9–2, shown at the bottom of that table, reflect a considerably more positive attitude toward the mentally ill on the part of person 1 (score = 26) than person 2 (score = 11). The summation feature of Likert scales makes it possible to make fine discriminations among people with different points of view. A single Likert question allows people to be put into only five categories. A six-item scale, such as the one in Table 9–2, permits much finer gradation—from a minimum possible score of 6 (6 × 1) to a maximum possible score of 30 (6 × 5).

Another technique for measuring attitudes is the **semantic differential** (SD). With the SD, the respondent is asked to rate a given concept (*e.g.,* primary nursing, team nursing) on a series of **bipolar adjectives,** such as good/bad, strong/weak, effective/ineffective, important/unimportant. Respondents are asked to place a check at the appropriate point on a seven-point scale that extends from one extreme of the dimension to the other. An example of the format for an SD is shown in Figure 9–1. The SD has the advantage of being flexible and easy to construct. The concept being rated can be virtually anything—a person, place, situation, abstract idea, controversial issue, and so forth. In most cases, several concepts are included on the same schedule so that comparisons can be made across concepts (*e.g.,* male nurse, female nurse, male physician, and female physician). The scoring procedure for SD responses is essentially the same as for Likert scales. Scores from 1 to 7 are assigned to each bipolar scale response, with higher scores generally associated with the positively worded adjective. Responses are then summed across the bipolar scales to yield a total score.

Another type of psychosocial measure that deserves special mention is the **visual analog scale** (VAS). The VAS has come into increased use in clinical settings

NURSE PRACTITIONERS

	7*	6	5	4	3	2	1	
competent								incompetent
worthless	1	2	3	4	5	6	7	valuable
important								unimportant
pleasant								unpleasant
bad								good
cold								warm
responsible								irresponsible
successful								unsuccessful

*The score values would not be printed on the form administered to actual subjects. The numbers are presented here solely for the purpose of illustrating how semantic differentials are scored.

Figure 9–1. Example of a semantic differential

to measure subjective experiences, such as pain, fatigue, nausea, and dyspnea. The VAS is a straight line, the end anchors of which are labeled as the extreme limits of the sensation or feeling being measured. Participants are asked to mark a point on the line corresponding to the amount of sensation experienced. Traditionally, the VAS line is 100 mm in length, which facilitates the derivation of a score from 0 to 100 through simple measurement of the distance from one end of the scale to the participant's mark on the line. An example of a VAS is presented in Figure 9–2.

Many social–psychological states and traits are of interest to those engaged in clinical nursing research, and many scales have been developed to measure them. As an actual research example, Ferketich and Mercer (1995) administered several scales in their study of paternal–infant attachment, including scales to measure paternal competence, father–infant attachment, self-esteem, mastery, marital adjustment, family functioning, depression, anxiety, social support, and life-events stress.

Scales permit researchers to efficiently quantify subtle gradations in the strength or intensity of individual characteristics. A good scale can be useful both for group-level comparisons (*e.g.,* comparing the stress levels of mastectomy patients before and after surgery) and for making individual comparisons (predicting that patient X will not need as much emotional support as patient Y because of scores on a coping scale). Scales can be administered either verbally or in writing and are, therefore, suitable for use with most people.

Scales are susceptible to several common problems, however, the most troublesome of which are referred to as **response set biases.** The most important biases include the following:

- **Social desirability response set bias** refers to the tendency of some people to misrepresent their attitudes or traits by giving answers that are consistent with prevailing social views.

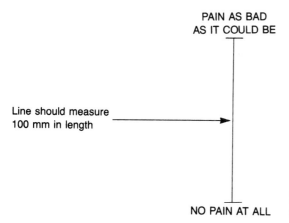

**PAIN AS BAD
AS IT COULD BE**

Line should measure
100 mm in length

NO PAIN AT ALL

Figure 9–2. Example of a visual analog scale

- **Extreme response set bias** results from the fact that some people consistently express themselves in terms of extreme response alternatives (*e.g.,* strongly agree), whereas others characteristically endorse middle-range alternatives. This response style is a distorting influence in that extreme responses may not necessarily signify the greatest intensity with regard to the phenomena under investigation.
- **Acquiescence response set bias** refers to the tendency of some people to agree with statements regardless of their content. In the research literature, these people are sometimes referred to as **yea-sayers.** A less common problem is the opposite tendency for other people, called **nay-sayers,** to disagree with statements independently of the question content.

These biases can be reduced through such strategies as **counterbalancing** positively and negatively worded statements, developing sensitively worded questions, creating a permissive, nonjudgmental atmosphere, and guaranteeing the confidentiality of responses.

Vignettes

Vignettes are brief descriptions of events or situations to which respondents are asked to react. The descriptions can be either fictitious or based on fact, but they are always structured to elicit information about respondents' perceptions, opinions, or knowledge about some phenomenon under study. The vignettes are usually written, narrative descriptions, but researchers have also begun to use videotaped vignettes that portray a specific situation. The questions posed to respondents after the vignettes may be either open-ended (*e.g.,* How would you recommend handling this situation?) or closed-ended (*e.g.,* On the nine-point scale below, rate how well you believe the nurse handled the situation).

Vignettes are an economical means of eliciting information about how people might behave in situations that would be difficult to observe in daily life. For example, we might want to assess how patients would react to or feel about nurses with different personal styles of interaction. In clinical settings, it would be difficult to expose patients to many nurses, all of whom have been evaluated as having different interaction styles. Another advantage of vignettes is that it is possible to experimentally manipulate the stimuli (the vignettes) by randomly assigning vignettes to participants (*e.g.,* vignettes describing homosexual versus heterosexual AIDS patients). Furthermore, vignettes can be incorporated into mailed questionnaires and are, therefore, an inexpensive data collection strategy.

The principal problem with vignettes is that of the validity of responses. If a respondent describes how he or she would react in a situation portrayed in the vignette, how accurate is that description of the respondent's actual behavior? Thus, although the use of vignettes can be profitable, the possibility of response biases should be recognized. Many examples of the use of vignettes may be found in the nursing research literature. For example, Gujol (1994) used vignettes to study critical care nurses' medication decisions in relation to surgical patients' ventilator status and time elapsed since surgery. McDonald and Bridge (1991) studied the effect of gender stereotyping on nursing care by experimentally manipulating the gender of patients as described in a vignette of a postoperative colostomy patient.

Projective Techniques

Most self-report methods depend on the respondents' capacities for self-insight and willingness to divulge personal information. **Projective techniques** include a variety of methods for obtaining psychological measurements through verbal self-report with only a minimum of participants' conscious cooperation. Projective methods give free play to the participants' imagination and fantasies by providing them with ambiguous stimuli that invite participants to read into them their own interpretations, thereby providing the researcher with information about their perception of the world. The rationale underlying the use of projective techniques is that the manner in which a person organizes and reacts to unstructured stimuli is a reflection of the person's needs, motives, attitudes, values, or personality traits.

Projective techniques are highly flexible because virtually any unstructured stimulus or situation can be used to induce projective responses, and the resulting data can often be analyzed either qualitatively or quantitatively. One class of projective methods uses pictorial materials. The Rorschach (ink blot) test is an example of a pictorial projective technique. Verbal projective techniques present participants with an ambiguous verbal stimulus rather than a pictorial one. For example, word-association methods present participants with a series of words to which participants respond with the first thing that comes to mind. A third class of projective measures falls into the category of expressive methods. The major expressive methods are play techniques, drawing and painting, and role playing. The assumption is that people express their feelings and emotions by working with or manipulating various materials.

Projective measures have been fairly controversial among researchers. Critics point out that a high degree of inference is required in gleaning information from projective tests, and the quality of the data depends heavily on the sensitivity and interpretive skill of the investigator or analyst. On the other hand, some people argue that projective methods probe the unconscious mind, encompass the whole personality, and provide data of breadth and depth unattainable by more traditional methods. One useful feature of projective instruments is that they are less susceptible to faking than self-report measures. Finally, some projective techniques are particularly useful with special groups, such as children or people with speech and hearing defects. For example, Cornman (1993) used a projective drawing technique (Kinetic Family Drawings) to study parents' and children's responses to childhood cancer.

Q Sorts

In a **Q sort,** the study participant is presented with a set of cards on which words, phrases, statements, or other messages are written. The participant is then asked to sort the cards according to a particular dimension, such as approval/disapproval or highest priority/lowest priority. The number of cards to be sorted is typically between 60 and 100. Usually, the participant sorts the cards into 9 or 11 piles, with the number of cards to be placed in each pile predetermined by the researcher.

The sorting instructions as well as the objects to be sorted in a Q-sort investigation vary according to the requirements of the research. The researcher can study personality by developing Q-sort cards on which personality characteristics are described. The participant can then be requested to sort items on a continuum from "very much like me" to "not at all like me." Other applications include asking patients to rate nursing behaviors on a continuum from most helpful to least helpful, asking cancer patients to rate various aspects of their treatment on a most distressing to least distressing continuum, and asking primiparas to rate various aspects of their labor and delivery experience in terms of a most problematic to least problematic dimension.

Q sorts can be a powerful tool, but, like other data collection techniques, this method also has drawbacks. On the positive side, Q sorts are versatile and can be applied to a wide variety of problems. The requirement that people place a predetermined number of cards in each pile virtually eliminates some of the biases that can occur in Likert-type scales. Furthermore, the task of sorting cards is sometimes more agreeable to participants than completing a paper-and-pencil task. On the other hand, it is difficult and time consuming to administer Q sorts to a large sample of people, and they cannot be administered by the mail. Some critics have argued that the forced procedure of distributing cards according to the researcher's specifications is artificial and actually excludes information about how the participants would ordinarily distribute their responses.

Several nurse researchers have used Q sorts to collect data. For example, Morse (1991) included a Q sort in her study of the structure and function of gift giving in the patient–nurse relationship. Von Essen and Sjoden (1993) compared the perceptions of psychiatric inpatients and nursing staff regarding the importance of various nurse caring behaviors.

Evaluation of Self-Report Methods

Verbal report instruments are strong with respect to the directness of their approach. If we want to know how people think or feel or what they believe, the most direct means of gathering this information is to ask them about it. Perhaps the strongest argument that can be made about the self-report method is that it frequently yields information that would be difficult, if not impossible, to gather by any other means. Behaviors can be directly observed, but only if the study participant is willing to manifest them publicly. For example, it may be impossible for a researcher to observe behaviors such as contraceptive practices or drug usage. Furthermore, observers can only observe behaviors occurring at the time of the study; self-report instruments can gather retrospective data about activities and events occurring in the past or about behaviors in which participants plan to engage in the future. Information about feelings, values, opinions, and motives can sometimes be inferred through observation, but behaviors and feelings do not always correspond exactly. People's actions do not always tell us about their states of mind. Self-report instruments can be designed to measure psychological characteristics through direct communication with the participants.

Despite these advantages, self-report methods share a number of weaknesses. The most serious issue is the question of the validity and accuracy of self-reports: How can we really be sure that respondents feel or act the way they say they do? How can we trust the information that respondents provide, particularly if the questions could potentially require them to admit to socially unpopular behavior or beliefs? Investigators often have no alternative but to assume that most of their respondents have been frank. Yet, we all have a tendency to want to present ourselves in the best light, and this may conflict with the truth. When reading research reports, you should be alert to potential biases introduced when participants are asked to describe themselves, particularly with respect to behaviors or feelings that our society judges to be controversial or wrong.

You should also be familiar with the advantages and disadvantages of unstructured and structured self-reports. In general, unstructured interviews are of greatest utility, from a researcher's point of view, when a new area of research is being explored. In such situations, an unstructured approach may allow the investigator to ascertain what the basic issues or problems are, how sensitive or controversial the topic is, how easy it is to secure respondents' cooperation in discussing the issues, how individuals conceptualize and talk about the problems, and what range of opinions or behaviors exists that are relevant to the topic. Unstructured methods may also help elucidate the underlying meaning of a pattern or relationship repeatedly observed in more structured research.

However, unstructured methods are extremely time consuming and demanding of the researcher's skill in analyzing and interpreting the resulting qualitative materials. Moreover, unstructured self-reports are not appropriate for capturing the measurable aspects of a phenomenon, such as incidence (*e.g.,* the percentage of infertile couples who elect in vitro fertilization), duration (*e.g.,* average time period during which pregnancy was attempted before infertility treatment was sought), or magnitude (*e.g.,* the average degree of stress experienced during infertility treatment). Structured self-reports are also especially appropriate when the researcher wants to rigorously test hypotheses concerning cause-and-effect relationships.

Self-reports are the most common method of data collection in nursing studies. Table 9–3 presents some examples of studies that have used unstructured and structured self-report methods.

Critiquing Self-Reports

One of the first questions a consumer must ask about the data collection method of a self-report study is whether the researcher made the correct decision in obtaining the data by means of self-report rather than by an alternative method.

Table 9–3. Examples of Studies Using Self-Reports

Research Question	Data Collection Approach
What is the experience of the lived body associated with discomfort? (Morse, Bottorff & Hutchinson, 1995)	Unstructured: Completely unstructured personal interviews
What are the social service concerns of women infected with HIV? (Seals, Sowell, Demi, Moneyham, Cohen & Guillory, 1995)	Unstructured: Focus group interviews
What is the process by which women progress in a healthy fashion through their experience of living with chronic pain? (Howell, 1994)	Unstructured: Critical incident diaries
What is the quality of life among women following a myocardial infarction? (Wingate, 1995)	Structured: Mailed questionnaires that included several psychosocial scales
What are the primary barriers to recruiting RNs in rural areas? (Stratton, Dunkin, Juhl & Geller, 1993)	Structured: Telephone interviews

Attention then should be paid to the adequacy of the actual methods used. Box 9–1 presents some guiding questions for critiquing self-reports.

It may be difficult to perform a thorough critique of self-report methods in studies that are reported in journals because a detailed description of the data collection methods may not be included. What the reader *can* expect is information about the following aspects of the self-report data collection:

- The degree of structure used in the questioning
- Whether interviews or questionnaires (or variants such as a projective method or Q-sort) were used
- Whether a composite scale was administered
- The length of time it took, on average, to collect data from each participant
- How the instruments were administered (*e.g.,* by telephone, in person, by mail, and so forth)
- The response rate

The degree of structure that the researcher imposes on the questioning is of special importance in assessing a data collection plan. The decision about an instrument's degree of structure should be based on a number of important considerations that the reader can often evaluate. For example, respondents who are not very articulate are more receptive to structured instruments with many closed-ended questions than to questioning that forces them to compose lengthy answers. Other considerations include the amount of time available (structured instruments are more efficient of participants' time); the expected size of the sample (open-

Box 9-1

Guidelines for Critiquing Self-Reports

1. Does the research question lend itself to a self-report method of data collection? Would an alternative method have been more appropriate?
2. Is the degree of structure of the researcher's approach consistent with the nature of the research question?
3. Given the research question and the characteristics of the respondents, did the researcher use the best possible mode for collecting the data (*i.e.,* personal interviews, telephone interviews, or self-administered questionnaires)?
4. Do the questions included in the instrument or topic guide adequately cover the complexities of the problem under investigation?
5. If a composite scale was used, does its use seem appropriate? Does the scale adequately capture the target research variable?
6. If a vignette, projective technique, or Q sort was used, does its use seem appropriate?

ended questions and unstructured interviews are difficult to analyze with large samples); the status of existing information on the topic (in a new area of inquiry, a structured approach may not be warranted); and, most important, the nature of the research question.

◩ OBSERVATIONAL METHODS

For some research questions, an alternative to self-reports is direct observation of people's behavior. Many kinds of information required by nurse researchers as evidence of nursing effectiveness or as clues to improving nursing practices can be obtained through direct observation. Suppose, for instance, that we were interested in studying nurses' willingness to interact with and listen to patients, or mental patients' methods of defending their personal territory, or children's reactions to the removal of a leg cast, or a patient's mode of emergence from anesthesia. These phenomena are all amenable to direct observation.

Within nursing research, observational methods have broad applicability, particularly for clinical inquiries. The nurse is in an advantageous position to observe, relatively unobtrusively, the behaviors and activities of patients, their families, and hospital staff. Observational methods can be used fruitfully to gather a variety of information, including information on characteristics and conditions of individuals (*e.g.,* the sleep–wake state of patients); verbal communication behaviors (*e.g.,* exchange of information at change-of-shift report); nonverbal communication behaviors (*e.g.,* facial expressions); activities (*e.g.,* geriatric patients' self-grooming activities); and environmental conditions (*e.g.,* architectural barriers in the homes of disabled people).

In observational studies, the researcher has flexibility with regard to several important dimensions:

- *The focus of the observation.* An observer cannot attend to every aspect of an event, interaction, or situation, and so a decision must be made regarding what will be observed. The focus can be broadly defined events, such as patient mood swings, or it can be small and highly specific behaviors, such as gestures or facial expressions.

- *Concealment.* As discussed in Chapter 5, researchers do not always tell people that they are being observed as part of a study. Concealment is controversial because of the ethical requirement for informed consent. However, people who know that are under observation often fail to behave normally, thereby jeopardizing the accuracy of the observations. The problem of behavioral distortions due to the known presence of an observer has been called a reactive measurement effect or, more simply, **reactivity.**

- *Duration of observation.* Some observations can be made in a relatively short period of time, such as when a researcher spends a week or two observing nurses' use of touch with patients. Other observations, particularly those in ethnographic and other field studies, may require months or even years of observation in the field.

- *Method of recording observations.* Observations can be made through the human senses and then recorded by traditional paper-and-pencil methods. Observations can also be done with the aid of highly sophisticated technical equipment, including video equipment, specialized microphones and audio recording equipment, and computers.

In summary, observational techniques can be used to measure a broad range of phenomena and are highly versatile along several important dimensions. Like self-report techniques, an important dimension for observational methods is the degree of structure the researcher imposes. Structured and unstructured observational techniques are described next.

Unstructured Observational Methods

Qualitative researchers who collect observational data about people and their environments do so with a minimum of structure and researcher-imposed interference. Qualitative researchers often use unstructured observation as a means of experiencing an aspect of a real-world situation first-hand. Skillful observation permits the researcher to see the world as the study participants see it, to develop a richer understanding and appreciation of the phenomena of interest on their own terms, to extract meaning from events and situations, and to grasp the subtleties of cultural variation.

Naturalistic observations often are made in field settings through a technique called **participant observation** (although it may be referred to as field observation or qualitative observation). A participant observer participates in the functioning of the group or institution that is under investigation, and strives to observe and record information within the contexts, experiences, structures, and symbols that are relevant to the study participants. By occupying a participating role within a setting, the observer may have insights that would have eluded a more passive or concealed observer.

The Observer–Participant Role

The role an observer plays in the social group under investigation is important because the social position of the observer determines what he or she is likely to see. That is, the behaviors that are likely to be available for observation will depend on the observer's position in a network of relations.

The extent of actual participation in the group being studied is better thought of as a continuum than as a participation–nonparticipation dichotomy. At one extreme of the continuum is complete immersion in the setting, with the researcher assuming the status of full participant; at the other extreme is complete separation, with the researcher assuming the status of an onlooker. The researcher may in some cases assume a fixed position on this continuum throughout the study. For example, a researcher studying the stress and coping of parents whose infant has died of sudden infant death syndrome (SIDS) might spend time observing the parents' interactions with each other and with other family members in their homes, but he or she would not likely end up participating in the life of the family as an actual family member.

On the other hand, the researcher's role as participant may evolve over the course of the field work. The researcher may begin primarily as a bystander, with participation in group activities increasing over time. In other cases it might be possible and profitable to become immersed in a social setting as quickly as possible, with participation diminishing over time to allow more time to be devoted to pure observation.

Leininger (1985) has offered the following four-phase strategy as a possible model for participant observation: (1) primarily observation; (2) primarily observation with some participation; (3) primarily participation with some observation; and (4) reflective observation. In the initial phase, the researcher observes and listens to those under study to obtain a broad view of the situation. This phase allows both observers and subjects to "size up" each other, to become acquainted, and to become more comfortable in interacting. In phase 2, observation is enhanced by a modest degree of participation. As the researcher participates more actively in the activities of the social group, the reactions of people to specific researcher behaviors can be more systematically studied. In phase 3, the researcher strives to become a more active participant, learning by the actual experience of doing rather than just watching and listening. In phase 4, the researcher reflects on the total process of what transpired and how people interacted with and reacted to the researcher.

The observer must overcome at least two major hurdles in assuming a satisfactory role vis-à-vis participants–informants. The first is to gain entrée into the social group under investigation; the second is to establish rapport and develop trust within the social group. Without gaining entrée, the study cannot proceed; but without the trust of the group, the researcher will typically be restricted to "front stage" knowledge (Leininger, 1985; *i.e.,* information that is distorted by the group's protective facades). The goal of the participant observer is to "get back stage"— to learn about the true realities of the group's experiences and behaviors. On the other hand, it should be recognized that being a fully participating member does not necessarily offer the best perspective for studying a phenomenon—just as being an actor in a play does not offer the most advantageous view of the performance.

Gathering Unstructured Observational Data

In gathering unstructured observational data, the researcher must decide what types of observations to make and where to make them. The participant observer typically places few restrictions on the nature of the data collected, in keeping with the goal of minimizing observer-imposed meanings and structure. Nevertheless, participant observers often do have a broad plan for the types of information to be gathered. Among the aspects of an observed activity likely to be considered relevant are the following:

1. *The physical setting—Where questions.* Where is the activity happening? What are the main features of the physical setting? What is the context within which human behavior unfolds?
2. *The participants—Who questions.* Who is present? What are the characteristics of those present? How many people are there? What are their roles? Who is given free access to the setting—who "belongs"? What brings these people together?
3. *Activities—What questions.* What is going on? What are the participants doing? Is there a discernible progression of activities? How do the participants interact with one another? What methods do they use to communicate, and how frequently do they do so? What type of affect is manifested during their interactions?
4. *Frequency and duration—When questions.* When did the activity or event begin and when is it scheduled to end? How much time has elapsed? Is the activity a recurring one and, if so, how regularly does it recur? How typical of such activities is the one that is under observation?
5. *Process—How questions.* How is the activity organized? How are people interacting and communicating? How does the event unfold?
6. *Outcomes—Why questions.* Why is the activity happening? What contributed to things happening in this manner? What kinds of things will ensue? What did *not* happen (especially if it ought to have happened) and why? What types of things were disruptive to the activity or situation?

The next decision is to identify a meaningful way to sample observations and to select observational locations. Researchers generally find it useful to use a combination of positioning approaches. **Single positioning** means staying in a single location for a period to observe behaviors and transactions in that location.

Multiple positioning involves moving around the site to observe behaviors from different locations. **Mobile positioning** involves following a person throughout a given activity or period.

Because participant observers cannot spend a lifetime in one site and because they cannot be in more than one place at a time, observation is almost always supplemented with information obtained in unstructured interviews or conversations. For example, an informant may be asked to describe what went on in a meeting that the observer was unable to attend, or informants may be asked to describe an event that occurred before the observer entered the field. In such a case, the informant functions as the observer's observer.

Recording Unstructured Observational Data

The most common forms of recordkeeping in participant observation studies are logs and field notes. A **log** is a daily record of events and conversations. **Field notes** may include the daily log but tend to be much broader, more analytic, and more interpretive than a simple listing of occurrences. Field notes represent the participant observer's efforts to record information and also to synthesize and understand the data.

Field notes are sometimes categorized according to the purpose they will serve during the analysis and integration of information. **Observational notes** are objective descriptions of events and conversations; information such as time, place, activity, and dialogue are recorded as completely and objectively as possible. **Theoretical notes** are interpretive attempts to attach meaning to observations. **Methodologic notes** are instructions or reminders about how subsequent observations will be made. **Personal notes** are comments about the researcher's own feelings during the research process.

The success of any participant observation study depends heavily on the quality of the logs and field notes. It is clearly essential for the researcher to record observations as quickly as possible, because memory is bound to fail if there is too long a delay. On the other hand, the participant observer cannot usually perform the recording function by openly carrying a clipboard, pens and paper or a tape recorder, because this action would undermine the observer's role as an ordinary participant of the group. The researcher, therefore, must develop the skill of making detailed mental notes that can later be committed to paper or recorded on tape through dictation. The use of portable computers with word processing capabilities can greatly facilitate the recording and organization of notes in the field.

Structured Observational Methods

Structured observation differs from the unstructured techniques in the specificity of behaviors or events selected for observation, in the advance preparation of observational forms, and in the kinds of activity in which the observer engages. The creativity of structured observation lies not in the observation itself but rather in the formulation of a system for accurately categorizing, recording, and encoding the observations and sampling the phenomena of interest.

Categories and Checklists

One approach to making structured observations of ongoing events and behaviors consists of the construction of a category system. A **category system** represents an attempt to designate in a systematic or quantitative fashion the qualitative behaviors and events transpiring within the observational setting. A category scheme essentially involves listing all those behaviors or characteristics that the observer is supposed to observe and record.

Some category systems are constructed so that *all* observed behaviors within a specified domain can be classified into one (and only one) category. An example of an exhaustive system is the modified coding system developed by Lee and Chiou (1995) for classifying nurses' postures. Their coding scheme was developed with the objective that *all* postures and joint positions could be classified. A contrasting technique is to develop a system in which only particular types of behavior are categorized. For example, if we were studying autistic children's aggressive behavior through structured observation, we might develop such categories as "strikes another child," "kicks or hits walls or floor," "throws objects around the room," and so on. In this nonexhaustive category system, many behaviors (all that are nonaggressive) would not be classified. Nonexhaustive systems are adequate for many research purposes, but they do run the risk of providing data that are difficult to interpret. When a large number of observed behaviors are not categorized, the investigator may have difficulty placing those that are categorized into proper perspective.

One of the most important requirements of a category system is the careful and explicit definition of the behaviors and characteristics to be observed. Each category must be explained in detail with an operational definition so that observers have relatively clearcut criteria for assessing the occurrence of the phenomenon in question. For example, Hurley and her colleagues (1992) developed an observational measure of discomfort in noncommunicative patients with advanced Alzheimer disease. An example of a behavioral indicator on this measure is "noisy breathing," which is defined as follows:

> Noisy breathing: negative sounding noise on inspiration or expiration; breathing looks strenuous, labored, or wearing; respirations sound loud, harsh, or gasping; difficulty breathing or trying at attempting to achieve good gas exchange; episodic bursts of rapid breaths or hyperventilation. (Hurley et al., p. 373)

Virtually all category systems require that some inferences be made on the part of the observer, but there is considerable variability on this dimension. Weiss' (1992) Tactile Interaction Index (TII) for observing patterns of interpersonal touch is an example of a system that requires a modest amount of inference. For example, one dimension of the TII concerns the part of a person's body that is being touched (*e.g.,* abdomen, arm, back, and so on). On the other hand, a category system such as the Abnormal Involuntary Movement Scale (AIMS) requires considerably more inference. The AIMS system, which was developed by the National Institute for Mental Health and used by Whall and associates (1989) for studying tardive dyskinetic movements over time during the day, contains such broad categories as "incapacitation due to abnormal movements." Even when these categories are accompanied by detailed definitions and descriptions, there is clearly a heavy inferential burden placed on the observer.

Once a category system has been developed, the researcher proceeds to construct a **checklist,** which is the instrument used by the observer to record observed phenomena. The checklist is generally formatted with the list of behaviors or events from the category system on the left and space for tallying the frequency or duration of occurrence of behaviors on the right. The task of the observer using an exhaustive category system is to place all observed behaviors in only one category for each element (*i.e.,* either an integral unit of behavior, such as a sentence in a conversation, or a time interval). Checklists based on exhaustive category systems are demanding of the observer because the recording task is continuous. The approach used with nonexhaustive category systems begins with a listing of categories of behaviors that may or may not be manifested by the participants. The observer's task is to watch for instances of the behaviors on the list. When a behavior occurs, the observer either places a check beside the appropriate behavior to designate its occurrence or makes a cumulative tally of the number of times the behavior was witnessed. With this type of checklist, the observer does not classify *all* the behaviors or characteristics of the people being observed, but rather identifies the occurrence and frequency of particular behaviors.

Rating Scales

Another approach to collecting structured observational data is through the use of **rating scales.** A rating scale is a tool that requires the observer to rate some phenomena in terms of points along a descriptive continuum. The observer may be required to make ratings of behavior or events at frequent intervals throughout the observational period in much the same way that a checklist would be used. Alternatively, the observer may use the rating scales to summarize an entire event or transaction after the observation is completed.

Rating scales can be used as an extension of checklists, in which the observer records not only the occurrence of some behavior but also some qualitative aspect of it, such as its magnitude or intensity. For example, Weiss' (1992) previously mentioned TII category scheme comprises four dimensions: location (part of body touched); action (type of gesture used, such as grabbing, hitting, patting, and so on); duration (temporal length of touch); and intensity. Observers using the index must both classify the nature and duration of the touch *and* rate the intensity on a four-point scale (light, moderate, strong, and deep). When rating scales are coupled with a category scheme in this fashion, considerably more information about the phenomena under investigation can be obtained. The disadvantage of this approach is that it places an immense burden on the observer, particularly if there is an extensive amount of activity.

Observational Sampling

The investigator must decide how and when the structured observational system will be applied. Observational sampling methods provide a mechanism for obtaining representative examples of the behaviors being observed without having to observe an entire event. The most frequently used system is **time sampling.** This procedure involves the selection of time periods during which the observations will take place. The time frames may be systematically selected (*e.g.*, every 30 seconds at 2-minute intervals) or may be selected at random.

   Event sampling, by contrast, selects integral behaviors or prespecified events for observation. Event sampling requires that the investigator either have some knowledge concerning the occurrence of events or be in a position to wait for (or precipitate) their occurrence. Examples of integral events that may be suitable for event sampling include shift changes of nurses in a hospital, cast removals of pediatric patients, epileptic seizures, and cardiac arrests in the emergency room. This sampling approach is preferable to time sampling when the events of principal interest are infrequent throughout the day and are at risk of being missed if specific time-sampling frames are established. When behaviors and events are relatively frequent, however, time sampling does have the virtue of enhancing the representativeness of the observed behaviors.

Evaluation of Observational Methods

The field of nursing is particularly well suited to observational research. Nurses are often in a position to watch people's behaviors and may, by training, be especially sensitive observers. Many nursing problems are better suited to an observational approach than to self-report techniques. Whenever people cannot be expected to describe adequately their own behaviors, observational methods may be needed. This may be the case when people are unaware of their own behavior (*e.g.*, manifesting preoperative symptoms of anxiety), when people are embarrassed to report their activities (*e.g.*, displays of aggression or hostility), when behaviors are emotionally laden (*e.g.*, grieving behavior among the bereaved), or when people are not capable of articulating their actions (*e.g.*, young children or the mentally ill). Observational methods have an intrinsic appeal with respect to their ability to directly capture a record of behaviors and events. Furthermore, virtually no other data collection method can provide the depth and variety of information as observation. With this approach, humans—the observers—are used as measuring instruments and provide a uniquely sensitive and intelligent (if fallible) tool.

   Several of the shortcomings of the observational approach have already been mentioned. These include possible ethical difficulties, reactivity of the observed when the observer is conspicuous, and lack of consent to being observed. Unquestionably, however, one of the most pervasive problems is the vulnerability of observational data to distortions and biases. A number of factors interfere with objective observations, including the following:

- Emotions, prejudices, attitudes, and values of the observer may result in faulty inference.
- Personal interest and commitment may color what is seen in the direction of what the observer wants to see.
- Anticipation of what is to be observed may affect what is observed.
- Hasty decisions before adequate information is collected may result in erroneous classifications or conclusions.

Observational biases probably cannot be eliminated completely, but they can be minimized through the careful training of observers.

As with self-reports, both unstructured and structured observational methods have advantages and disadvantages. Unstructured observational methods have the potential of yielding a deeper and richer understanding of human behaviors and social situations than is possible with more structured procedures. With a skillful observer, participant observation can help the researcher "get inside" a particular situation and lead to a more complete understanding of its complexities. Furthermore, unstructured observational approaches are inherently flexible and, therefore, permit the observer freedom to reconceptualize the problem after becoming familiar with the situation. On the other hand, observer bias may pose a threat: once the researcher begins to participate in a group's activities, the possibility of emotional involvement becomes a salient issue. The researcher in the new role of member may fail to attend to certain aspects of the situation or may develop a myopic view on issues of importance to the group. Another potential problem is that unstructured observational methods are highly dependent on the observational and interpersonal skills of the observer.

Researchers generally choose an approach that matches the research problem—and their paradigmatic orientation. Unstructured observational methods appear to be extremely profitable for in-depth research in which the investigator wishes to establish an adequate conceptualization of the important issues in a social setting or to develop a set of hypotheses. The more structured observational methods are generally better suited to the formal testing of research hypotheses regarding specific human behaviors. Table 9–4 briefly describes several nursing studies in which structured and unstructured observational methods were used to collect data.

Critiquing Observational Methods

As in the case of self-reports, the first question you should ask when critiquing an observational study is whether the data should have been collected by some other approach. The advantages and disadvantages of observational methods, discussed previously, should be helpful in considering the appropriateness of using direct observation.

Table 9–4. Examples of Studies Using Observation

Research Question	Type of Observation	Phenomena Observed
What are the patterns of transitions in nurse–patient interactions? (Bottorff & Varcoe, 1995)	Unstructured	Nurse–patient interactions
What are the differences between official and lay definitions of maternal and child health needs in Northern Ireland and Jamaica? (Mason, 1994)	Participant observation	Health-related behaviors and health-care systems
What is the effectiveness of a special program to teach children with disabilities about handwashing? (Day, Arnaud & Monsma, 1993)	Structured checklist	Children's handwashing
What are the motor performance correlates of functional dependence in long-term care residents? (Glick & Swanson, 1995)	Structured ratings	Motor performance of long-term care residents

Some additional guidelines for critiquing observational studies are presented in Box 9–2. A journal article should usually document the following aspects of the observational plan:

- The degree of structure in the observational plan
- The basic focus of the observations
- The degree to which the observer was concealed during data collection and the effect of the arrangement on reactivity problems
- For unstructured methods, how entry into the observed group was gained, the relationship between the observer and those observed, the time over which data were collected, and the method of recording data
- For structured methods, a description of the category system or rating scales, the settings in which observations took place, and the length of the observation sessions
- The plan for sampling events and behaviors to observe

▧ BIOPHYSIOLOGIC MEASURES

The trend in nursing research has been toward increased clinical, patient-centered investigations. One result of this trend is greater use of biophysiologic and physical variables that require specialized technical instruments and equipment for their measurement. Clinical nursing studies involve biophysiologic instruments both for

---

Guidelines for Critiquing Observational Methods

Box 9-2

1. Does the research question lend itself to an observational approach? Would an alternative method have been more appropriate?
2. Is the degree of structure of the observational method consistent with the nature of the research question?
3. To what degree were observers concealed during data collection? If there was no concealment, what effect might the observers' presence have had on the behaviors and events they were observing?
4. What was the focus of the observation? How much inference was required on the part of the observers, and to what extent did this lead to the potential for bias?
5. Where did the observations actually take place? To what extent did the setting influence the naturalness of the behaviors observed?
6. How were data actually recorded (*e.g.*, on field notes, checklists)? Did the recording procedure appear appropriate?
7. What was the plan by which events or behaviors were sampled for observation? Did this plan appear appropriate?
8. What steps were taken to minimize observer biases?

---

creating independent variables (*e.g.*, an intervention using biofeedback equipment) and for measuring dependent variables. For the most part, our discussion focuses on the use of biophysiologic measures as dependent variables.

Uses of Biophysiologic Measures in Nursing Research

Most nursing studies in which biophysiologic measures have been used fall into one of five classes:

1. *Studies of basic biophysiologic processes that have relevance for nursing care.* These studies involve participants who are healthy and normal or some subhuman animal species. For example, Heitkemper and Bond (1995) studied the effects of ovarian hormones on gastric motility in rats.
2. *Explorations of the ways in which nursing actions affect the health outcomes of patients.* For example, Verderber, Gallagher, and Severino (1995) studied the effect of three common nursing actions (nurse-administered bed bath, passive range-of-motion exercises, and turning from side to side) on transcutaneous oxygen and carbon dioxide tensions.
3. *Evaluations of a specific nursing procedure or intervention.* These studies differ from the studies in the preceding category in that they involve a test of a *new* nursing procedure hypothesized to improve biophysiologic

outcomes among patients. For example, Rogers and Aldrich (1993) used electroencephalogram (EEG), electrooculogram (EOG), and electromyogram (EMG) recordings as outcome measures in their evaluation of the effectiveness of nap therapy for narcoleptic patients.

4. *Studies to improve the measurement and recording of biophysiologic information regularly gathered by nurses.* For example, Klein and her colleagues (1993) compared tympanic membrane temperature with pulmonary artery and rectal temperature to determine consistency among the measures.

5. *Studies of the correlates of physiologic functioning in patients with health problems.* For example, Medoff-Cooper, Verklan, and Carlson (1993) examined the physiologic correlates (heart rate, oxygen saturation, blood pressure) of nutritive sucking patterns in very-low-birthweight babies.

The physiologic phenomena that have been of interest to nurse researchers run the full gamut of available measures.

Types of Biophysiologic Measures

Biophysiologic measures can be classified in one of two major categories. **In vivo measures** are those performed directly within or on living organisms. An example of an in vivo measure is blood flow determination through radiography. In vivo instruments have been developed to measure all bodily functions, and technologic improvements continue to advance our ability to measure biophysiologic phenomena more accurately, more conveniently, and more rapidly than ever before.

With **in vitro measures,** data are gathered from participants by extracting some biophysiologic material from them and subjecting it to laboratory analysis. The analysis is normally done by specialized laboratory technicians. Several classes of laboratory analysis have been used in studies by nurse researchers, including the following:

Chemical measures, such as the measurement of hormone levels, sugar levels, or potassium levels

Microbiologic measures, such as bacterial counts and identification

Cytologic or histologic measures, such as tissue biopsies

Some examples of how in vivo and in vitro measures have been used by nurse researchers are presented in Table 9–5.

Evaluation of Biophysiologic Measures

Biophysiologic measures offer a number of advantages to nurse researchers, including the following:

- Biophysiologic measures tend to be relatively accurate, precise, and sensitive, especially when compared with devices for obtaining psychological

Table 9–5. Examples of Studies Using Biophysiologic Measures

Research Question	Biophysiologic Measures
What is the effect of supplemental dietary calcium on the development of DOCA-salt hypertension in weanling rats? (Perry, 1995)	In vivo: Systolic blood pressure, body weight; in vitro: total serum calcium levels
What are the respiratory responses to unsupported arm exercise lifts paced in phase with expiration? (Breslin & Garoutte, 1995)	In vivo: diaphragm recruitment (electromyographic amplitude); pattern of thoracoabdominal motion
What is the ventilatory efficiency of different modes of mechanical ventilation used to achieve full ventilatory support in normal subjects? (Shelledy, Rau & Thomas-Goodfellow, 1995)	In vivo: respiratory rate, minute volume, average tidal volume, oxygen consumption, ventilatory equivalent
What are the changes in composition and bacterial contamination of blood salvaged from the cardiopulmonary bypass circuit of pediatric patients over an 18-hour period? (Hishon, Ryan, Lithgow & Butt, 1995)	In vitro: bacterial contamination and biochemical/hematologic alterations in salvaged blood

measurements, such as self-report measures of anxiety, pain, attitudes, and so forth.

- A major strength of biophysiologic measures is their objectivity. Nurse A and nurse B, reading from the same spirometer output, are likely to record the same or highly similar tidal volume measurements for a patient. Furthermore, barring the possibility of equipment malfunctioning, two different spirometers are likely to produce identical tidal volume readouts.
- Patients are unlikely to be able to distort measurements of biophysiologic functioning deliberately.
- Biophysiologic instrumentation provides valid measures of the targeted variables: thermometers can be depended on to measure temperature and not blood volume, and so forth. For nonbiophysiologic measures, the question of whether an instrument is really measuring the target concept is a continuously perplexing problem.
- Because equipment for obtaining biophysiologic measurements is available in hospital settings, the cost to nurse researchers of collecting biophysiologic data may be low or nonexistent.

Biophysiologic measures also have some disadvantages:

- The measuring tool may affect the variables it is attempting to measure. The presence of a sensing device, such as a transducer, located in a blood vessel partially blocks that vessel and, hence, alters the pressure–flow characteristics being measured.

- There are normally interferences that create artifacts in biophysiologic measures. For example, noise generated within a measuring instrument interferes with the signal being produced.
- There is a high degree of interaction among the major biophysiologic systems, and these interrelationships can result in problems if the stimulation of one system leads to responses in other systems.
- Energy must often be applied to the organism when taking the biophysiologic measurements. The energy requirements mean that extreme caution must continually be exercised to avoid the risk of damaging cells by high-energy concentrations.

In summary, biophysiologic measures are plentiful, tend to be accurate and valid, and are extremely useful in clinical nursing studies. However, in using them, great care must be exercised with regard to practical, ethical, medical, and technical considerations.

Critiquing Biophysiologic Measures

Biophysiologic measures offer the nurse researcher many advantages, as discussed previously, and their shortcomings are relatively minor. As always, however, the most important consideration in evaluating a researcher's data collection strategy is the appropriateness of the measures for the research question, and this is also true for biophysiologic measures. Their objectivity, accuracy, and availability are of little significance if an alternative data collection strategy would have resulted in a better measurement of the key research concepts. Stress, for example, is a concept that could be measured in various ways: through self-report (*e.g.,* through the use of a standardized scale such as the State-Trait Anxiety Inventory); through direct observation of participants' behavior during exposure to stressful stimuli; or by measuring heart rate, blood pressure, or levels of adrenocorticotropic hormone (ACTH) in urine samples. The choice of which measure to use, however, must be linked to the way in which stress is conceptualized in the research problem.

Additional criteria for assessing the use of biophysiologic measures are presented in Box 9–3. The general questions to consider are these: Did the researcher select the *correct* biophysiologic measure? Was care taken in the collection of the data? Did the researcher competently interpret the data?

▨ IMPLEMENTING THE DATA COLLECTION PLAN

In addition to selecting or devising methods and instruments for collecting research data, researchers must develop and implement a plan for actually gathering the data. This involves a number of decisions that could affect the quality of the data being collected.

Guidelines for Critiquing Biophysiologic Methods

Box 9–3

1. Does the research question lend itself to a biophysiologic approach? Would an alternative method have been theoretically more appropriate?
2. Was the proper instrumentation used to obtain the biophysiologic measurements? Would an alternative instrument or method have been more appropriate?
3. Does the researcher appear to have the skills necessary for proper interpretation of the biophysiologic measures?

One important decision concerns who will actually collect the data. In many studies, the researcher hires assistants to collect data rather than doing it personally. This is especially likely to be the case in large-scale quantitative interview and observational studies. In other studies, nurses or other health-care providers are asked to assist in the collection of data as a supplement to their regular job responsibilities. From a consumer's perspective, the critical issues are whether the people responsible for collecting data might have introduced any biases and whether they are able to produce data that are accurate, thorough, and believable. In any research endeavor, adequate training of data collectors is essential.

Another issue concerns the circumstances under which data have been gathered. For example, it may be critical to ensure total privacy to participants. In most cases, it is important for the researcher to create a nonjudgmental atmosphere in which participants are encouraged to be candid or behave naturally. Again, you as a consumer must ask whether there is anything about the way in which the data were collected that could have introduced bias or otherwise affected data quality.

In evaluating the data collection plan of a study, then, you should critically appraise not only the actual methods chosen, but also the manner in which the data were collected. Box 9–4 provides some specific guidelines for critiquing the procedures used to collect research data.

◈ WHAT TO EXPECT IN THE RESEARCH LITERATURE

The collection of data is an important and time-consuming activity in a research investigation. It is also an activity in which there is considerable room for creativity and critical thinking—and for differences of opinion, because the variables of interest to nurse researchers can often be conceptualized or measured in many different ways. Here are some hints on what consumers can expect to find in the research literature with respect to data collection plans:

Box 9–4

Guidelines for Critiquing
Data Collection Procedures

1. Who collected the research data? Were the data collectors appropriate, or is there something about them (*e.g.,* their professional role, their relationship with study participants) that could undermine the collection of unbiased, high-quality data?
2. How were the data collectors trained? Does the training appear adequate?
3. Where and under what circumstances were the data gathered? Were other people present during the data collection? Could the presence of others have created any distortions?
4. Did the collection of data place any undue burdens (in terms of time or stress) on participants? How might this have affected data quality?

- Researchers describe their data collection plan in the methods section of a research report. In a report for a quantitative study, the specific data collection methods are often described in a subsection with the heading "Measures" or "Instruments." The actual steps taken to collect the data are sometimes described in a separate subsection with the heading "Procedures."
- Descriptions of any instruments used to collect data tend to be fairly brief due to space constraints in professional journals. Therefore, it is not always possible to evaluate thoroughly whether the selected data collection plan was sound. For example, if a study involved the administration of a measure of depression (*e.g.,* the Center for Epidemiological Studies Depression Scale, or CES-D), the research report most likely would not describe individual items on this scale—although the report *should* provide a reference to the appropriate source. Moreover, there is typically insufficient space in journals for the researcher to offer a rationale for the plan (*e.g.,* a rationale for why the CES-D was chosen instead of the Beck Depression Scale, or why depression was not measured through an approach other than structured self-report). Because of these facts, it may be difficult for consumers to undertake a detailed critique of the data collection plan.
- Most nursing studies reported in nursing journals use a data collection plan that is structured and quantitative, but increasing numbers of nurses are undertaking qualitative studies. Among the methods described in this chapter, self-reports are the most frequently used by nurse researchers. Most studies that collect self-report data incorporate one or more social–psychological scale.
- Many nursing studies integrate a variety of data collection approaches. In quantitative studies, structured self-reports combined with biophysiologic measures are especially common. Qualitative studies are especially likely to

combine unstructured observations and self-reports. Studies that integrate qualitative and quantitative data are also gaining in popularity.

RESEARCH EXAMPLES

In this and the following two sections, we present summaries of actual nursing studies. Use the guidelines presented in this chapter to evaluate the researchers' data collection plans, referring to the original articles if necessary.

Example of Scales and Biophysiologic Measures

Topf (1992) used an experimental design to test whether sleep was affected by a person's ability to control hospital noises. Subjects were randomly assigned to three groups: (1) those who received instruction in control over critical care unit (CCU) sounds and were subjected to a noisy condition, (2) those who received no instruction and were subjected to a noisy condition, and (3) those who were subjected to a quiet condition. Data were collected in a sleep laboratory that simulated a CCU environment so that actual noise levels could be controlled.

The participants' subjective stress due to hospital noise was measured by the 31-item self-report measure, the Disturbance Due to Hospital Noise Scale. The items consisted of tape-recorded CCU sounds, which participants rated on a five-point scale in terms of how bothered they were by the sounds (from not at all bothered to extremely bothered). A total score for stress due to hospital noise was calculated by computing the average rating across items. Subjects also completed a self-report scale designed to assess social desirability response set bias (*i.e.,* the subjects' tendency to describe themselves in favorable terms to gain others' approval).

Various measures of sleep were obtained through polysomnographic equipment, which included EEG, EMG, and EOG recordings. The physiologic measures included sleep efficiency; minutes in bed, asleep and awake, in various sleep stages; and number of stage shifts, intrasleep awakenings, and rapid-eye-movement periods. The actual measures were derived through scoring by a polysomnographic specialist; a second polysomnographic specialist scored some records to establish interscorer agreement. Agreement between the two scorers ranged from 78% to 94%. Subjects were also asked the morning after the session to rate, on a 10-point scale, how well they had slept the previous night.

The findings indicated that sleep patterns were strongly related to whether there was noise in the laboratory, but they were not related to receipt of instruction in control over CCU sounds.

Example of Participant Observation and Unstructured Self-Report

Chase (1995) conducted an ethnographic study of the "culture" of the CCU to examine the social context within which nurses' critical care clinical judgment occurs. Field work was done over a 2-year period, primarily in an 11-bed open heart surgical intensive care unit (ICU).

Participant observations were conducted approximately twice weekly over the 2 years of the study. Although initially the observations were fairly general, more focused observations were undertaken later in the field work in response to initial observations about communication patterns. The early observations also led the researcher to conduct observations for several months in a 10-bed general surgical ICU, for comparison purposes. Extensive field notes were recorded at each observational session.

In-depth, unstructured interviews were also conducted with 10 nurses who were followed extensively. The in-depth interviews, which were conducted in private and audiotaped, began with broad questions such as the following: "Can you recall a time when you have been unsure of what to do for a patient? What did you have to consider?" Additional on-the-spot interviews were conducted with 20 nurses and 10 physicians.

Chase concluded that parallel hierarchies for nurses and physicians allowed for checks on clinical judgment both within and across professional lines. Such rituals as the nursing report and physician rounds provided a context for a critique of judgment processes. Communication of judgment, which was frequently an open and casual conversation, was viewed as contributing to better patient outcomes.

Example of Structured Interview, Scales, and Records

Yates and Belknap (1991) used a variety of structured data collection procedures in a study designed to identify predictors of physical functioning after a cardiac event. Physical functioning, the dependent variable, was measured both objectively (scores on a symptom-limited exercise test for functional aerobic impairment) and subjectively (by a four-item VAS). A VAS was also used to measure perceived physical recovery.

Self-report data were collected 9 weeks after the cardiac event in the participants' homes during a 90-minute structured interview. As part of the interview, participants completed several self-administered psychological scales, including measures of depression, self-esteem, and mastery. Study participants were also asked a number of questions regarding their activity levels in the previous month. Finally, various pieces of data used in the analyses were obtained from hospital records (*e.g.,* number of coronary arteries with occlusions greater than 70%, number of arteries bypassed).

The findings suggested that a person's return to greater activity levels after a cardiac illness was associated with lower levels of depression and higher levels of objective physical functioning, physical recovery, and self-esteem.

▨ SUMMARY

Some researchers use existing data in their studies—for example, those doing **historical research,** a **secondary analysis,** or an analysis of **records**—but most collect new data. Data collection methods vary along four important dimensions: structure, quantifiability, researcher obtrusiveness, and objectivity. The three principal data collection approaches for nurse researchers are self-report, observation, and biophysiologic measures.

Self-report data are collected by means of an oral interview or written questionnaire. Unstructured self-reports are the primary means of data collection in qualitative studies. Methods of collecting unstructured or loosely structured self-report data include (1) **completely unstructured interviews,** which are conversational discussions on the topic of interest; (2) **focused interviews,** guided by a broad **topic guide;** (3) **focus group interviews,** which involve discussions with small groups; (4) **life histories,** which encourage respondents to narrate their life experiences regarding some theme; (5) the **critical incidents technique,** which involves probes about the circumstances surrounding a behavior that is critical to some outcome of interest; and (6) **diaries,** in which respondents are asked to maintain daily records about some aspects of their lives.

Structured self-reports usually employ a formal **instrument**—a **questionnaire** or **interview schedule,** which may contain a combination of **open-ended questions** (which permit respondents to respond in their own words) and **closed-ended questions** (which offer respondents fixed alternatives from which to choose). Questionnaires are less costly and time consuming than interviews, offer the possibility of anonymity, and run no risk of interviewer bias. However, interviews yield a higher response rate, are suitable for a wider variety of people, and provide richer data than questionnaires.

Social–psychological **scales** are self-report tools for quantitatively measuring the intensity of such characteristics as personality traits, attitudes, needs, and perceptions. **Likert scales** (also known as **summated rating scales**) present the respondent with a series of **items** worded either favorably or unfavorably toward some phenomenon. Responses indicating level of agreement or disagreement with each statement are then combined to form a composite score. The **semantic differential** (SD) technique consists of a series of scales involving **bipolar adjectives** (*e.g.,* good/bad) along which respondents are asked to rate their reaction toward some phenomenon. A **visual analog scale** (VAS) often is used to measure, along a bipolar continuum, subjective experiences, such as pain and nausea. Scales are versatile and powerful but are susceptible to **response set biases,** which concern the tendency of certain persons to respond to items in characteristic ways, independently of the item's content.

Vignettes, another special form of self-report, are brief descriptions of some event, person, or situation to which respondents are asked to react. **Projective techniques** encompass a variety of data collection methods that rely on the participant's projection of psychological traits or states in response to vaguely structured stimuli. **Q sorts** involve having the participant sort a set of statements into piles according to specified criteria. Self-report methods are indispensable as a means of collecting data on human beings but are susceptible to errors of reporting.

Observational methods are techniques for acquiring data through the direct observation of phenomena. Observational techniques vary along a continuum from tightly structured procedures to unstructured procedures. One type of **unstructured observation** is referred to as **participant observation.** The researcher in a participant observation study gains entry into the social group of interest and participates to varying degrees in its functioning. This approach places relatively few restrictions on the types or amount of data collected. **Logs** of daily events and **field notes** of the observer's experiences and interpretations constitute the major data collection instruments.

Structured observational methods dictate what the observer should observe. In this approach, observers often use **checklists,** which are tools for recording the appearance, frequency, or duration of prespecified behaviors, events, or characteristics. Checklists are based on the development of **category systems** for encoding the observed phenomena. Alternatively, the observer may use a **rating scale** to rate some phenomenon according to points along a dimension that is typically bipolar (*e.g.,* passive/aggressive). Most structured observations make use of some form of sampling plan (such as **time sampling** or **event sampling**) for selecting the behaviors, events, and conditions to be observed. Observational techniques are versatile and offer an important alternative to self-report techniques. Nevertheless, human perceptual and judgmental errors can pose a serious threat to the validity and accuracy of observational information.

Data may also be derived from **biophysiologic measures,** which can be classified as either **in vivo measurements** (those performed within or on living organisms) or **in vitro measurements** (those performed outside the organism's body, such as blood tests). Biophysiologic measures have the advantage of being objective, accurate, and precise.

STUDY SUGGESTIONS

Chapter 9 of the accompanying *Study Guide to Accompany Essentials of Nursing Research*, 4th edition offers various exercises and study suggestions for reinforcing the concepts presented in this chapter.

Suggested Readings

Methodologic References

Frank-Stromberg, M. (Ed.). (1988). *Instruments for clinical nursing research.* Norwalk, CT: Appleton and Lange.
Kerlinger, F. N. (1986). *Foundations of behavioral research* (3rd ed.). New York: Holt, Rinehart and Winston.

Leininger, M. M. (Ed.). (1985). *Qualitative research methods in nursing.* New York: Grune & Stratton.

Lofland, J., & Lofland, L. (1984). *Analyzing social settings: A guide to qualitative observation and analysis.* Belmont, CA: Wadsworth.

Polit, D. F., & Hungler, B. P. (1995). *Nursing research: Principles and methods* (5th ed.) Philadelphia: J. B. Lippincott.

Rew, L., Bechtel, D., & Sapp, A. (1993). Self-as-instrument in qualitative research. *Nursing Research, 42,* 300–301.

Waltz, C. F., Strickland, O. L., & Lenz, E. R. (1991). *Measurement in nursing research* (2nd ed.). Philadelphia: F. A. Davis.

Substantive References

Bottorff, J. L., & Varcoe, C. (1995). Transitions in nurse-patient interactions. *Qualitative Health Research, 5,* 315–331.

Breslin, E. H., & Garoutte, B. C. (1995). Respiratory responses to unsupported arm lifts paced during expiration. *Western Journal of Nursing Research, 17,* 91–100.

Chase, S. K. (1995). The social context of critical care clinical judgment. *Heart & Lung, 24,* 154–162.

Cornman, B. J. (1993). Childhood cancer: Differential effects on the family members. *Oncology Nursing Forum, 20,* 1559–1566.

Day, R. A., Arnaud, S. S., & Monsma, M. (1993). Effectiveness of a handwashing program. *Clinical Nursing Research, 2,* 24–40.

Ferketich, S. L., & Mercer, R. T. (1995). Paternal-infant attachment of experienced and inexperienced fathers during infancy. *Nursing Research, 44,* 31–37.

Glick, O. J., & Swanson, E. A. (1995). Motor performance correlates of functional dependence in long-term care residents. *Nursing Research, 44,* 4–8.

Gujol, M. C. (1994). A survey of pain assessment and management practices among critical care nurses. *American Journal of Critical Care, 3,* 123–128.

Heitkemper, M. M., & Bond, E. F. (1995). Gastric motility in rats with varying ovarian hormone status. *Western Journal of Nursing Research, 17,* 9–19.

Hishon, M. L., Ryan, A., Lithgow, P., & Butt, W. (1995). An evaluation of changes in composition and contamination of salvaged blood from the cardiopulmonary bypass circuit of pediatric patients. *Heart & Lung, 24,* 307–311.

Howell, S. L. (1994). A theoretical model for caring for women with chronic, nonmalignant pain. *Qualitative Health Research, 4,* 94–122.

Hurley, A. C., Volicer, B. J., Hanrahan, P. A., Houde, S., & Volicer, L. (1992). Assessment of discomfort in advanced Alzheimer patients. *Research in Nursing & Health, 15,* 369–377.

Klein, D. G., Mitchell, C., Petrinec, A., Monroe, A., Oblak, M., Ross, B., & Youngblut, J. M. (1993). A comparison of pulmonary artery, rectal, and tympanic membrane measurement in the ICU. *Heart & Lung, 22,* 435–441.

Lee, Y. H., & Chiou, W. K. (1995). Ergonomic analysis of working posture in nursing personnel: Example of modified Ovako Working Analysis System application. *Research in Nursing & Health, 18,* 67–75.

Logan, J., & Jenny, J. (1990). Deriving a new nursing diagnosis through qualitative research: Dysfunctional ventilatory weaning response. *Nursing Diagnosis, 1,* 37–43.

Mason, C. (1994). Maternal and child health needs in Northern Ireland and Jamaica: Official and lay perspectives. *Qualitative Health Research, 4,* 74–93.

McDonald, D. D., & Bridge, R. G. (1991). Gender stereotyping and nursing care. *Research in Nursing & Health, 14,* 373–378,

Medoff-Cooper, B., Verklan, T., & Carlson, S. (1993). The development of sucking patterns and physiologic correlates in very-low-birth-weight infants. *Nursing Research, 42,* 100–105.

Micelli, D. L., Waxman, H., Cavalieri, T., & Lage, S. (1994). Prodromal falls among older nursing home residents. *Applied Nursing Research, 7,* 18–27.

Morse, J. M. (1991). The structure and function of gift giving in the patient–nurse relationship. *Western Journal of Nursing Research, 13,* 597–615.

Morse, J. M., Bottorff, J. L., & Hutchinson, S. (1995). The paradox of comfort. *Nursing Research, 44,* 14–19.

Perry, P. A. (1995). Effect of supplemental dietary calcium on the development of DOCA-salt hypertension in weanling rate. *Western Journal of Nursing Research, 17,* 63–75.

Rajan, L. (1994). The impact of obstetric procedures and analgesia/anaesthesia during labour and delivery on breast feeding. *Midwifery, 10,* 87–103.

Rogers, A. E., & Aldrich, M. S. (1993). The effect of regularly scheduled naps on sleep attacks and excessive daytime sleepiness associated with narcolepsy. *Nursing Research, 42,* 111–117.

Seals, B. F., Sowell, R. L., Demi, A. S., Moneyham, L., Cohen, L., & Guillory, J. (1995). Falling through the cracks: Social service concerns of women infected with HIV. *Qualitative Health Research, 5,* 496–515.

Shelledy, D. C., Rau, J. L., & Thomas-Goodfellow, L. (1995). A comparison of the effects of assist-control, SIMV, and SIMV with pressure support on ventilation, oxygen consumption, and ventilatory equivalent. *Heart & Lung, 24,* 67–75.

Stratton, T. D., Dunkin, J. W., Juhl, N., & Geller, J. M. (1993). Recruiting registered nurses to rural practice settings. *Applied Nursing Research, 6,* 64–70.

Topf, M. (1992). Effects of personal control over hospital noise on sleep. *Research in Nursing & Health, 15,* 19–28.

Verderber, A., Gallagher, K. J., & Severino, R. (1995). The effect of nursing interventions on transcutaneous oxygen and carbon dioxide tensions. *Western Journal of Nursing Research, 17,* 76–90.

von Essen, L., & Sjoden, P. (1993). Perceived importance of caring behaviors to Swedish psychiatric inpatients and staff, with comparisons to somatically-ill samples. *Research in Nursing & Health, 16,* 293–303.

Weiss, S. J. (1992). Measurement of the sensory qualities in tactile interaction. *Nursing Research, 41,* 82–86.

Whall, A. L., Booth, D., Kosinski, J., Donbroski, D., Zakul-Krupa, I., & Weissfeld, L. (1989). Tardive dyskinetic movements over time. *Applied Nursing Research, 2,* 128–134.

Widerquist, J. G. (1992). The spirituality of Florence Nightingale. *Nursing Research, 41,* 49–55.

Wingate, S. (1995). Quality of life for women after a myocardial infarction. *Heart & Lung, 24,* 467–473.

Yates, B. C., & Belknap, D. C. (1991). Predictors of physical functioning after a cardiac event. *Heart & Lung, 20,* 383–390.

Data Quality Assessments

Student Objectives

On completion of this chapter, the student will be able to:

- describe the major characteristics and advantages of measurement
- describe the components of an imperfect (obtained) score
- identify several major sources of measurement error
- describe three different aspects of reliability and specify how each aspect can be assessed
- interpret the meaning of reliability coefficients
- describe three different aspects of validity and specify how each aspect can be assessed
- describe the four dimensions used in establishing the trustworthiness of qualitative data
- identify several methods of enhancing and documenting data credibility in qualitative studies
- describe four types of triangulation
- evaluate the overall quality of a measuring tool or data collection approach used in a research study
- define new terms in the chapter

New Terms

Audit trail
Coefficient alpha
Concurrent validity
Confirmability
Construct validity
Content validity
Credibility
Criterion-related validity
Cronbach's alpha
Data source triangulation
Dependability
Equivalence
Error of measurement
Face validity
Factor
Factor analysis
Inquiry audit
Internal consistency
Interobserver reliability
Interrater reliability

Investigator triangulation
Known-groups technique
Measurement
Member check
Method triangulation
Negative case analysis
Obtained score
Peer debriefing
Persistent observation
Predictive validity
Prolonged engagement
Psychometric evaluation
Quantification
Reliability
Reliability coefficient
Researcher credibility
Split-half technique
Stability
Stepwise replication
Test–retest reliability

Theory triangulation
Thick description
Transferability
Triangulation

True score
Trustworthiness of data
Validity
Validity coefficient

Data collection methods vary considerably in their ability to capture adequately the constructs in which nurse researchers are interested. An ideal data collection procedure is one that results in gauges of the constructs that are credible, accurate, unbiased, and sensitive. For most concepts of interest to nurse researchers, few, if any, data collection procedures match this ideal. In this chapter, we discuss criteria for evaluating the quality of data obtained in both quantitative and qualitative research projects.

MEASUREMENT AND THE ASSESSMENT OF QUANTITATIVE DATA

In a quantitative study, the data take the form of *measures* of an abstract construct. Most social scientists agree that measurement constitutes one of the most perplexing and enduring problems in quantitative research. Before describing criteria for assessing quantitative measures, we must briefly discuss the concept of measurement.

Measurement

Definition of Measurement

Measurement involves rules for assigning numeric values to *qualities* of objects to designate the *quantity* of the attribute. No attribute *inherently* has a numeric value; human beings invent the rules to quantitatively measure concepts. An often-quoted statement by an early American psychologist, L. L. Thurstone, advances a position assumed by many quantitative researchers: "Whatever exists, exists in some amount and can be measured." The notion underlying this statement is that attributes of objects are not constant: they vary from day to day, from situation to situation, or from one object to another. This variability is capable of a numeric expression that signifies *how much* of an attribute is present in the object. **Quantification** is used to communicate that amount. The purpose of assigning numbers, then, is to differentiate among people or objects that possess varying degrees of the critical attribute.

This definition of measurement also indicates that numbers must be assigned to objects according to rules rather than haphazardly. Quantification in the absence of rules would be meaningless. The rules for measuring temperature, weight, blood pressure, and other physical attributes are widely known and accepted. Rules for measuring many variables for nursing research studies, however, have to be invented. What are the rules for measuring patient satisfaction? Pain? Depression? Whether the data are collected through observation, self-report, a projective test, or some other method, the researcher must specify the criteria according to which numeric values are to be assigned.

Advantages of Measurement

One of the principal strengths of measurement is that it removes much of the guesswork in gathering information. Consider how handicapped nurses and doctors would be in the absence of measures of body temperature, blood pressure, and so on. Because measurement is based on explicit rules, the information tends to be objective: two people measuring the weight of a subject using the same scale would be likely to get identical results. Two people scoring a standardized self-report stress scale would be likely to arrive at identical scores. Not all quantitative measures are completely objective, but most are likely to incorporate rules for minimizing subjectivity.

An additional advantage is that quantitative measurement makes it possible to obtain reasonably precise information. Instead of describing Nathan as rather tall, for example, we can depict him as a man who is 6 feet 2 inches tall. If we chose, or if the research requirements demanded it, we could obtain even more precise height measurements. Because of the possibility for precision, the researcher's task of differentiating among objects that possess different degrees of an attribute becomes considerably easier.

Finally, measurement constitutes a language of communication. Numbers are much less vague than words and, therefore, are capable of communicating information to a broad audience. If a researcher reported that the average oral temperature of a sample of postoperative patients was somewhat high, different readers might develop different conceptions about the physiologic state of the sample. If the researcher reported an average temperature of 99.6°F, however, there is no possibility of ambiguity and subjective interpretations.

Errors of Measurement

Researchers almost always work with fallible measures. Values and scores obtained from even the best measuring instruments have a certain margin of error. One can think of every obtained score or piece of quantitative data as consisting of two parts: an error component and a true component. This can be written as an equation, as follows:

$$\text{Obtained score} = \text{True score} \pm \text{Error}$$

The **obtained** (or **observed**) **score** could be, for example, a patient's heart rate or score on a scale of subjective pain. The **true score** is the true value that would be obtained if it were possible to have an infallible measure of the target attribute. The true score is a hypothetical entity; it can never be known because measures are *not* infallible. The final term in the equation is the **error of measurement.** The difference between true and obtained scores is the result of extraneous factors that affect the measurement and result in distortions.

Many factors contribute to errors of measurement. Among the most common are the following:

- *Situational contaminants.* Measurements can be affected by the conditions under which they are produced (*e.g.,* people's awareness of an observer's presence can affect a measure; environmental factors, such as temperature, humidity, lighting, or time of day, can represent sources of measurement error).
- *Response-set biases.* A number of relatively enduring characteristics of the respondents can interfere with accurate measures of the target attribute (see Chapter 9).
- *Transitory personal factors.* Temporary personal factors (*e.g.,* fatigue, hunger, anxiety, mood) can influence people's motivation to cooperate, act naturally, or do their best.
- *Administration variations.* Alterations in the methods of collecting data from one person to the next can affect obtained scores (*e.g.,* if some biophysiologic measures are taken before a feeding and others are taken postprandially, then measurement errors might occur).
- *Instrument clarity.* If the directions for obtaining measures are vague or poorly understood, then scores may reflect this ambiguity and misunderstanding.
- *Item sampling.* Sometimes errors are introduced as a result of the sampling of items used to measure an attribute. For example, a nursing student's score on a 100-item test of general nursing knowledge will be influenced to a certain extent by *which* 100 questions are included on the test.

This list is not exhaustive, but it does illustrate that data are susceptible to measurement error from a variety of sources.

Reliability of Measuring Instruments

The **reliability** of a quantitative measure is a major criterion for assessing its quality. Essentially, the reliability of an instrument is the degree of consistency with which the instrument measures the attribute. If a spring scale gave a reading of 120 lb for a person's weight one minute and a reading of 150 lb the next minute, we would naturally be wary of using that scale because the information would be unreliable. The less variation an instrument produces in repeated measurements of an attribute, the higher is its reliability.

Another way of defining reliability is in terms of accuracy. An instrument can be said to be reliable if its measures accurately reflect the true measures of the attribute under investigation (*i.e.*, an instrument is reliable to the extent that errors of measurement are absent from obtained scores). A reliable measure is one that maximizes the true score component and minimizes the error component.

Three aspects of reliability are of interest to researchers collecting quantitative data: stability, internal consistency, and equivalence.

Stability

The **stability** of a measure refers to the extent to which the same scores are obtained when the instrument is used with the same people on separate occasions. Assessments of the stability of a measuring tool are derived through procedures referred to as **test–retest reliability.** The researcher administers the same measure to a sample of people on two occasions and then compares the scores obtained.

To illustrate this procedure, suppose we were interested in the stability of a self-report scale that measured self-esteem in adolescents. Because self-esteem is presumably a fairly stable attribute that would not change markedly from one day to the next, we would expect a reliable measure of it to yield consistent scores on two separate tests. As a check on the instrument's stability, we might arrange to administer the scale 3 weeks apart to a sample of teenagers. Fictitious data for this example are presented in Table 10–1. It can be seen that, on the whole, the differences in the scores on the two tests are not large. Researchers generally use an objective procedure for determining exactly how small the differences are. Researchers compute a **reliability coefficient,** which is a numeric index of how reliable the test is. Reliability coefficients (usually designated as r) range from a

Table 10–1. Fictitious Data for Test–Retest Reliability of Self-Esteem Scale

Subject Number	Time 1	Time 2	
1	55	57	
2	49	46	
3	78	74	
4	37	35	
5	44	46	
6	50	56	
7	58	55	
8	62	66	
9	48	50	
10	67	63	$r = .95$

low of .00 to a high of 1.00.[1] The higher the value, the more reliable (stable) is the measuring instrument. In the example shown in Table 10–1, the computed reliability coefficient is .95, which is quite high. For most purposes, reliability coefficients above .70 are considered satisfactory, but coefficients in the .85 to .95 range are far preferable.

The test–retest approach to estimating reliability has certain disadvantages. The major problem is that many traits of interest *do* change over time, independently of the stability of the instrument. Attitudes, mood, knowledge, physical condition, and so forth can be modified by intervening experiences between the two measurements. Thus, stability indexes are most appropriate for relatively enduring characteristics, such as personality and abilities.

Internal Consistency

Ideally, scales designed to measure an attribute are composed of a set of items that are all measuring the critical attribute and nothing else. On a scale to measure empathy in nurses, it would be inappropriate to include an item that is a better measure of diagnostic competence than empathy. An instrument may be said to have **internal consistency reliability** to the extent that all its subparts are measuring the same characteristic. This approach to reliability is the best means of assessing an important source of measurement error in multi-item measures, namely the sampling of items.

Procedures for estimating a scale's internal consistency are economical in that they require only one administration. One of the oldest methods for assessing internal consistency is the **split-half technique.** In this approach, the items comprising a test or scale are split into two groups and scored independently, and the scores on the two half-tests are used to compute a reliability coefficient. If the two half-tests are really measuring the same attribute, the reliability coefficient will be high. To illustrate this procedure, the fictitious scores from the first administration of the self-esteem scale are reproduced in the second column of Table 10–2. Let us suppose that the total scale consists of 20 items. To compute a split-half reliability coefficient, the items must be divided into two groups of 10, such as odd items versus even items. One half-test, therefore, consists of items 1, 3, 5, 7, 9, 11, 13, 15, 17, and 19, whereas the remaining items comprise the second half-test. The scores on the two halves for our example are shown in the third and fourth columns of Table 10–2. The reliability coefficient computed on the fictitious data is .80, suggesting a reasonably high correspondence between the odd and even items, and further suggesting that the items on the test are measuring the same attribute.[2]

More sophisticated and accurate methods of computing internal consistency

---

[1] Computation procedures for reliability coefficients are not presented in this textbook, but formulas can be found in the references cited at the end of this chapter. Although reliability coefficients can, technically, be negative (*i.e.*, less than .00), they are usually a positive number between .00 and 1.00.

[2] The value of the coefficient is the value after a correction using the Spearman-Brown formula.

Table 10–2. Fictitious Data for Split-Half Reliability of the Self-Esteem Scale

Subject Number	Total Score	Odd-Numbers Score	Even-Numbers Score	
1	55	28	27	
2	49	26	23	
3	78	36	42	
4	37	18	19	
5	44	23	21	
6	50	30	20	
7	58	30	28	
8	62	33	29	
9	48	23	25	
10	67	28	39	$r = .80$

estimates are now in use, most notably, **Cronbach's alpha** or **coefficient alpha.** This method gives an estimate of the split-half correlation for *all possible* ways of dividing the measure into two halves, not just odd versus even items. As with test–retest reliability coefficients, indexes of internal consistency range in value between 0.00 and 1.00. The higher the reliability coefficient, the more accurate (internally consistent) the measure.

Equivalence

The **equivalence** approach to estimating reliability—used primarily when different observers or raters are using an instrument to measure the same phenomena—seeks to determine the consistency or equivalence of the instrument in yielding measurements of the same traits in the same subjects. This approach is often used to assess the reliability of structured observational instruments. As noted in Chapter 9, a potential weakness of direct observation is the risk of observer error. The degree of error can be assessed through **interrater** (or **interobserver**) **reliability,** which is estimated by having two or more trained observers watch some event simultaneously and independently record the relevant information. The resulting data can then be used to calculate an index of equivalence or agreement. That is, a reliability coefficient can be computed to demonstrate the strength of the relation between the ratings of the two observers. As with other reliability coefficients, the values range from .00 to 1.00, with higher values indicating a greater degree of equivalence. When two independent observers score some phenomenon in a congruent fashion, there is a strong likelihood that the scores are accurate and reliable.

Interpretation of Reliability Coefficients

Reliability coefficients can be used as an important indicator of the quality of an instrument. A measure with low reliability interferes with an adequate testing of a researcher's hypothesis. If data fail to confirm a research hypothesis, one possibility is that the measuring tools were unreliable—not necessarily that the expected relationships do not exist. Thus, knowledge of the reliability of an instrument is useful in the interpretation of research results.

Reliability estimates vary according to the procedure used to obtain them. As shown in Table 10–3, which presents examples of reliability efforts by nurse researchers, estimates of reliability computed by different procedures for the same instrument are not identical. Test–retest reliability coefficients tend to decline as the time between administrations increases, even when the trait being measured is fairly enduring. It also should be noted that the reliability of an instrument is related in part to the heterogeneity of the sample. The more homogeneous the sample (*i.e.,* the more similar the scores on the measure), the *lower* the reliability coefficient will be. This is because instruments are designed to measure differences among those being measured. If the members of the sample are fairly similar to one another, then it is more difficult for the instrument to discriminate reliably among those who possess varying degrees of the attribute being measured.

Validity of Measuring Instruments

The second important criterion by which the quality of a quantitative instrument is evaluated is its validity. **Validity** refers to the degree to which an instrument measures what it is supposed to be measuring. When a researcher develops an instrument to measure patients' perceived susceptibility to illness, how can he or she really know that the resulting scores validly reflect this variable and not something else?

The reliability and validity of an instrument are not totally independent qualities. *A measuring device that is not reliable cannot possibly be valid.* An instrument cannot validly be measuring the attribute of interest if it is erratic, inconsistent,

Table 10–3. Example of Reliability Assessments by Nurse Researchers

Instrument	Type of Reliability	Reliability Coefficient
Smoking and Women Questionnaire (SWQ): a 14-item self-report scale (Gulick & Escobar-Florez, 1995)	Test–retest (1–3 weeks)	.84
	Cronbach's alpha	.83
Discomfort Scale for Alzheimer patients (DS-DAT): a 9-item observational scale (Hurley, Volicer, Hanrahan, Houde & Volicer, 1992)	Test–retest	.60
	Cronbach's alpha	.87
	Interrater reliability	.90
Miller Intuitiveness Instrument (MII): a 5-subscale self-report instrument (Miller, 1995)	Test–retest (15 days)	.85
	Cronbach's alpha	.94

and inaccurate. An instrument can be reliable, however, without being valid. Suppose we had the idea to measure anxiety in patients by measuring the circumference of their wrists. We could obtain highly accurate, consistent, and precise measurements of their wrist circumferences, but such measures would not be valid indicators of anxiety. Thus, the high reliability of an instrument provides no evidence of its validity for an intended purpose; the low reliability of a measure *is* evidence of low validity.

Like reliability, validity has a number of different aspects and assessment approaches. One aspect is known as face validity. **Face validity** refers to whether the instrument looks as though it is measuring the appropriate construct. Although it is often useful for an instrument to have face validity, three other aspects of validity are of greater importance in assessments of an instrument: content validity, criterion-related validity, and construct validity.

Content Validity

Content validity is concerned with the sampling adequacy of the content area being measured. Content validity is of particular relevance to people designing tests of knowledge in a specific content area. In such a context, the validity question being asked is: How representative are the questions on this test of the universe of all questions that might be asked on this topic? As an example, suppose we were interested in testing the knowledge of a group of lay people about the danger signals of cancer identified by the American Cancer Society. To be representative, or content valid, the questions on the test should include items from each of the seven danger signals (represented by the acronym, CAUTION):

Change in bowel or bladder habits

A sore that does not heal

Unusual bleeding or discharge

Thickening or lump in breast or elsewhere

Indigestion or difficulty in swallowing

Obvious change in wart or mole

Nagging cough or hoarseness

Content validity is also a relevant issue in measures of complex psychosocial traits. For example, Frank-Stromberg (1989) made efforts to make her scale, the Reaction to the Diagnosis of Cancer Questionnaire, content valid. Before developing the scale, she asked 340 cancer patients the following open-ended question: "What do you remember of your feelings when first told you had cancer?" Prevalent themes that emerged in the responses to this question were then incorporated into items in the scale, thus reflecting the major content areas experienced by cancer patients.

The content validity of an instrument is necessarily based on judgment. There are no totally objective methods for ensuring the adequate content coverage of an instrument. Experts in the content area are often called on to analyze the items' adequacy in representing the hypothetical content universe in the correct proportions. It is also possible to calculate a content validity index that indicates the extent of agreement among the experts, but ultimately the experts' subjective judgments must be relied on.

Criterion-Related Validity

Criterion-related validity assessment is a pragmatic approach in which the researcher seeks to establish the relationship between the scores on the instrument in question and some external criterion. In this approach, the researcher is not seeking to ascertain how well the tool is measuring a theoretical trait. The instrument, whatever abstract attribute it is measuring, is said to be valid if its scores correspond strongly with scores on some criterion.

One requirement of the criterion-related approach to validation is the availability of a reasonably reliable and valid criterion with which the measures on the target instrument can be compared. This, unfortunately, is seldom easy. If we were developing an observational instrument to measure nursing effectiveness, we might use supervisory ratings as our criterion. But how can we be sure that these ratings are valid and reliable? Usually the researcher must be content with less-than-perfect criteria.

Once the criterion is established, the validity can be estimated easily. A **validity coefficient** is computed by using a mathematic formula that correlates the scores on the instrument with scores on the criterion variable. The magnitude of the coefficient represents the indicator of how valid the instrument is. Again, these coefficients (r) typically range between .00 and 1.00, with higher values indicating greater criterion-related validity. For example, a validity coefficient of .83 between scores on a measure of birth control effectiveness and the number of subsequent pregnancies (the criterion) would indicate a fairly high degree of criterion-related validity.

Sometimes a distinction is made between two types of criterion-related validity. The distinction is not critical, but the terms are used frequently enough to warrant their mention. **Predictive validity** refers to the ability of an instrument to differentiate between the performances or behaviors of people on some future criterion. When a school of nursing correlates students' incoming SAT scores with their subsequent grade-point averages, the predictive validity of the SATs for nursing school performance is being evaluated. **Concurrent validity** refers to the ability of an instrument to distinguish among people who differ in their present status on some criterion. For example, a psychological test to differentiate between those patients in a mental institution who can and cannot be released could be correlated with current behavioral ratings of health-care personnel. The difference between predictive and concurrent validity, then, is the difference in the timing of obtaining measurements on a criterion.

Construct Validity

Validating an instrument in terms of **construct validity** is one of the most difficult and challenging tasks that a researcher faces. Construct validity is concerned with the following question: What construct is the instrument *actually* measuring? Unfortunately, the more abstract the concept, the more difficult it is to establish the construct validity of the measure; at the same time, the more abstract the concept, the less suitable it is to validate a measure by the criterion-related approach. What objective criterion is there for concepts such as empathy, grief, role conflict, and separation anxiety?

Construct validation is addressed in several ways, but there is always an emphasis on logical analysis and the testing of relationships predicted on the basis of theoretical considerations. Constructs are usually explicated in terms of other concepts; therefore, the researcher needs to be in a position to make predictions about the manner in which the construct will function in relation to other constructs.

One common approach to construct validation is the **known-groups technique.** In this procedure, groups that are expected to differ on the critical attribute because of some known characteristic are administered the instrument. For instance, in validating a measure of fear of the labor experience, one might contrast the scores of primiparas and multiparas. Because one would expect that women who had never given birth would experience more fears and anxiety than women who had already had children, one might question the validity of the instrument if such differences did not emerge. There is not necessarily an expectation that the differences would be great. Some primiparas probably would feel minimal anxiety, whereas some multiparas might express many fears. On the whole, however, it would be anticipated that some group differences would be reflected in the scores.

Another method of construct validation consists of an examination of relationships based on theoretical predictions. A researcher might reason as follows: According to theory, construct X is related to construct Y; instrument A is a measure of construct X, and instrument B is a measure of construct Y; scores on A and B are related to each other, as predicted by the theory; therefore, it is inferred that A and B are valid measures of X and Y. This logical analysis is fallible and does not constitute proof of construct validity, but, nevertheless, it is important as a type of evidence.

Another approach to construct validation employs a statistical procedure known as **factor analysis,** which is a method for identifying clusters of related variables or items on a scale. Each cluster, called a **factor,** represents a relatively unitary attribute. The procedure is used to identify and group together different measures of some underlying attribute (*e.g.,* different items on a scale) and to distinguish them from measures of different attributes.

In summary, construct validation employs both logical and empirical procedures. Like content validity, construct validity requires a judgment pertaining to what the instrument is measuring. Unlike content validity, however, the logical operations required by construct validation are typically linked to a conceptual framework. Construct validity and criterion-related validity share an empirical component, but, in the latter case, there is usually a pragmatic, objective criterion with which to compare a measure rather than a second measure of an abstract theoretical construct.

Interpretation of Validity

Like reliability, validity is not an all-or-nothing characteristic of an instrument. An instrument cannot really be said to possess or lack validity; it is a question of degree. Like all tests of hypotheses, the testing of an instrument's validity is not proved or established but rather is supported by a greater or lesser degree of evidence.

Strictly speaking, a researcher does not validate an instrument per se but rather some application of the instrument. A measure of anxiety may be valid for presurgical patients on the day before the operation but may not be valid for nursing students on the morning of a final examination. In a sense, validation is a never-ending process. The more evidence that can be gathered that an instrument is measuring what it is supposed to be measuring, the greater the confidence the researcher can have in its validity.

Nurse researchers have become increasingly sophisticated in assessing the validity of measures. Table 10–4 presents some examples of validation efforts by nurse researchers.

ASSESSMENT OF QUALITATIVE DATA

The methods of assessment described thus far are relevant primarily to structured data collection instruments that yield quantitative scores. For the most part, these procedures cannot be meaningfully applied to such qualitative materials as re-

Table 10–4. Examples of Validity Assessments by Nurse Researchers

Instrument	Type of Validity	Procedure
Sense of Belonging Instrument (SOBI): a 27-item self-report scale (Hagerty & Patusky, 1995)	Content	Review by a panel of seven experts
	Construct	Known groups (contrasting scores of students, depressed patients, and nuns); factor analysis; correlation with other similar measures
The Pain-O-Meter: A device for recording sensory and affective components of pain (Gaston-Johansson, Franco & Zimmerman, 1992)	Construct	Known groups (scores before and after pain-relieving analgesics)
	Criterion	Relation to scores on other pain measures
Mastery of Stress Instrument: A 60-item self-report scale for adults (Younger, 1993)	Content	Review by a panel of 18 experts
	Concurrent	Correlation with Mastery Scale scores
	Construct	Relation to other personal characteristics; factor analysis

sponses in unstructured interviews or narrative descriptions from a participant observer's field notes. This does not imply, however, that qualitative researchers are unconcerned with the quality of their data collection techniques. The central question underlying the concepts of validity and reliability is: Do the measures used by the researcher yield data reflecting the *truth?* Certainly, qualitative researchers are as eager as quantitative researchers to have their findings reflect the true state of human experience.

Many qualitative nurse researchers seek to evaluate the quality of their data and their findings through procedures that have been outlined by Lincoln and Guba (1985), two proponents of the naturalistic paradigm of inquiry. These researchers have suggested four criteria for establishing the **trustworthiness** of qualitative data and the ensuing analysis: credibility, dependability, confirmability, and transferability. Table 10–5 presents some examples of qualitative nursing studies that have used various techniques to establish the trustworthiness of the data.

Credibility

Careful qualitative researchers take steps to improve and evaluate the **credibility** of their data and conclusions, which refers to confidence in the truth of the data. Lincoln and Guba point out that the credibility of an inquiry involves two aspects: first, carrying out the investigation in such a way that the believability of the findings

Table 10–5. Examples of Trustworthiness Assessments by Nurse Researchers

Research Question	Procedure
What is the essential structure of spiritual care as viewed by Christian patients? (Conco, 1995)	Member checks Peer debriefings Thick description Triangulation: Data source and method
What is the personal or subjective experience of forgetfulness among elders? (Cromwell, 1994)	Member checks Peer debriefing Partial audit Thick description Triangulation: Data source
What is the experience of therapeutic reading offered through bibliotherapy? (Cohen, 1994)	Member checks Peer debriefing Negative case analysis Independent audit Triangulation: Data source

is enhanced and, second, taking steps to demonstrate credibility. Credibility of qualitative data and the resulting findings is the aspect of data quality on which most methodologic attention has focused. Lincoln and Guba suggest a variety of techniques for improving and documenting the credibility of qualitative research. A few that are especially relevant to the evaluation of qualitative studies by consumers are mentioned here.

Prolonged Engagement and Persistent Observation

Lincoln and Guba recommend several activities that make it more likely that credible data and interpretations will be produced. A first and very important step is **prolonged engagement**—the investment of sufficient time in the data collection activities to have an in-depth understanding of the culture, language, or views of the group under study and to test for misinformation and distortions. Prolonged engagement is also essential for building trust and rapport with informants.

Credible data collection in naturalistic inquiries also involves **persistent observation,** which concerns the salience of the data being gathered and recorded. Persistent observation refers to the researcher's focus on the characteristics or aspects of a situation or a conversation that are relevant to the phenomena being studied. As Lincoln and Guba note, "If prolonged engagement provides scope, persistent observation provides depth" (p. 304).

Triangulation

The technique known as **triangulation** is also used to improve the likelihood that qualitative findings will be credible. Triangulation refers to the use of multiple referents to draw conclusions about what constitutes the truth. Denzin (1989) has identified four types of triangulation:

1. **Data source triangulation:** the use of multiple data sources in a study (*e.g.,* interviewing multiple key informants about the same topic)
2. **Investigator triangulation:** the use of multiple individuals to collect, analyze, and/or interpret a single set of data
3. **Theory triangulation:** the use of multiple perspectives to interpret a single set of data
4. **Method triangulation:** the use of multiple methods to address a research problem (*e.g.,* observations plus interviews)

The purpose of using triangulation is to provide a basis for convergence on the truth. In other words, by using multiple methods and perspectives, it is hoped that true information can be sorted out from information with errors.

External Checks: Peer Debriefing and Member Checks

Two other techniques that Lincoln and Guba recommend for establishing credibility involve activities that provide an external check on the inquiry process. **Peer debriefing** is a session held with one or more objective peers to review and explore various aspects of the inquiry. Peer debriefing is a process that exposes the researcher to the searching questions of others who are experienced in either naturalistic inquiry or in the phenomenon being studied (or both). These sessions can also be useful to the researcher interested in testing some working hypotheses or in exploring avenues to pursue in the emerging research design.

Member checks refers to providing feedback to the study participants regarding the data and the researcher's emerging findings and interpretations, and securing the participants' reactions. Member checking with study participants can be carried out both informally in an ongoing way as data are being collected and more formally after data have been collected and analyzed. Lincoln and Guba consider member checking the most important technique for establishing the credibility of qualitative data.

Searching for Disconfirming Evidence

The credibility of a data set can be enhanced by the researcher's systematic search for data that will challenge an emerging categorization or descriptive theory. The search for disconfirming evidence occurs through purposive sampling methods but is facilitated through other processes already described here, such as prolonged engagement and peer debriefings. The purposive sampling of individuals that can offer conflicting accounts or points of view can greatly strengthen a comprehensive description of a phenomenon.

Lincoln and Guba refer to a similar activity of **negative case analysis**—a process by which the researcher revises his or her hypotheses through the inclusion of cases that appear to disconfirm earlier hypotheses. The goal of this procedure is to continuously refine a hypothesis or theory until it accounts for *all* cases without exception.

Researcher Credibility

Another aspect of credibility discussed by Patton (1990) is **researcher credibility** (*i.e.,* the faith that can be put in the researcher). In qualitative studies, the researcher *is* the data collecting instrument—as well as the creator of the analytic process—and, therefore, the researcher's training, qualifications, and experience are important in establishing confidence in the data.

From a consumer's point of view, the research report should contain information about the researcher, including information about credentials. In addition, the report should make clear the personal connections the researcher had to the people, topic, or community under study. For example, it is relevant for a reader of a report on AIDS patients' coping mechanisms to know that the researcher is HIV positive. Patton argues that the researcher should report "any personal and professional information that may have affected data collection, analysis and interpretation— negatively or positively. . ." (p. 472).

Dependability

The **dependability** of qualitative data refers to the stability of data over time and over conditions. It might be said that credibility (in qualitative studies) is to validity (in quantitative studies) what dependability is to reliability. Like the reliability-validity relationship in quantitative research, there can be no credibility in the absence of dependability.

One approach to assessing the dependability of data is to undertake a procedure referred to as **stepwise replication.** This approach, which is conceptually similar to the conventional split-half technique, involves having a research group of two or more people who can be divided into two teams. These teams deal with data sources separately and conduct, essentially, independent inquiries through which data can be compared. Ongoing, regular communication between the teams is essential for the success of this procedure.

Another technique relating to dependability is the **inquiry audit.** An inquiry audit involves a scrutiny of the data and relevant supporting documents by an external reviewer, an approach that also has a bearing on the confirmability of the data, as we discuss next.

Confirmability

Confirmability refers to the objectivity or neutrality of the data, such that there would be agreement between two or more independent people about the data's relevance or meaning. In qualitative studies, the issue of confirmability does not focus on the characteristics of the researcher (is he or she objective and unbiased?) but rather on the characteristics of the data (*i.e.,* are the data confirmable?).

Inquiry audits can be used to establish both the dependability and confirmability of the data. In an inquiry audit, the investigator must develop an **audit trail** (*i.e.,* a systematic collection of materials and documentation that will allow an independent auditor to come to conclusions about the data). Six classes of records are of special interest in creating an adequate audit trail: (a) the raw data (*e.g.,* field notes, interview transcripts); (b) data reduction and analysis products (*e.g.,* theoretical notes, documentation on working hypotheses); (c) process notes (*e.g.,* methodologic notes, notes from member check sessions); (d) materials relating to intentions and dispositions (*e.g.,* personal notes on intentions); (e) instrument development information (*e.g.,* pilot forms); and (f) data reconstruction products (*e.g.,* drafts of the final report).

Once the audit trail materials are assembled, the inquiry auditor proceeds to audit, in a fashion analogous to a financial audit, the trustworthiness of the data and the meanings attached to them. Although the auditing task is complex, it can serve as an invaluable tool for persuading others that qualitative data are worthy of confidence.

Transferability

In Lincoln and Guba's framework, **transferability** refers essentially to the generalizability of the data (*i.e.,* the extent to which the findings from the data can be transferred to other settings or groups). This is, to some extent, a sampling and design issue rather than an issue relating to the soundness of the data per se. As

Lincoln and Guba note, however, the responsibility of the investigator is to provide sufficient descriptive data in the research report so that consumers can evaluate the applicability of the data to other contexts: "Thus the naturalist cannot specify the external validity of an inquiry; he or she can provide only the thick description necessary to enable someone interested in making a transfer to reach a conclusion about whether transfer can be contemplated as a possibility" (p. 316).

Thick description, a widely used term among qualitative researchers, refers to a rich and thorough description of the research setting or context, and the transactions and processes observed during the inquiry. Thus, if there is to be transferability, the burden of proof rests with the investigator to provide sufficient information to permit judgments about contextual similarity.

ASSISTANCE TO CONSUMERS OF NURSING RESEARCH

What to Expect in the Research Literature

Consumers need information on the quality of the data collection methods and procedures to interpret the findings of a study. Here is what to expect in the research literature with respect to data quality issues:

- The amount of detail about data quality that appears in a research report varies considerably. Some articles have virtually no information. In a few situations, such information may not be needed (*e.g.,* when biophysiologic instrumentation with a proven and widely known record for accuracy and validity is used). Most research reports, however, *should* provide some evidence that data quality was sufficiently high to merit the testing of the research hypotheses or the answering of the research questions. Most studies provide a modest amount of information about data quality, normally in the methods section of the report.
- Unfortunately, for many types of data it is difficult, if not impossible, to ascertain data quality. For example, if a survey asked about the smoking and drinking habits of respondents, their self-reports would typically have to be accepted at face value.
- In some reports, the *focus* of the study is on data quality. Many methodologic studies examine the validity and reliability of quantitative instruments that could be used by other nurse researchers or practitioners. In these **psychometric evaluations,** information about data quality is carefully documented, and relevant information appears throughout the report.
- In many quantitative studies that involve the use of structured self-report scales or observational scales, the research report mentions validity and reliability information that was previously reported in a separate report, usually by the researcher who developed the measure. If the characteristics

of the samples in the original study and the new research study are similar, the citation provides valuable information about data quality in the new study. Increasingly, researchers are also reporting reliability information for the actual research sample (typically internal consistency or interrater reliability). When the reliability coefficients obtained with the actual sample are high, the researcher can be more confident that the measures are accurately capturing the research variables.

- If a research report provides information on the reliability of a quantitative scale without specifying the type of reliability measure used, it is probably safe to assume that internal consistency reliability was assessed via the Cronbach alpha method.

- Qualitative studies are especially uneven in the amount of information they provide about data quality. Some do not address data quality issues at all, whereas others elaborate in great detail the steps the researcher took to confirm that the data were trustworthy. The total absence of relevant information makes it difficult for consumers to come to conclusions about the believability of qualitative findings.

- Because the process of assessing data quality in qualitative studies may be inextricably linked to the analysis of the data, discussions of data quality are sometimes included in the results section of the report. In some cases, the text will not explicitly point out that data quality issues are being discussed. Readers may have to be alert to evidence of triangulation or other verification techniques in such statements as, "Informants' reports of experiences of serious illness were accepted only if they could be checked against records by local health-care providers."

Critiquing Data Quality

If the data used in a study are seriously flawed, the findings are not likely to be meaningful. Therefore, it is important for consumers to consider whether the researcher has taken appropriate steps to operationalize the research variables and to collect data that accurately reflect reality. In both qualitative and quantitative studies, careful consumers have the right—indeed the obligation—to ask: Can I really trust the data? Do the data accurately reflect the true state of the phenomenon under study?

In quantitative studies, you should expect some discussion of the reliability and validity of the measures—preferably, information collected directly with the sample under study (rather than evidence from other studies). You should be wary about the results of quantitative studies when the researcher has either failed to provide information about data quality or when the report suggests unfavorable reliability or validity. Also, data quality deserves special scrutiny when the research hypotheses are not confirmed. There may be many reasons that hypotheses are not supported by data (*e.g.,* too small a sample or a faulty theory), but the quality of the measures is generally an important area of concern. When hypotheses are not supported, one distinct possibility is that the instruments were not sufficiently good measures of the constructs under study. Box 10–1 provides some guidelines for critiquing data quality in quantitative studies.

Information about data quality is equally important in qualitative studies. You should be particularly alert to information on data quality when a single researcher has been responsible for collecting, analyzing, and interpreting all the data, as is frequently the case. Some guidelines for critiquing the trustworthiness of data in qualitative studies are presented in Box 10–2.

▨ RESEARCH EXAMPLES

In this section, we present examples of the efforts researchers took to assess data in a quantitative and a qualitative study. Use the relevant guidelines in Boxes 10–1 and 10–2 to evaluate the researchers' activities.

Example From a Quantitative Study

Prescott and colleagues (1991) undertook several activities to develop and refine the Patient Intensity for Nursing Index (PINI). The PINI is a 10-item scale for nurses to use in evaluating the intensity of nursing care and the nursing skill level needed by individual patients. The PINI includes items relating to severity of illness, dependency, complexity of care, and time.

Box 10–1

Guidelines for Evaluating Data Quality in Quantitative Studies

1. Does there appear to be a strong congruence between the research variables as conceptualized (*i.e.,* as discussed in the introduction) and as operationalized (*i.e.,* as described in the methods section)?
2. Do the rules for the measurement of the variables seem sensible? Were the data collected in such a way that measurement errors were minimized?
3. Does the report provide any evidence of the reliability of the data? Does the evidence come from the research sample itself, or is it based on a prior study? If the latter, is it reasonable to believe that reliability would be similar for the research sample (*e.g.,* are the sample characteristics similar)?
4. If there is reliability information, what method of estimating reliability was used? Was this method appropriate? Is the reliability sufficiently high?
5. Does the report provide evidence of the validity of the measures? Does the evidence come from the research sample itself, or is it based on a prior study? If the latter, is it reasonable to believe that validity would be similar for the research sample (*e.g.,* are the sample characteristics similar)?
6. If there is validity information, what validity approach was used? Was this method appropriate? Does the validity of the instrument appear to be adequate?

Box 10-2

Guidelines for Evaluating Data Quality in Qualitative Studies

1. Does the research report discuss efforts the researcher made to enhance or evaluate the trustworthiness of the data? If so, is the description sufficiently detailed and clear?
2. Which techniques (if any) did the researcher use to enhance and appraise the credibility of the data? Was the investigator in the field an adequate amount of time? Was triangulation used, and, if so, of what type? Did the researcher search for disconfirming evidence? Were there peer debriefings and/or member checks? Do the researcher's qualifications enhance the credibility of the data?
3. Which techniques (if any) did the researcher use to enhance and appraise the dependability, confirmability, and transferability of the data?
4. Were the procedures used to enhance and document data quality adequate? Given the procedures used (if any), what can you conclude about the trustworthiness of the data?

After an initial development study, the research team performed an extensive psychometric evaluation. Interrater reliability was assessed by having day and evening RNs from one unit in each of five hospitals use the PINI on the same 150 patients as closely in time as possible (*i.e.,* late in the shift for day nurses, early in the shift for night nurses). The overall interrater reliability was 0.62. The internal consistency of the PINI, using the Cronbach alpha method, was 0.85.

Four substudies were undertaken for the validity testing, using data on 6445 patients collected by 487 RNs. The nurses worked in various clinical units of five hospitals in several states. The first substudy involved a factor analysis, which suggested that the PINI measures three underlying constructs: severity of illness, dependency, and complexity. The second substudy involved the testing of six hypotheses that predicted the relationship between PINI scores and other existing measures, such as length of hospital stay and scores on the hospital patient classification. All the hypotheses were supported. The third substudy involved comparing PINI scores for two groups of patients with different requirements, based on diagnostic-related groups (DRG) ratings. The low- and high-intensity nursing groups had substantially different PINI scores, as predicted. Finally, the fourth substudy involved comparing nurses' ratings of one item on the PINI—hours of care—with observer-recorded time data. Although nurses completing the PINI tended to overestimate time requirements, agreement between the nurses and the observers was reasonably high. The researchers concluded that "the psychometric evaluation of the PINI as a measure of nursing intensity has been very positive" (p. 219).

Example From a Qualitative Study

Gagliardi (1991) conducted an in-depth inquiry to investigate the experience of families living with a child with Duchenne muscular dystrophy. Three families that had a young boy (aged 7 to 9) with Duchenne were included in the study. The researcher visited each family weekly over a 10-week period and engaged in participant observation, including involvement in play activities, trips to summer camps, watching television with family members, and participation in family conversations. Logs of the observations were maintained the same day. Periodically, the researcher wrote analytic memoranda that were used to examine the researcher's emotions, biases, and conflicts.

In-depth unstructured interviews were also conducted; the interviews were taped and later transcribed. Interviews were conducted twice over the 10-week period, and then a third time 1 year later.

Gagliardi used several procedures to evaluate data quality. First, triangulation was used: data triangulation was achieved by interviewing multiple members of the family, and method triangulation was achieved by collecting both observational and self-report data. Member checks were undertaken by having family members verify themes emerging in the data during the second and third interviews. The grouping of narrative materials into themes was also verified by having two external auditors and several colleagues independently categorize a sample of the data, resulting in a 90% rate of agreement. The researcher met with her colleagues every 3 weeks to explore areas of disagreement and to help further reduce bias.

Six themes emerged as primary descriptors of the family's experience in Gagliardi's analysis of the data: (1) Disillusionment—the erosion of the hope for normalcy; (2) Society confirms the impossibility of normalcy; (3) Dynamics of the family—who's disabled anyway?; (4) A smaller world; (5) Letting go or hanging on; and (6) Things must change.

SUMMARY

In quantitative studies, assessments of data quality involve consideration of measurement issues. **Measurement** involves a set of rules according to which numeric values are assigned to objects to represent varying degrees of some attribute. Few, if any, measuring instruments used by researchers are infallible. The **obtained scores** from the measuring tools may be decomposed into two parts: a true score and an error component. The **true score** is a hypothetical entity that represents the value that would be obtained if it were possible to arrive at a perfect measure of the attribute. The error component, or **error of measurement,** represents the inaccuracies present in the measurement process. Sources of measurement error include situational contaminants, response-set biases, and transitory personal factors, such as fatigue.

One important characteristic of a quantitative instrument is its **reliability,** which refers to the degree of consistency or accuracy with which an instrument measures an attribute. The higher the reliability of an instrument, the lower the amount of error present in the obtained scores. There are different methods for assessing various aspects of an instrument's reliability. The **stability** aspect, which concerns the extent to which the instrument yields the same results on repeated administrations, is evaluated by **test–retest procedures.** The **internal consistency** aspect of reliability refers to the extent to which all the instrument's subparts or items are measuring the same attribute. Internal consistency is assessed using either the **split-half reliability technique** or, more likely, **Cronbach's alpha method.** When the focus of a reliability assessment is on establishing **equivalence** between observers in rating or coding behaviors, estimates of **interrater** (or **interobserver**) **reliability** are obtained.

Validity refers to the degree to which an instrument measures what it is supposed to be measuring. **Content validity** is concerned with the sampling adequacy of the content being measured. **Criterion-related validity** focuses on the relationship or correlation between the instrument and some outside criterion. **Construct validity** refers to the adequacy of an instrument in measuring the abstract construct of interest. One approach to assessing the construct validity of a measuring tool is the **known-groups technique,** which contrasts the scores of groups that are presumed to differ on the attribute. Another is **factor analysis,** a statistical procedure for identifying unitary clusters of items or measures.

Data quality is equally important in qualitative and quantitative research. In both, the fundamental issue is whether one can have confidence that the data represent the true state of the phenomena under study. The criteria often used to assess the **trustworthiness** of qualitative data are credibility, dependability, confirmability, and transferability. **Credibility,** roughly analogous to validity in a quantitative study, refers to the believability of the data. Various techniques and activities can be used to improve and document the credibility of qualitative data, including **prolonged engagement,** which strives for adequate scope of data coverage, and **persistent observation,** which is aimed at achieving adequate depth. **Triangulation** is the process of using multiple referents to draw conclusions about what constitutes the truth. The four major forms include **data triangulation, investigator triangulation, theoretical triangulation,** and **method triangulation.** Two especially important tools for establishing credibility are **peer debriefings,** wherein the researcher obtains feedback about data quality and interpretive issues from peers, and **member checks,** wherein informants are asked to comment on the data and on the researcher's interpretations.

Dependability of qualitative data refers to the stability of data over time and over conditions, and is somewhat analogous to the concept of reliability in quantitative studies. **Confirmability** refers to the objectivity or neutrality of the data. Independent **inquiry audits** by external auditors can be used to assess and document dependability and confirmability. **Transferability** refers to the extent to which findings from the data can be transferred to other settings or groups. Transferability can be enhanced by the use of **thick descriptions** of the context of the data collection.

Suggested Readings

Methodologic References

Brink, P. J. (1991). Issues of reliability and validity. In J. M. Morse (Ed.). *Qualitative nursing research: A contemporary dialogue.* Newbury Park, CA: Sage.

Denzin, N. K. (1989). *The research act* (3rd ed.). New York: McGraw-Hill.

Guilford, J. P. (1964). *Psychometric methods* (2nd ed.). New York: McGraw-Hill.

Kerlinger, F. N. (1986). *Foundations of behavioral research* (3rd ed). New York: Holt, Rinehart, and Winston.

Lincoln, Y. S., & Guba, E. G. (1985). *Naturalistic inquiry.* Newbury Park, CA: Sage.

Nunnally, J. (1978). *Psychometric theory.* New York: McGraw-Hill.

Patton, M. Q. (1990). *Qualitative evaluation and research methods.* Newbury Park, CA: Sage.

Waltz, C. F., Strickland, O. L., & Lenz, E. R. (1991). *Measurement in nursing research* (2nd ed.). Philadelphia: F. A. Davis.

Substantive References

Cohen, L. J. (1994). What is the experience of therapeutic reading? *Western Journal of Nursing Research, 16,* 426–437.

Conco, D. (1995). Christian patients' views of spiritual care. *Western Journal of Nursing Research, 17,* 266–276.

Cromwell, S. L. (1994). The subjective experience of forgetfulness among elders. *Qualitative Health Research, 4,* 444–462.

Frank-Stromberg, M. (1989). Reaction to the Diagnosis of Cancer Questionnaire: Development and psychometric evaluation. *Nursing Research, 38,* 364–369.

Gagliardi, B. A. (1991). The family's experience of living with a child with Duchenne muscular dystrophy. *Applied Nursing Research, 4,* 159–164.

Gaston-Johansson, F., Franco, T., & Zimmerman, L. (1992). Pain and psychological distress in patients undergoing autologous bone marrow transplantation. *Oncology Nursing Forum, 19,* 41–48.

Gulick, E. E., & Escobar-Florez, L. (1995). Reliability and validity of the Smoking and Women Questionnaire among three ethnic groups. *Public Health Nursing, 12,* 117–126.

Hagerty, B. M., & Patusky, K. (1995). Developing a measure of sense of belonging. *Nursing Research, 44,* 9–13.

Hurley, A. C., Volicer, B. J., Hanrahan, P. A., Houde, S., & Volicer, L. (1992). Assessment of discomfort in advanced Alzheimer patients. *Research in Nursing and Health, 14,* 213–221.

Miller, V. G. (1995). Characteristics of intuitive nurses. *Western Journal of Nursing Research, 17,* 305–316.

Prescott, P. A., Ryan, J. W., Soeken, K. L., Castorr, A. H., Thompson, K. O., & Phillips, C. Y. (1991). The Patient Intensity for Nursing Index: A validity assessment. *Research in Nursing and Health, 14,* 213–221.

Younger, J. B. (1993). Development and testing of the Mastery of Stress instrument. *Nursing Research, 42,* 68–73.

Analysis of Research Data

PART V

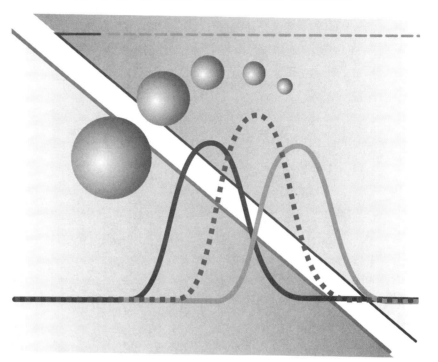

11

Quantitative Analysis

Student Objectives

On completion of this chapter, the student will be able to:

- identify the four levels of measurement and describe and compare the characteristics of each
- distinguish descriptive and inferential statistics
- describe the characteristics of frequency distributions
- identify different shapes of distributions
- describe the concepts of central tendency and variability
- identify and compare measures of central tendency and variability
- describe the meaning and interpretation of a standard deviation
- interpret a correlation coefficient
- evaluate a researcher's choice of descriptive statistics in presenting study results
- describe the principle of a sampling distribution
- describe the logic and purpose of the null hypothesis
- distinguish between Type I and Type II errors
- describe the purpose of tests of statistical significance
- distinguish the characteristics and uses of parametric and nonparametric statistical tests
- describe hypothesis testing procedures
- specify the appropriate applications for t-tests, analysis of variance, chi-squared, and correlation coefficients and interpret the meaning of the calculated statistics
- describe the applications and principles of multiple regression, analysis of covariance, and factor analysis
- understand the results of simple statistical procedures described in a research report
- evaluate a researcher's presentation of statistical information in a report
- define new terms in the chapter

New Terms

Alpha level
Analysis of covariance (ANCOVA)
Analysis of variance (ANOVA)
Bell-shaped curve
Bimodal distribution
Bivariate statistics
Canonical analysis
Canonical correlation coefficient
Causal modeling
Central tendency
Chi-squared test

Contingency table
Correlation
Correlation coefficient
Correlation matrix
Covariate
Cross-tabulation
Degrees of freedom
Dependent groups t-test
Descriptive statistics
Discriminant function analysis
Estimation procedures

F ratio
Factor analysis
Factor extraction
Factor matrix
Factor rotation
Frequency distribution
Frequency polygon
Hypothesis testing
Independent groups t-test
Inferential statistics
Interaction effects
Interval measurement
Inverse relationship
Laws of probability
Level of significance
Level of measurement
Linear structural relations analysis
    (LISREL)
Logistic regression
Logit analysis
Main effects
Mean
Mean square
Median
Mode
Multimodal distribution
Multiple comparison procedures
Multiple correlation analysis
Multiple correlation coefficient
Multiple regression analysis
Multivariate analysis of covariance
    (MANCOVA)
Multivariate analysis of variance
    (MANOVA)
Multivariate statistics
N
n
Negative relationship
Negative skew
Nominal measurement
Nonsignificant result
Normal distribution
Nonparametric test
Null hypothesis

Odds
Odds ratio
Ordinal measurement
p value
Paired t-test
Parameter
Parametric test
Path analysis
Pearson's r
Perfect relationship
Positive relationship
Positive skew
Post hoc tests
Product–moment correlation
    coefficient
r
R
R^2
R_c
Range
Ratio measurement
Sampling distribution
Sampling error
Scientific hypothesis
Skewed distribution
Spearman's rank-order correlation
    (Spearman's rho)
Standard deviation
Standard error of the mean
Statistic
Statistical test
Statistically significant
Sum of squares between groups
Sum of squares within groups
Symmetric distribution
Test statistic
t-test
Type I error
Type II error
Unimodal distribution
Univariate statistics
Variability
Variance

The data collected in the course of a research project do not in and of themselves answer the research questions or test the research hypotheses. The research data need to be processed and analyzed in some systematic fashion so trends and patterns of relationships can be detected. This chapter describes statistical procedures for analyzing quantitative data, and Chapter 12 discusses the analysis of qualitative data.

◩ LEVELS OF MEASUREMENT

A quantitative measure can be classified according to its **level of measurement.** This classification system is important primarily because the types of statistical analysis that can be performed with quantitative data depend on the measurement level employed. There are four major classes, or levels, of measurement:

1. **Nominal measurement,** the lowest level of measurement, involves using numbers simply to classify characteristics into categories. Examples of variables that are amenable to nominal measurement include gender, blood type, and nursing specialty. The numbers assigned in nominal measurement are not intended to convey quantitative information. If we establish a rule to code males as 1 and females as 2, the numbers in and of themselves have no meaning. The number 2 here clearly does not mean more than 1. Nominal measurement provides no information about an attribute except that of equivalence or nonequivalence. The numbers used in nominal measurement cannot be treated mathematically. It is nonsensical, for example, to compute the average gender of the sample by adding the numeric values and dividing by the number of participants.

2. **Ordinal measurement** permits the numeric ranking of objects on the basis of their standings relative to each other on a specified attribute. If a researcher were to rank order people from the heaviest to the lightest, then we would say that an ordinal level of measurement had been used. As another example, consider this ordinal scheme for measuring a patient's ability to perform activities of daily living: 1 = is completely dependent; 2 = needs another person's assistance; 3 = needs mechanical assistance; and 4 = is completely independent. The numbers signify incremental ability to perform independently the activities of daily living. Ordinal measurement does not, however, tell us anything about how much greater one level of an attribute is than another level. We do not know if being completely independent is twice as good as needing mechanical assistance, for example. Ordinal measurement only tells us the relative ranking of the levels of the attribute. As with nominal measures, the types of mathematic operation permissible with ordinal-level data are restricted.

3. **Interval measurement** occurs when the researcher can specify both the rank ordering of objects on an attribute and the distance between those

objects. Most educational and psychological tests (*e.g.,* the Scholastic Assessment Test, or SAT) are based on interval scales. A score of 550 on the SAT is higher than a score of 500, which, in turn, is higher than 450. Moreover, the difference between 550 and 500 on the test is presumed to be equivalent to the difference between 500 and 450. The use of interval scales greatly expands the researcher's analytic possibilities. Interval-level data can be averaged meaningfully, for example. Many sophisticated statistical procedures used by nurse researchers require that measurements be made on an interval scale.

4. **Ratio measurement** is the highest level of measurement. Ratio scales have a rational, meaningful zero. Interval scales, because of the absence of a rational zero point, fail to provide information about the absolute magnitude of the attribute. The Fahrenheit scale for measuring temperature, an example of interval measurement, illustrates this point. The assignment of numbers to temperature on the Fahrenheit scale involves an arbitrary zero point. Zero on the thermometer does not signify a total absence of heat. Because of this property, it would not be appropriate to say that 60°F is twice as hot as 30°F. Many physical measures, however, do have a rational zero and are, therefore, considered ratio-level measures. A person's weight, for example, is measured on a ratio scale. It is perfectly acceptable to say that someone who weighs 200 lb is twice as heavy as someone who weighs 100 lb. All the statistical procedures suitable for interval data are also appropriate for ratio-level data.

The four levels of measurement constitute a hierarchy, with ratio scales at the pinnacle and nominal measurement at the base. Researchers generally strive to use the highest levels of measurement possible because higher levels yield more information and are amenable to more powerful and sensitive analytic procedures than lower levels. Table 11–1 presents examples of concepts that nurse researchers have operationalized at different levels of measurement.

◩ DESCRIPTIVE STATISTICS

Without the aid of statistics, the quantitative data collected in a research project would be little more than a chaotic mass of numbers. Statistical procedures enable the researcher to reduce, summarize, organize, evaluate, interpret, and communicate numeric information.

Statistics are classified as either descriptive or inferential. **Descriptive statistics** are used to describe and synthesize data. Averages and percentages are examples of descriptive statistics. Actually, when such indexes are calculated on data from a population, they are referred to as **parameters.** A descriptive index from a sample is called a **statistic.** Most scientific questions are about parameters, but researchers calculate statistics to estimate these parameters.

Table 11–1. Examples of Variables Measured at Different Levels of Measurement

Research Questions	Role of Variable	Level of Measurement	IV or DV*
What are the linkages between sexual risk taking, substance use, and AIDS knowledge among pregnant adolescents and young mothers? (Koniak-Griffin & Brecht, 1995)	Frequency of substance use	Ordinal	IV
	AIDS knowledge	Ratio	DV
	Number of sexual partners	Ratio	IV
	Use of condoms vs. nonuse	Nominal	DV
What is the effect of a slow stroke effleurage back rub on older adults' anxiety salivary secretory immunoglobulin (s-IgA) and anxiety? (Groër, Mozingo, Droppleman, Davis, Jolly, Boynton, Davis & Kay, 1994)	Treatment group (experimental vs. control)	Nominal	IV
	Scores on STAI anxiety scale	Interval	DV
	S-IgA concentrations	Ratio	DV
What factors are related to body satisfaction in edentulous complete-denture-wearing clients? (Rudy, Guckes, Li, McCarthy & Brahim, 1993)	Chronic illness status (chronic vs. not chronic)	Nominal	IV
	Education (high school, college, graduate school)	Ordinal	IV
	Body image scale scores	Interval	DV

* IV = independent variable; DV = dependent variable.

Frequency Distributions

Data that are not analyzed or organized are overwhelming. It is not even possible to discern general trends until some order or structure is imposed on the data. Consider the 60 numbers presented in Table 11–2. Let us assume that these numbers represent the scores of 60 high school students on a 30-item test to measure knowledge about AIDS—scores that we will assume to be measured on an interval scale. Visual inspection of the numbers in this table is not very helpful in understanding how the students performed.

Frequency distributions represent a method of imposing some order on a mass of numeric data. A **frequency distribution** is a systematic arrangement of numeric values from the lowest to the highest, together with a count (or percentage) of the number of times each value was obtained. The fictitious test scores of the 60 students are presented as a frequency distribution in Table 11–3. This organized

Table 11–2. AIDS Knowledge Test Scores

22	27	25	19	24	25	23	29	24	20
26	16	20	26	17	22	24	18	26	28
15	24	23	22	21	24	20	25	18	27
24	23	16	25	30	29	27	21	23	24
26	18	30	21	17	25	22	24	29	28
20	25	26	24	23	19	27	28	25	26

arrangement makes it convenient to see at a glance what are the highest and lowest scores, where the scores tend to cluster, what is the most common score, and how many students were in the sample (total sample size is typically designated as **N** in research reports). None of this was easily discernible before the data were organized.

Some researchers display frequency data graphically. Graphs have the advantage of being able to communicate a lot of information almost instantaneously. One type of graph is known as a **frequency polygon,** an example of which is presented

Table 11–3. Frequency Distribution of AIDS Knowledge Test Scores

Score	Frequency	Percentage
15	1	1.7
16	2	3.3
17	2	3.3
18	3	5.0
19	2	3.3
20	4	6.7
21	3	5.0
22	4	6.7
23	5	8.3
24	9	15.0
25	7	11.7
26	6	10.0
27	4	6.7
28	3	5.0
29	3	5.0
30	2	3.3
	$N = 60$	100.0

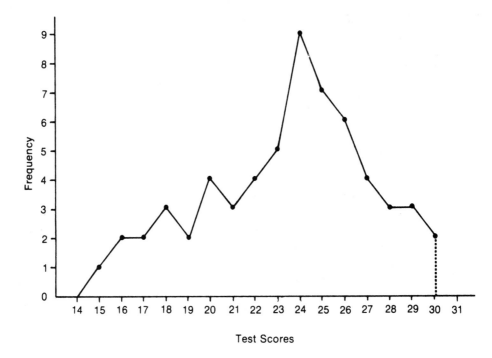

Figure 11–1. Frequency polygon of AIDS knowledge test scores

in Figure 11–1. In frequency polygons, scores are placed on the horizontal line (with the lowest value on the left), and the vertical line is used to indicate the frequency count or, alternatively, percentages. Distributions of data values are sometimes described by their shapes. A distribution is said to be **symmetric** in shape if, when folded over, the two halves of a frequency polygon would be superimposed, such as the distributions in Figure 11–2. Asymmetric distributions are de-

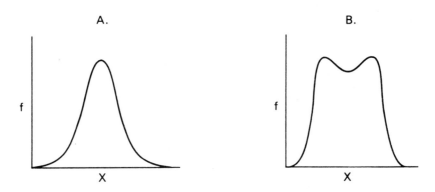

Figure 11–2. Examples of symmetric distributions

scribed as being **skewed.** In skewed distributions, the peak is off-center, and one tail is longer than the other. Distributions that are skewed can be described in terms of the direction of the skew. When the longer tail is pointed toward the right, the distribution is said to be **positively skewed.** The first part of Figure 11–3 depicts a positively skewed distribution. If, on the other hand, the tail points to the left, the distribution is **negatively skewed,** as illustrated in the second graph in Figure 11–3. An example of an attribute that is positively skewed is personal income. Most people have low to moderate incomes, with only a few people in high-income brackets at the right-hand end of the distribution. An example of a negatively skewed attribute is age at death. Here, the bulk of people are at the far right end of the distribution, with relatively few people dying at an early age.

A second aspect of a distribution's shape has to do with how many peaks or high points it has. A **unimodal distribution** is one that has only one peak, whereas a **multimodal distribution** has two or more peaks (two or more values of high frequency). The most common type of multimodal distribution is one with two peaks, which is called a **bimodal distribution.** Graph A in Figure 11–2 is unimodal, as are both graphs in Figure 11–3. A bimodal distribution is illustrated in graph B of Figure 11–2.

Some distributions are encountered so frequently that special labels are used to designate them. Of particular interest in statistical analysis is the **normal distribution** (sometimes called a **bell-shaped curve**). A normal distribution is one that is symmetric, unimodal, and not very peaked, as illustrated by the distribution in graph A of Figure 11–2. Many physical and psychological attributes of humans have been found to approximate a normal distribution. Examples include height, intelligence, and grip strength.

For variables measured on a nominal or ordinal scale, researchers generally describe the data by reporting their distributions in terms of percentages. For

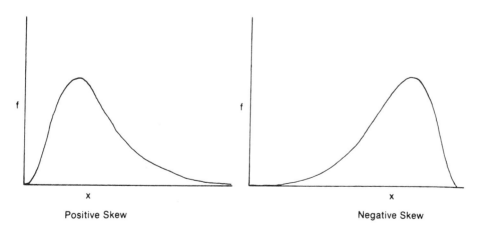

Figure 11–3. Examples of skewed distributions

example, Table 11–4 presents distribution information on sample characteristics from a study that examined physical functioning and psychosocial adjustment in survivors of sudden cardiac death (Sauvé, 1995). This table shows both the frequency (*N*) and percentage of patients in various categories for selected background characteristics.

Central Tendency

For variables measured on an interval or ratio scale, the distribution of data is usually of less interest than an overall summary of the sample's scores. The researcher asks such questions as: What was the average blood pressure of the patients after the intervention? How satisfied was the typical patient with his or her nursing care? These questions seek a single number that best represents a whole distribution of values. Such indexes of typicalness are referred to as measures of **central tendency.** To lay people, the term *average* is normally used to designate central tendency. There are three commonly used kinds of averages, or indexes of central tendency: The mode, the median, and the mean.

- **Mode:** The mode is the number in a distribution that occurs most frequently. In the following distribution of numbers the mode is 53:

Table 11–4. Example of Table Showing Frequency Distribution Information: Sample Characteristics in Study of People with Sudden Cardiac Death

Category	*N*	%
Race		
White	58	95.1
Nonwhite	3	4.9
Marital Status		
Married	45	73.8
Widowed	8	13.1
Separated/divorced	8	13.1
Education		
<12 years	18	29.5
≥12 years	32	70.5
Time to awakening		
≤1 hour	18	29.5
2 to 24 hours	28	45.9
25 to 48 hours	10	16.4
≥49 hours	5	8.2

Adapted from Sauvé (1995), with permission. Originally part of Table I of the report, titled *Demographics and Features of the Cardiac Arrest (N = 61)*.

50 51 51 52 53 53 53 53 54 55 56

The value of 53 was obtained four times, a higher frequency than for any other number. The mode of the AIDS knowledge test scores was 24 (see Table 11–3). The mode, in other words, identifies the most popular value. The mode is used primarily for describing typical or high-frequency values for nominal-level measures. For example, in the study by Sauvé (see Table 11–4), we could make the following statement: The typical (modal) patient was white, married, had at least 12 years of education, and awakened from the cardiac arrest within 2 to 24 hours.

- **Median:** The median is that point in a distribution above which and below which 50% of the cases fall. Consider the following set of values:

2 2 3 3 4 5 6 7 8 9

The value that divides the cases exactly in half is midway between 4 and 5; thus, 4.5 is the median for this set of numbers. The median for the AIDS knowledge test scores is 24. An important characteristic of the median is that it does not take into account the quantitative values of individual scores; it is insensitive to extreme values. In the above set of values, if the value of 9 were changed to 99, the median would remain unchanged at 4.5. Because of this property, the median is the preferred index of central tendency when the distribution is highly skewed and when one is interested in finding a single typical value. In research reports, the median may be abbreviated as **Md** or **Mdn.**

- **Mean:** The mean is equal to the sum of all values divided by the number of participants—in other words, what people refer to as the average. The mean of the AIDS knowledge test scores is 23.42 (1405 ÷ 60). As another example, consider the following weights of eight people:

85 109 120 135 158 177 181 195

In this example, the mean is 145. Unlike the median, the mean is affected by the value of every score. If we were to exchange the 195-lb person for one weighing 275 lb, the mean weight would increase from 145 to 155. A substitution of this kind would leave the median unchanged. In research reports, the mean is often symbolized as **M** or $\bar{X}$ (*e.g.*, $\bar{X} = 145$).

The mean is unquestionably the most widely used measure of central tendency. When researchers work with interval-level or ratio-level measurements, the mean, rather than the median or mode, is almost always the statistic reported. Of the three indexes of central tendency, the mean is the most stable: If repeated samples were drawn from a given population, the means would vary or fluctuate less than the modes or medians. Because of its stability, the mean is the best estimate of the central tendency of the population. When a distribution is highly skewed, however, the mean does not do a good job of designating the center of the distribution, and in such situations, the median is preferred. For example, the median is a better measure of central tendency for designating average income in the United States because income is positively skewed.

Variability

Measures of central tendency do not give a total picture of a distribution. Two sets of data with identical means could be quite different from one another. The characteristic of concern in this section is how spread out or dispersed the data are (*i.e.*, how different the people in the sample are from one another on the attribute of interest). The **variability** of two distributions could be different even when the means are identical.

Consider the two distributions in Figure 11–4, which represent the hypothetical scores of students from two high schools on the SAT. Both distributions have an average score of 500, but the two groups of students are clearly different. In school A, there is a wide range of obtained scores—from scores below 300 to some above 700. This school has many students who performed among the best, but it also has students who did relatively poorly. In school B, on the other hand, there are few low scorers but also few outstanding students on the test. School A is said to be more heterogeneous (*i.e.*, more variable) than school B, whereas school B may be described as more homogeneous than school A.

To describe a distribution fully, researchers use one or more indexes of vari-

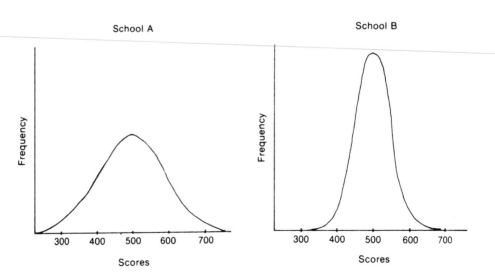

Figure 11–4. Two distributions of different variability

ability that summarize the extent to which scores differ from one another. Several such indexes have been developed, the most important of which are the range and the standard deviation.

- **Range:** The range is simply the highest score minus the lowest score in a given distribution. In the example of the AIDS knowledge test scores, the range is 15 (30 − 15). In the examples shown in Figure 11–4, the range for school A is 500 (750 − 250), whereas the range for school B is 300 (650 − 350). The chief virtue of the range is the ease with which it can be computed. Because it is based on only two scores, however, the range is a highly unstable index. From sample to sample drawn from the same population, the range tends to fluctuate considerably. Moreover, the range completely ignores variations in scores between the two extremes. In school B of Figure 11–4, suppose that a single student obtained a score of 250 and another obtained a score of 750. The range of both schools would then be 500, despite obvious differences in the heterogeneity of scores. For these reasons, the range is used largely as a gross descriptive index.

- **Standard deviation:** With interval- or ratio-level data, the most widely used measure of variability is the standard deviation. Like the mean, the standard deviation is calculated based on every value in a distribution. The standard deviation summarizes the average amount of deviation of values from the mean. In the AIDS knowledge test example, the standard deviation is 3.725.[1] In research reports, the standard deviation is often abbreviated as *s* or **SD.** Occasionally, the standard deviation is simply shown in relation to the mean without a formal label, such as $M = 4$ (1.5) or $M = 4 \pm 1.5$, where 4.0 is the mean and 1.5 is the standard deviation.[2]

A standard deviation is typically more difficult for students to interpret than the range. With regard to the AIDS knowledge test, one might well ask, 3.725 *what?* What does the number mean? We will try to answer these questions from several vantage points. First, as we already know, the standard deviation is an index of how variable the values in a distribution are. If two different groups of students had means of 23 on the AIDS knowledge test, but one group had a standard deviation of 7 whereas the other had a standard deviation of 3, we would immediately know that the second group of nursing students was more homogeneous (*i.e.,* their scores were more similar to one another).

As noted above, the standard deviation is a kind of average of the deviations from the mean. The mean tells us the single best point for summarizing an entire

---

[1] Formulas for computing the standard deviation, as well as other statistics discussed in this chapter, are not shown in this textbook. The emphasis here is on helping readers to understand the statistics and their applications. References at the end of the chapter can be consulted for computation formulas.

[2] Occasionally, a research report will make a reference to an index of variability known as the **variance.** The variance is simply the value of the standard deviation squared. In the example of the AIDS knowledge test scores, the variance is 3.725^2, or 13.876.

distribution, whereas a standard deviation tells us how much, on average, the scores deviate from that mean. In the AIDS test example, they deviated by an average of just under 4 points. A standard deviation might thus be interpreted as an indication of our degree of error when we use a mean to describe an entire data set.

When the distribution of scores is normal (or nearly normal), it is possible to say even more about the standard deviation. There are roughly three standard deviations above and below the mean with normally distributed data. To illustrate some further characteristics, suppose we have a normal distribution of scores in which the mean is 50 and the standard deviation is 10. Such a distribution is shown in Figure 11–5. In a normal distribution such as this, a fixed percentage of cases fall within certain distances from the mean. Sixty-eight percent of all cases fall within one standard deviation above and below the mean. In this example, nearly 7 of every 10 scores fall between 40 and 60. Ninety-five percent of the scores in a normal distribution fall within two standard deviations from the mean. Only a handful of cases—about 2% at each extreme—lie more than two standard deviations from the mean. Using this figure, we can see that a person who obtained a score of 70 achieved a higher score than about 98% of the sample.

Nurse researchers usually present summary descriptive statistics in their research reports, often in tables. Some measures of central tendency and variability from an actual nursing study are presented in Table 11–5. This study (Redeker,

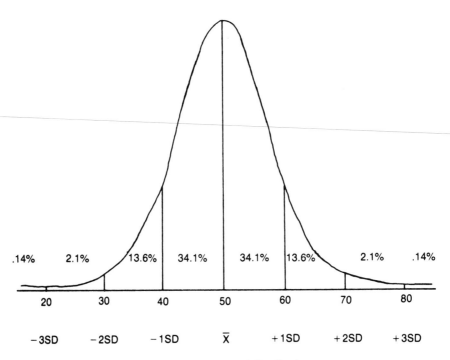

Figure 11–5. Standard deviations in a normal distribution

Table 11–5. Example of Table Showing Central Tendency and Variability Measures: Study of Uncertainty in Illness Among Coronary Bypass Surgery Patients

Subscale of MUIS	1 Week After Surgery				6 Weeks After Surgery			
	Mean	SD	Range	Possible Range	Mean	SD	Range	Possible Range
Ambiguity	36.4	10.8	16–55	18–80	33.6	10.2	15–63	15–75
Complexity	23.1	6.1	12–39	12–60	24.5	5.7	13–43	12–60

Adapted from Redeker (1992), with permission. Originally part of Table 1 of the report, titled *Means, Standard Deviations, and Ranges of MUIS and WCCL Subscales for Surveys 1 and 2 (N = 129)*.

1992) examined the concept of uncertainty in illness among coronary bypass surgery patients. The table shows scores on the two subscales of the Mishel Uncertainty in Illness (MUIS) scale, a Likert-type scale administered 1 week (survey 1) and 6 weeks (survey 2) after the surgery. The table presents the means, standard deviations, and observed ranges on the two subscales for the two administrations as well as the potential ranges (*i.e.,* the minimum and maximum value theoretically possible for people answering all items in the extremes). Looking at the values for the Complexity subscale, we learn the following: (1) the average score increased over time (from 23.1 to 24.5), indicating that perceptions of complexity rose over the period of convalescence; (2) the scores, on average, became more similar over time (the standard deviations decreased from 6.1 to 5.7), indicating that there was greater agreement about perceived complexity later in the convalescent period; and (3) the obtained scores clustered closer to the bottom part of the possible range (the highest obtained score was 43, although a score of 60 was theoretically possible), indicating that perceived complexity was not as high as it might have been.

Bivariate Descriptive Statistics

So far, our discussion has focused on descriptive indexes of single variables. The mean, mode, standard deviation, and so forth are all used to describe data for one variable at a time. We have been examining what is referred to as **univariate** (one-variable) **descriptive statistics.** Research usually is concerned, however, with relationships between variables. What is needed, then, is some method of describing these relationships. In this section, we look at **bivariate** (two-variable) **descriptive statistics.**

Contingency Tables

A **contingency table** is a two-dimensional frequency distribution in which the frequencies of two variables are **cross-tabulated.** Suppose we have data on participants' genders and responses to a question on whether they are nonsmokers, light

Table 11–6. Contingency Table for Gender and Smoking Status Relationship

Gender	Smoking Status			
	Nonsmoker	Light Smoker	Heavy Smoker	Total
Female	10 (45% of females)	8 (35% of females)	4 (18% of females)	22 (50% of sample)
Male	6 (27% of males)	8 (35% of males)	8 (36% of males)	22 (50% of sample)
TOTAL	16 (36% of sample)	16 (36% of sample)	12 (27% of sample)	44 (100% of sample)

smokers, or heavy smokers. We might be interested in learning if there is a tendency for men to smoke more heavily than women or vice versa. Some fictitious data on these two variables are presented in a contingency table in Table 11–6. Six cells are created by placing one variable (gender) along the vertical dimension and the other variable (smoking status) along the horizontal dimension. After all subjects have been placed in the appropriate cells, percentages can be computed. This simple procedure allows us to see at a glance that, in this particular sample, women were more likely than men to be nonsmokers (45% versus 27%) and less likely to be heavy smokers (18% versus 36%). Contingency tables usually are used with nominal data or ordinal data that have few levels or ranks. In the present example, gender is a nominal measure, and smoking status is an ordinal measure.

Table 11–7 presents a cross-tabulation table from an actual study (Anderson,

Table 11–7. Example of a Cross-tabulation Table: Study of Men and Women With HIV Infection

Source of HIV Infection	Men		Women		Total	
	n	%	n	%	n	%
Gay/bisexual contacts	54	70.1	0	0.0	54	42.5
Heterosexual contacts	3	3.9	31	62.0	34	26.8
Blood transfusion	4	5.2	7	14.0	11	8.7
Intravenous drug use	16	20.8	12	24.0	28	22.0
TOTAL	77	(100.0)	50	(100.0)	127	(100.0)

Adapted from Anderson (1995), with permission. Originally part of Table 2 of the report, titled *Sociodemographic Differences Between Men and Women.*

1995) in which the investigator examined interrelationships among personality, socioeconomic status, and appraisal in men and women with HIV infection. In this table, the source of the HIV infection is cross-tabulated with the patients' gender. Overall, 42.5% of the sample reported gay or bisexual contacts as the source of the infection, whereas 26.8% of the sample cited heterosexual contacts as the source. However, there were powerful gender differences: 70.1% of the men but none of the women reported gay or bisexual contacts as the source; women, by contrast, were more likely to cite heterosexual contacts (62.0% versus 3.9% for men).

A comparison of Tables 11–6 and 11–7 illustrates that cross-tabulated data can be presented in one of two ways (*i.e.*, percentages within the cells can be computed on the basis of either row totals or column totals). In Table 11–6, the number 10 in the first cell (female nonsmokers) was divided by the *row* total (*i.e.*, by the total number of females—22) to arrive at the percentage (45%) of females who were nonsmokers. (The table might well have shown 63% in this cell—the percentage of nonsmokers who were female.) In Table 11–7, the number 54 in the first cell (men citing gay/bisexual contacts) was divided by the *column* total (*i.e.*, by the total number of men—77) to yield the percentage of males with a gay/ bisexual contact as the HIV source (70.1%). Either approach is acceptable— although the latter is generally preferred because then the percentages in a column total 100%. You may need to spend an extra minute when examining cross-tabulation tables to determine which total was used as the basis for calculating percentages.

Correlation

The most common method of describing the relationship between two measures is through **correlation** procedures. The correlation question is: To what extent are two variables related to each other? For example, to what degree are anxiety test scores and blood pressure measures related? This question can be answered quantitatively by the calculation of an index that describes the intensity and direction of the relationship: The **correlation coefficient.**

Two variables that are obviously related to one another are height and weight. On average, tall people tend to weigh more than short people. We would say that the relationship between height and weight was a **perfect relationship** if the tallest person in the world was the heaviest, the second tallest person was the second heaviest, and so forth. The correlation coefficient summarizes how perfect a relationship is. The possible values for a correlation coefficient range from -1.00 through .00 to $+1.00$. If height and weight were perfectly correlated, the correlation coefficient expressing this relationship would be 1.00. Because the relationship exists but is not perfect, the correlation coefficient is probably in the vicinity of .50 or .60. The relationship between height and weight is called a **positive relationship** because increases in height tend to be associated with increases in weight.

When two variables are totally unrelated, the correlation coefficient is equal to zero. One might anticipate that a woman's dress size is unrelated to her intelligence. Large women are as likely to perform well on tests of mental ability as small women. The correlation coefficient summarizing such a relationship would presumably be in the vicinity of .00.

Correlation coefficients running between .00 and −1.00 express what is known as a **negative,** or **inverse, relationship.** When two variables are inversely related, increments in one variable are associated with decrements in the second variable. Let us suppose that there is an inverse relationship between adult patients' ages and the number of questions they ask before surgery. This means that, on average, the older the patient, the fewer the questions. If the relationship were perfect (*i.e.,* if the oldest patient asked the fewest questions and so on), then the correlation coefficient would be equal to −1.00. In actuality, the relationship between age and number of questions is likely to be modest—perhaps in the vicinity of −.20 or −.30. A correlation coefficient of this magnitude describes a weak relationship wherein older patients tend to ask few questions and younger patients tend to be more inquisitive. It should be noted that the higher the absolute value of the coefficient (*i.e.,* the value disregarding the sign), the stronger the relationship. A correlation of −.80, for instance, is much stronger than a correlation of +.20.

The most commonly used correlation index is the **product–moment correlation coefficient,** also referred to as the **Pearson's *r*.** This coefficient is computed when the variables being correlated have been measured on either an interval or ratio scale. The correlation index generally used for ordinal-level measures is **Spearman's rank-order correlation** (r_s) sometimes referred to as **Spearman's rho**.

Perfect correlations (+1.00 and −1.00) are rare in research with humans. It is difficult to offer guidelines on what should be interpreted as strong or weak relationships. This determination depends, to a great extent, on the nature of the variables. If we were to measure patients' body temperatures both orally and rectally, a correlation (*r*) of .70 between the two measurements would be low. For most psychosocial variables (*e.g.,* stress and severity of illness), however, an *r* of .70 would be rather high.

In research reports, correlation coefficients are often reported in tables displaying a two-dimensional **correlation matrix,** in which every variable is displayed in both a row and a column. To read a correlation matrix, one finds the row for one of the variables and reads across until the row intersects with the column for the second variable. Table 11–8 presents a portion of a correlation matrix from the previously mentioned study of coronary bypass surgery patients (Redeker, 1992). This table lists, on the left, the two subscales of the Uncertainty in Illness scale as well as three subscales (Avoidance, Blamed Self, and Problem-Focused) of an instrument that measures different styles of coping with stress. The numbers in the top row, from 1 to 5, correspond to the five subscales: 1 is Ambiguity, 2 is Complexity, and so forth. The correlation matrix shows, in the first row, the value of the correlation coefficient between Ambiguity on the one hand and all five variables on the other. At the intersection of row 1 and column 1, we find the value 1.00, which simply indicates that scores on the Ambiguity subscales are perfectly correlated with themselves. The next entry represents the correlation between the

Table 11–8. Example of a Correlation Matrix: Study of Uncertainty in Illness and Coping Among Bypass Surgery Patients

	1	2	3	4	5
1. Ambiguity	1.00	.66	.31	.13	−.09
2. Complexity		1.00	.20	.06	−.03
3. Avoidance			1.00	.55	.40
4. Blamed self				1.00	.33
5. Problem-focused					1.00

Adapted from Redeker (1992), with permission. Originally part of Table 2, titled *Correlations Between Uncertainty and Coping Variables for Surveys 1 and 2.*

Ambiguity and Complexity scores; the value of .66 (which can be read as +.66) indicates a fairly high and positive relationship between the two subscales of the MUIS. Ambiguity scores are more modestly (but still positively) related to Avoidance and Blamed Self subscales scores. Finally, there was a slight tendency for people with high scores on the Ambiguity subscale to have low scores on the Problem-Focused subscale ($r = -.09$). The next row presents the values of the correlation coefficients between Complexity scores and the remaining variables, and so on. The strongest correlation in the matrix is between scores on the two MUIS subscales ($r = .66$), and the weakest correlation is between scores on the Complexity and Problem-Focused subscales ($r = -.03$).

 # INTRODUCTION TO INFERENTIAL STATISTICS

Descriptive statistics are useful for summarizing empirical information, but usually the researcher needs to do more than simply describe the sample data. **Inferential statistics,** which are based on the **laws of probability,** provide a means for drawing conclusions about a population, given data obtained from a sample. This is precisely what most researchers want to be able to do.

Sampling Distributions

If a sample is to be used as a basis for making estimates of population characteristics, then it is clearly advisable to obtain as representative a sample as possible. As we saw in Chapter 8, random samples (*i.e.,* probability samples) are the most effective means of securing representative samples. Inferential statistical procedures are based on the assumption of random sampling from populations, although this assumption is widely violated and ignored.

Even when random sampling is used, however, it cannot be expected that the sample characteristics will be identical with those of the population. Suppose we have a population of 30,000 nursing school applicants who have taken the SAT. By using descriptive statistics on the scores, we find that the mean for the entire population is 500 and that the standard deviation is 100. Now, let us suppose that we do not know these parameters, but that we must estimate them by using the scores from a random sample of 25 students. Should we expect to find a mean of *exactly* 500 and a standard deviation of 100 for this sample? It would be extremely improbable to obtain identical values. Let us say that, instead, we calculated a mean of 505. If a completely new random sample were drawn and another mean computed, we might obtain a value such as 497. Sample statistics often fluctuate and are unequal to the value of the corresponding population parameter because of **sampling error.** The challenge for a researcher is to determine whether sample values are good estimates of population parameters.

A researcher works with only one sample on which statistics are computed and inferences made. However, to understand inferential statistics, we must perform a small mental exercise. With the population of 30,000 nursing school applicants, consider drawing a sample of 25 students, calculating a mean, replacing the 25 students, and drawing a new sample. Each mean computed in this fashion will be considered a separate piece of data. If we draw 5000 such samples, we will have 5000 means or data points, which could then be used to construct a frequency polygon, as shown in Figure 11–6. This kind of distribution is called a **sampling distribution of the mean.** A sampling distribution is a theoretical rather than an actual distribution because in practice one does not draw consecutive samples from a population and plot their means.

Statisticians have been able to demonstrate that sampling distributions of means follow a normal distribution—a fact that is helpful in determining the probability that sample values are good estimates of parameters. It can be shown mathematically that the mean of a sampling distribution composed of an infinite number of sample means is equal to the population mean. In the present example, the mean of the sampling distribution is 500, the same value as the mean of the population.

Earlier in this chapter, we discussed the standard deviation in terms of percentages of cases falling within a certain distance from the mean. When scores are normally distributed, 68% of the cases fall between $+1$ SD and -1 SD from the mean. Because a sampling distribution of means is normally distributed, we can make a similar statement. The probability is 68 out of 100 that any randomly drawn sample mean lies within the range of values between $+1$ SD and -1 SD of the mean on the sampling distribution. The problem, then, is to determine the value of the standard deviation of the sampling distribution.

The standard deviation of a theoretical distribution of sample means is called the **standard error of the mean** (often abbreviated **SEM**). The word *error* signifies that the various sample means comprising the distribution contain some error

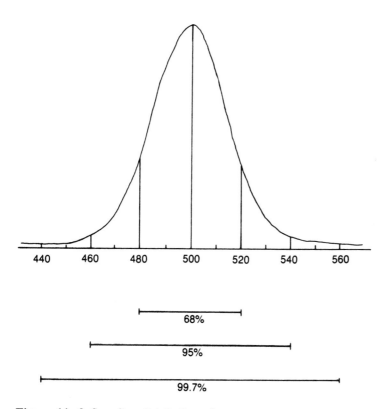

Figure 11–6. Sampling distribution of a mean.

in their estimates of the population mean. The term *standard* indicates the magnitude of a standard, or average, error. The smaller the standard error (*i.e.,* the less variable the sample means), the more accurate are those means as estimates of the population value.

Because one does not ever actually construct a sampling distribution, how can its standard deviation be computed? Fortunately, there is a formula for estimating the standard error of the mean from the data from a single sample, using two pieces of information: The sample's standard deviation and sample size. In the present example, the SEM has been calculated as 20, as shown in Figure 11–6. This statistic represents an estimate of how much sampling fluctuation or sampling error there would be from one sample mean to another in samples of 25 students.

We can now use these calculations to estimate the probability of drawing a sample with a certain mean. With a sample size of 25 and a population mean of 500, the chances are about 95 out of 100 that a sample mean would fall between the values of 460 and 540. Only five times out of 100 would the mean of a randomly selected sample exceed 540 or be less than 460. In other words, only five times out of 100 would we be likely to draw a sample whose mean deviates from the population mean by more than 40 points.

Because the value of the standard error of the mean is partly a function of sample size, we need only increase sample size to increase the accuracy of our estimate of the population mean. Suppose that instead of using a sample of 25 nursing school applicants to estimate the average SAT score of the population, we use a sample of 100 students. With this many students, the standard error of the mean would be 10 rather than 20. In this situation, the probability of obtaining a sample whose mean is greater than 520 or less than 480 would be about 5 in 100. The chances of drawing a sample with a mean very different from that of the population are reduced as the sample size increases because large numbers promote the likelihood that extreme cases will cancel each other out.

You may be wondering why you need to learn about these abstract statistical notions. Consider, though, that what we are talking about concerns how likely it is that the researcher's results are accurate. As an intelligent consumer of nursing research, you need to evaluate critically how believable and valid research results are so that you can decide whether to incorporate the findings into the practice of nursing. The concepts embodied in the standard error are important in such an evaluation and are related to considerations we stressed in Chapter 8 on sampling. First, the more homogeneous the population is on the critical attribute (*i.e.*, the smaller the standard deviation), the more likely it is that results calculated from a sample will be accurate. Second, the larger the sample size, the greater is the likelihood of accuracy. The concepts discussed in this section are also important for you to understand because they are the basis for statistical hypothesis testing.

Hypothesis Testing

Statistical inference consists of two major types of technique: Estimation of parameters and hypothesis testing. **Estimation procedures** are used to estimate a single population characteristic, such as the mean value of some attribute (*e.g.*, the mean creatinine level of patients 24 hours after a kidney transplantation). Estimation procedures, however, are not particularly common because researchers typically are more interested in relationships between two or more variables than in estimating the accuracy of a single sample value. For this reason, we focus here on hypothesis testing.

Statistical **hypothesis testing** provides researchers with objective criteria for deciding whether their hypotheses should be accepted as true or rejected as false. Suppose a nurse researcher hypothesizes that maternity patients exposed to a teaching film on breastfeeding will breastfeed longer than mothers who do not see the film. The researcher subsequently learns that the mean number of days of breastfeeding is 131.5 for 25 experimental-group subjects and 112.1 for 25 control-group subjects. Should the researcher conclude that the hypothesis has been supported? True, the group differences are in the predicted direction, but the results might simply be due to sampling fluctuations. In other words, the two groups might

happen to be different, regardless of their exposure to the film; perhaps in another sample the groups would be nearly identical. Statistical hypothesis testing helps researchers to make objective decisions about the results of their studies. Researchers need such a mechanism to help them decide which outcomes are likely to reflect only chance differences between groups and which are likely to reflect true hypothesized effects.

The procedures used in testing hypotheses are based on rules of negative inference. This logic often seems somewhat awkward and peculiar to beginning students, so we will try to convey the concepts with a concrete illustration. In the above example, a nurse researcher showed the teaching film to only half the mothers and found that, on average, those who had seen the film breastfed longer than those who had not. There are two possible explanations for this outcome: (1) the experimental treatment was successful in encouraging breastfeeding or (2) the difference was due to chance factors (*e.g.,* differences in the characteristics of the two groups even before the film was shown).

The first explanation is the researcher's **scientific hypothesis,** but the second explanation is known as the **null hypothesis.** The null hypothesis, it may be recalled, is a statement that there is no actual relationship between the independent variable and the dependent variable and that any such observed relationship is only a function of chance or sampling fluctuations. The need for a null hypothesis lies in the fact that statistical hypothesis testing is basically a process of disproof or rejection. It is not possible to demonstrate directly that the first explanation—the scientific hypothesis—is correct. But it is possible to show, using theoretical sampling distributions, that the null hypothesis has a high probability of being incorrect, and such evidence lends support to the scientific hypothesis.

The rejection of the null hypothesis, then, is what the researcher seeks to accomplish through **statistical tests.** Although null hypotheses are accepted or rejected on the basis of sample data, the hypothesis is made about population values. The real interest in testing hypotheses, as in all statistical inference, is to use a sample to draw conclusions about a population.

Type I and Type II Errors

The researcher's decision about whether to accept or reject the null hypothesis is based on a consideration of how probable it is that observed group differences are due to chance alone. Because information about the entire population is not available, it is not possible to assert flatly that the null hypothesis is or is not true. The researcher must be content with the knowledge that the hypothesis is either probably true or probably false. We make statistical inferences based on incomplete information, so there is always a risk of making an error.

A researcher can make two types of error: (1) erroneous rejection of a true null hypothesis and (2) erroneous acceptance of a false null hypothesis. The possible outcomes of a researcher's decision are summarized in Figure 11–7. An investigator makes a **Type I error** by rejecting the null hypothesis when it is, in fact, true. For instance, if we concluded that the experimental treatment was effective in promot-

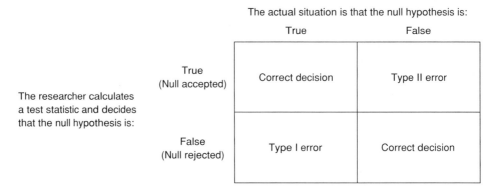

Figure 11–7. Outcomes of statistical decision making

ing breastfeeding when, in actuality, observed group differences were due only to sampling fluctuations, then we would have made a Type I error. In the reverse situation, we might conclude that observed differences in number of days of breastfeeding were due to random sampling fluctuations when, in fact, the experimental treatment *did* have an effect. This situation, in which a false null hypothesis is accepted, is an example of a **Type II error.**

Level of Significance
The researcher does not know when an error in statistical decision making has been committed. The truth or falseness of a null hypothesis could only be definitively ascertained by collecting information from the entire population, in which case there would be no need for statistical inference.

The degree of risk in making a Type I error is controlled by the researcher. The selection of a **level of significance** determines the chance of making this type of error. Level of significance is the phrase used to signify the probability of making a Type I error.

The two most frequently used levels of significance (often referred to as **alpha,** or α) are .05 and .01. If we say we are using a .05 significance level, this means that we are accepting the risk that out of 100 samples, a true null hypothesis would be rejected five times. In 95 out of 100 cases, however, a true null hypothesis would be correctly accepted. With a .01 significance level, the risk of making a Type I error is *lower:* In only one sample out of 100 would we erroneously reject the null hypothesis. By convention, the minimal acceptable level for α in scientific research generally is .05.

Naturally, researchers would like to reduce the risk of committing both types of error. Unfortunately, lowering the risk of making a Type I error increases the risk of making a Type II error. The stricter the criterion we use for rejecting a null hypothesis, the greater the probability that we will accept a false null hypothesis.

Thus, there is a trade-off that the researcher must consider in establishing criteria for statistical decision making. However, researchers can often reduce the risk of a Type II error simply by increasing the size of their samples.[3]

Tests of Statistical Significance

Within a hypothesis testing framework, the researcher uses the data collected in a study to compute a **test statistic.** For every test statistic, there is a related theoretical sampling distribution, analogous to the sampling distribution of means discussed previously. Hypothesis testing uses theoretical distributions to establish probable and improbable values for the test statistics, which are, in turn, used as a basis for accepting or rejecting the null hypothesis.

A simple example will illustrate the process. Suppose a researcher wants to test the hypothesis that the average SAT score for students applying to nursing schools is higher than that for all other students taking the SAT, whose mean score is 500. The null hypothesis is that there is no difference in the mean population scores of students who do or do not apply to nursing school. Let us say that the mean score for a sample of 100 nursing school applicants is 525, with a standard deviation of 100. Using statistical procedures, we can assess the likelihood that a mean of 525 represents a chance deviation from the population mean of 500 (*i.e.,* a random fluctuation resulting in sampling error).

In hypothesis testing, one assumes that the null hypothesis is true and then gathers evidence to disprove it. Assuming a mean of 500 for the nursing school applicant population, a sampling distribution can be constructed with a mean of 500 and a standard deviation equal to about 10. In this example, 10 is the standard error of the mean, calculated from a formula that used the standard deviation of 100 in the sample. This is shown in Figure 11–8. Based on our knowledge of normal distribution characteristics, we can determine probable and improbable values of sample means drawn from the nursing school applicant population. If, as is assumed, the population mean is actually 500, then 95% of all sample means would fall between 480 and 520, because in a normal distribution, 95% of the cases are within two standard deviations from the mean. The obtained sample mean of 525 lies in the region considered improbable if the null hypothesis is correct, assuming that our criterion of improbability is a significance level of .05. The improbable range beyond 2 *SD*s corresponds to only 5% (100% − 95%) of the sampling distribution. We would thus reject the null hypothesis that the mean of the nursing school applicant population equals 500. We would not be justified in saying that we have *proved* the research hypothesis because the possibility of having made a Type I error remains.

Researchers reporting the results of hypothesis tests often state that their findings are **statistically significant.** As noted earlier in this book, the word

---

[3] The risk of committing a Type II error can be estimated through power analysis. In many nursing studies, the risk of a Type II error is high because of small sample size, suggesting a need for greater use of power analysis among nurse researchers.

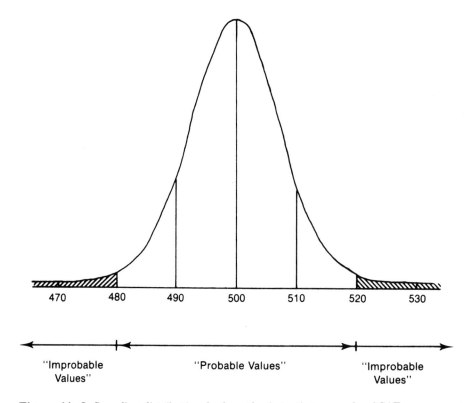

Figure 11–8. Sampling distribution for hypothesis testing example of SAT scores

significant should not be read as *important* or *meaningful.* In statistics, the term *significant* means that the obtained results are not likely to have been due to chance, at some specified level of probability. A **nonsignificant result** means that any observed difference or relationship could have been the result of a chance fluctuation.

Parametric and Nonparametric Tests

A distinction can be made between two classes of statistical tests. The bulk of the tests that we discuss in this chapter—and also most tests used by researchers— are called **parametric tests.** Parametric tests are characterized by three attributes: (1) they focus on population parameters; (2) they require measurements on at least an interval scale; and (3) they involve several other assumptions about the variables under consideration, such as the assumption that the variables are normally distributed in the population.

Nonparametric tests may be contrasted with parametric tests in terms of several of these characteristics. This second class of statistical tests is not based on the estimation of parameters. Nonparametric methods also involve less restrictive assumptions about the shape of the distribution of the critical variables. Finally, nonparametric tests are usually applied when the data have been measured on a nominal or ordinal scale.

Parametric tests are more powerful and offer more flexibility than nonparametric tests and are, for these reasons, generally preferred when variables are measured on at least the interval scale. Nonparametric tests are most useful when (1) the data under consideration cannot in any manner be construed as interval-level measures or (2) the distribution of data is markedly nonnormal.

Overview of Hypothesis Testing Procedures

In the next section, various types of statistical procedures for testing research hypotheses are discussed. The emphasis throughout is on explaining applications of statistical tests and on interpreting the meaning of test results rather than on describing actual computations. You may well wish to pursue other texts for a fuller explanation of statistical techniques. In this basic textbook on research methods, our primary concern is to alert you to the potential use (or misuse) of statistical tests for different purposes.

Each of the statistical tests described in this chapter has a particular application and can be used only with particular kinds of data; however, the overall process of testing hypotheses is basically the same for all tests. The steps that a researcher takes are essentially the following:

1. *Determination of which test statistic to use.* The researcher must consider such factors as whether a parametric test is justified, which levels of measurement were used for the measures, and, if relevant, how many groups are being compared.
2. *Selection of the level of significance.* An α level of .05 is usually acceptable, but, in some cases, the level is set more stringently at .01 or .001.
3. *Computation of a test statistic.* The researcher then calculates a test statistic based on the actual collected data, using appropriate computation formulas.
4. *Calculation of the degrees of freedom.* The term **degrees of freedom** (df) is a concept used throughout hypothesis testing to refer to the number of observations free to vary about a parameter. The concept is too complex for full elaboration here, but the computation of degrees of freedom is extremely easy.
5. *Comparison of the test statistic to a tabled value.* Theoretical distributions have been developed for all test statistics, and values for these distributions are available in statistical tables. The theoretical distributions enable the researcher to discover whether obtained values of the test statistic are beyond the range of what is probable if the null hypothesis is true. The researcher examines a table appropriate for the test used, obtains the tabled value by entering the table at a point corresponding to the relevant degrees of freedom and significance level, and compares the tabled value

to that of the computed test statistic. If the tabled value is smaller than the absolute value of the computed test statistic, then the results are statistically significant. If the tabled value is larger, then the results are nonsignificant.

When a computer is used to perform the calculations, the researcher follows only the first step and then gives the necessary commands to the computer. The computer will calculate the test statistic, the degrees of freedom, and the *actual* probability that the relationship being tested is due to chance. For example, the computer may print that the probability (p) of an experimental group doing better on a measure of postoperative recovery than the control group on the basis of chance alone is .025. This means that fewer than 3 times out of 100 (or only 25 times out of 1000) would a difference between the two groups as large as the one obtained reflect haphazard sampling differences rather than differences resulting from an experimental intervention. This computed probability level can then be compared with the investigator's desired level of significance. In the present example, if the significance level desired were .05, the results would be said to be significant because .025 is more stringent than .05. If .01 were the desired significance level, the results would be nonsignificant (sometimes abbreviated *NS*). Any computed probability level greater than .05 (*e.g.,* .20) indicates a nonsignificant relationship (*i.e.,* one that could have occurred on the basis of chance in more than 5 out of 100 samples). In the section that follows, a number of specific statistical tests and their applications are described.

▨ BIVARIATE STATISTICAL TESTS

You will find that researchers use a wide variety of statistical tests to analyze their research data and to make inferences about the validity of their hypotheses. Some of the most frequently used bivariate tests are briefly described and illustrated below.

t-Tests

A common research situation is the comparison of two groups of people with regard to the dependent variable. For instance, we might wish to compare the scores of an experimental group with those of a control group of patients on a measure of physical functioning. Or we might be interested in contrasting the average heart rate of cardiac patients before and after an exercise stress test. The appropriate analytic procedure for testing the statistical significance of a difference between the means of two groups is the parametric test known as the *t*-**test**.

Suppose a researcher wanted to test the effect of early discharge of maternity patients on their perceived maternal competence. The researcher administers a scale of perceived maternal competence 1 week after delivery to 10 primiparas who were discharged early (*i.e.*, within 24 hours of delivery) and to 10 primiparas who remained in the hospital for longer periods. Some hypothetical data for this example are presented in Table 11–9. The mean scores for these two groups are 19.0 and 25.0, respectively. Is this difference a true population difference—is it likely to be replicated in other samples of early-discharge and later-discharge mothers? Or is the group difference just the result of chance fluctuations? The 20 scores—10 for each group—vary from one person to another. Some of that variability can be attributed to individual differences in perceived maternal competence. Some of the variability could also be due to measurement error (unreliability of the researcher's scale), whereas some could be the result of the participants' moods on that particular day, and so forth. The research question is: Can a significant portion of the variability be attributed to the independent variable—time of discharge from the hospital? The *t*-test allows the researcher to answer this question in an objective fashion.

The formula for computing the *t* statistic essentially involves using information about the group means, sample size, and variability to generate a value for *t*. In the present example, the computed value of *t* is 2.86. The researcher would then calculate the degrees of freedom. Here, the degrees of freedom are equal to the total sample size minus 2 ($df = 20 - 2 = 18$). Then the researcher would look in a table to determine the tabled value for *t* with 18 degrees of freedom. For an α level of .05, the tabled value of *t* is 2.10. This value establishes an upper limit to what is probable if the null hypothesis is true. Thus, the calculated *t* of 2.86 is improbable (*i.e.*, statistically significant). We are now in a position to say that the primiparas

Table 11–9. Fictitious Data for *t*-Test Example: Scores on a Perceived Maternal Competence Scale for Two Groups of Mothers

Regular-Discharge Mothers	Early-Discharge Mothers
30	23
27	17
25	22
20	18
24	20
32	26
17	16
18	13
28	21
29	14
Mean = 25.0	Mean = 19.0; $t = 2.86$;
	$df = 18, p < .05$

discharged early had significantly lower perceptions of maternal competence than those who were not discharged early. The difference in perceived maternal competence between the two groups was sufficiently large that it is improbable that it reflects merely chance fluctuations. In fewer than 5 out of 100 samples would a difference this great be found by chance alone.

The situation we just described calls for an **independent groups *t*-test**: The study participants in the two groups were different people, independent of each other. There are certain situations for which this type of *t*-test is not appropriate. For example, if means for a single group of people measured before and after an intervention were being compared, then the researcher would compute a **paired *t*-test** (also known as a **dependent groups *t*-test**), using a different formula.

Table 11–10 presents the results of four independent *t*-tests from an actual study in which women with stage I breast cancer were compared with a matched comparison group of women who had not experienced breast cancer, in terms of four psychosocial characteristics (Nelson, 1991). The women who had breast cancer had higher scores on a question about perceived health (they perceived themselves as less healthy). This difference was not statistically significant, however, and could thus have been the result of random fluctuations in the sample. Similarly, the two groups did not differ significantly on the Self-Esteem or Health-Promoting Lifestyles scales. The two groups differed significantly only in terms of the Benefits and Barriers to Exercise scale, indicating significantly more perceived barriers (and fewer benefits) to exercise among those in the breast cancer group.

Table 11–10. Example of a Table with *t*-Tests: Psychosocial Variables by Breast Cancer Group Status

Variables	Group with Breast Cancer ($n = 54$)		Matched Cohorts ($n = 54$)		t	p
	$\bar{X}$	SD	$\bar{X}$	SD		
Perceived Health	2.1	.9	1.9	.7	1.48	NS
Self-Esteem	31.2	4.7	31.4	3.7	−.18	NS
Health-Promoting Lifestyle Profile	141.3	18.6	141.7	17.5	−.11	NS
Benefits and Barriers to Exercise	104.9	18.9	123.2	27.3	−2.40	<.05

Reprinted from the *Oncology Nursing Forum* with permission from the Oncology Nursing Press, Inc. Nelson, Jenenne P. Perceived Health, Self-Esteem, Health Habits, and Perceived Benefits and Barriers to Exercise in Women Who Have and Who Have Not Experienced Stage I Breast Cancer. *Oncology Nursing Forum* 18(7):1191–1197, 1991.

Analysis of Variance

The procedure known as **analysis of variance (ANOVA)** is another parametric procedure used to test the significance of mean group differences. ANOVA, unlike the *t*-test, is not restricted to two-group situations; the means of three or more groups can be compared. The statistic computed in an ANOVA test is the **F ratio**. ANOVA decomposes the total variability of a set of data into two components: (1) variability attributable to the independent variable and (2) variability due to all other sources, such as individual differences and measurement error. Variation *between* the groups being compared is contrasted with variation *within* groups to yield an F ratio.

Suppose that a researcher were interested in comparing the effectiveness of different instructional techniques to teach high school students about AIDS. One group of students is exposed to a film on AIDS. A second group is given a special lecture. A third group serves as a control group and receives no special instruction. The dependent variable in this study is the student's score on the AIDS knowledge test the day after the intervention. The null hypothesis for this study is that the population means for AIDS knowledge test scores will be the same for all three groups, whereas the research hypothesis predicts that the mean test scores will be different in the three groups.

The 60 test scores shown in Table 11–2 are reproduced in Table 11–11, according to treatment group. As this table shows, there is variation from one student to the next within a group, but there are also group differences. The mean test scores are 25.35, 24.75, and 20.15 for groups A, B, and C, respectively. These

Table 11–11. Fictitious Data for One-Way ANOVA: Instructional Mode Effects on AIDS Knowledge Test Scores

	Film Group (A)		Lecture Group (B)		Control Group (C)		
	26	25	22	24	15	22	
	20	29	24	25	26	19	
	16	30	27	21	24	20	
	25	27	23	27	18	22	
	25	29	23	25	20	18	$F = 18.64$
	23	28	26	21	20	24	$df = 2, 57$
	26	26	22	24	19	18	$p < .001$
	25	25	24	29	21	23	
	24	27	24	28	17	20	
	23	28	30	26	17	24	
Mean	25.35		24.75		20.15		

means are different, but are they significantly different? Or are the differences attributable to random fluctuations?

If we applied ANOVA to these data, we would find an F ratio of 18.64. Two types of degree of freedom must be calculated: Between groups, which is the number of groups minus 1, and within groups, which is the total number of subjects minus the number of groups. In this example, then, $df = 2$ and 57. In a table of values for a theoretical F distribution, we would find that the value of F for 2 and 57 df, for an alpha of .05, is 3.16. Because our obtained F value of 18.64 exceeds 3.16, we reject the null hypothesis that the population means are equal. The differences between groups in average test scores are well beyond chance expectations. Differences of this magnitude would be obtained by chance alone in fewer than 5 samples out of 100. (Actually, the probability of achieving an F of 18.64 by chance alone is less than 1 in 1000.)

The data support the hypothesis that the instructional interventions affect students' knowledge about AIDS. The ANOVA procedure does not allow us to say, however, that each group differed significantly from all other groups. We cannot tell from these results if treatment A was significantly more effective than treatment B. Statistical analyses known as **multiple comparison procedures** (also called **post hoc tests**) should be used in these situations. The function of these procedures is to isolate the comparisons between group means that are responsible for the rejection of the overall ANOVA null hypothesis. Note that it is *not* appropriate to use a series of t-tests (Group A versus B, A versus C, and B versus C) in this situation because this would increase the risk of a Type I error.

ANOVA also can be used to test the effect of two (or more) independent variables on a dependent variable (*e.g.*, when a factorial experimental design or a blocking design have been used). Let us suppose we were interested in determining whether the two instructional techniques discussed previously were equally effective in helping both freshmen and sophomore high school students acquire knowledge about AIDS. We could set up a design in which freshmen and sophomores would be randomly assigned, separately, to the two modes of instruction. Some hypothetical data for the four groups are shown in Table 11–12. The data in this table reveal the following about two **main effects:** On average, people in the film group scored higher than those in the lecture group (25.35 versus 24.75); and sophomore students scored higher than freshmen (26.20 versus 23.90). In addition, there is an **interaction effect:** Freshmen scored higher when exposed to the lecture, whereas sophomores scored higher when exposed to the film. By performing a two-way ANOVA on these data, it would be possible to ascertain the statistical significance of these differences.

In research reports, tables displaying ANOVA results are sometimes organized in a fashion similar to that used in Table 11–10 for t-tests, with descriptive statistics on the dependent variables for the groups being compared, followed by the value of the test statistic (F) and the probability level. Other researchers, however, present ANOVA results somewhat differently. One example is shown in Table 11–13. This table is from a study of the sexual development of adolescents with

Table 11–12. Fictitious Data for Two-Way (2×2) ANOVA Example: Instructional Mode and Year in School in Relation to Test Scores

Year in School	Instructional Mode					
	Film			Lecture		
Freshman	26 20	$\bar{X} = 23.3$		22 24	$\bar{X} = 24.5$	Freshman mean = 23.90
	16 25			27 33		
	25 23			23 26		
	26 25			22 24		
	24 23			24 30		
Sophomore	25 29	$\bar{X} = 27.4$		24 25	$\bar{X} = 25.0$	Sophomore mean = 26.20
	30 27			21 27		
	29 28			27 25		
	26 25			21 24		
	27 28			28 26		
	Film group mean = 25.35			Lecture group mean = 24.75		Grand mean = 25.05

physical disabilities (Meeropol, 1991). It displays the results of an ANOVA in which scores on a scale of self-perceived peer sexual similarity were analyzed in relationship to the nature of the disability. The degrees of freedom for the analysis are shown in the first column: There were 6 *df* between groups (*i.e.*, there were seven diagnostic groups) and 43 *df* within groups. The next two columns are headed *SS* and *MS*, which are abbreviations for sum of squares and mean square, respectively. The values in these columns represent intermediary calculations performed to derive the *F* statistic. The **sum of squares between groups** is the amount of variability in scores that can be attributed to group differences, whereas the **sum of squares within groups** is the amount of variability from one person to another *within* a diagnostic group. When the *SS* is divided by *df* to arrive at average

Table 11–13. Example of an ANOVA Summary Table: ANOVA for Peer Similarity Means, by Type of Diagnosis

Source	*df*	*SS*	*MS*	*F*	*p*
Between groups	6	14.436	2.406	2.811	.021
Within groups	43	36.802	0.856		
TOTAL	49	51.238			

SS, sum of squares; MS, mean square.
Adapted from Meeropol (1991), with permission. Originally part of Table 5 of the report, titled *ANOVA for Peer Similarity Scale Means.*

variability, the value is referred to as the **mean square.** The ratio of the MS between groups, divided by the MS within groups, yields the F ratio. In this example, the value of F (2.811) with 6 and 43 df, is statistically significant ($p < .05$), indicating that perceived peer sexual similarity among adolescents with physical handicaps differs for those with different types of handicaps (adolescents with scoliosis had especially low scores, suggesting they perceive themselves as more different from their peers than other handicapped adolescents).

Chi-Squared Test

The **chi-squared** (χ^2) **test** is a nonparametric test used when there are categories of data and hypotheses about the proportion of cases that fall into the various categories, as when a contingency table has been created. Consider the following example. A researcher is interested in studying the effect of planned nursing instruction on patients' compliance with a self-medication regimen. The experimental group of patients is instructed by nurses who are implementing a new instructional approach based on Orem's Self-Care Model. A second (control) group of patients is cared for by nurses who continue their usual mode of instruction. The hypothesis being tested is that a higher proportion of people in the experimental group than in the control group will comply with the regimen. Some hypothetical data for this example are presented in Table 11–14.

The chi-squared statistic is computed by summing differences between the observed frequencies in each cell and the frequencies that would be expected if there were no relationship between the independent variable and the dependent variable. In this example, the value of the computed χ^2 statistic is 18.18. As usual, the researcher would need to compare this test statistic with the value from a theoretical chi-squared distribution. For the chi-squared statistic, the degrees of freedom are equal to the number of rows minus 1 times the number of columns minus 1. In the present case, $df = 1 \times 1$, or 1. With one degree of freedom, the value that must be exceeded to establish significance at the .05 level is 3.84. The obtained value of 18.18 is substantially larger than would be expected by chance.

Table 11–14. Observed Frequencies
for a Chi-Squared Example on Patient Compliance

	Experimental	**Control**	**Total**
Compliance	60	30	90
Noncompliance	40	70	110
TOTAL	100	100	200

$\chi^2 = 18.18$; $df = 1$; $p < .001$

Thus, we can conclude that a significantly larger proportion of patients in the experimental group than in the control group complied with the self-medication instructions.

Earlier in this chapter, we presented an example of a cross-tabulation table from a study of HIV-positive men and women, cross-tabulating gender with source of the HIV infection (see Table 11–7). The value of the chi-squared statistic computed from the data in that table is 76.15. With 3 df, this χ^2 value is significant at the .001 level: Men and women were significantly different with respect to source of the HIV infection.

Correlation Coefficients

We explained previously the purpose and interpretation of Pearson's product–moment correlation coefficient. Pearson's r is both descriptive and inferential. As a descriptive statistic, the correlation coefficient summarizes the magnitude and direction of a relationship between two variables. As an inferential statistic, r is used to test hypotheses about population correlations. In a correlation situation, the null hypothesis is that there is no relationship between two variables of interest.

Suppose we were studying the relationship between patients' self-reported level of stress (higher scores imply more stress) and the pH level of their saliva. With a sample of 50 patients, we find that $r = -.29$. This value implies that there was a tendency for people who received high stress scores to have lower pH levels than those with low stress scores. But we need to question whether this finding can be generalized to the population. Does the coefficient of $-.29$ reflect a random fluctuation, observed only in the particular group of participants sampled, or is the relationship significant? Degrees of freedom for correlation coefficients are equal to the number of participants minus 2, or 48 in this example. In a statistical table for correlation coefficients, the tabled value for r with $df = 48$ and a .05 level of significance is .282. Because the *absolute* value of the calculated r is .29, the null hypothesis can be rejected. We may conclude that there is a significant relationship between a person's self-reported level of stress and the acidity of his or her saliva. (In the correlation matrix presented earlier in Table 11–8, all correlations greater than .12 are significant at or beyond the .05 level.)

Guide to Bivariate Statistical Tests

The selection and use of a statistical test depends on several factors, such as the number of groups and the levels of measurement of the research variables. To aid you in evaluating the appropriateness of statistical procedures used by researchers in the literature, a chart summarizing the major features of several commonly used parametric and nonparametric tests is presented in Table 11–15. This table does not include every test that you may encounter in research reports, but it does include the bivariate statistical tests most often used by nurse researchers.

Table 11–15. Guide to Widely Used Bivariate Statistical Tests

Name	Test Statistic	Purpose	Measurement Level*	
			IV	DV
Parametric Tests				
t-test for independent groups	*t*	To test the difference between two independent group means	Nominal	Interval, Ratio
t-test for dependent groups	*t*	To test the difference between two dependent group means	Nominal	Interval, Ratio
Analysis of variance—ANOVA	*F*	To test the difference among the means of 3+ independent groups, or of more than one independent variable	Nominal	Interval, Ratio
Repeated measures ANOVA	*F*	To test the difference among means of 3+ related groups or sets of scores	Nominal	Interval, Ratio
Pearson's *r*	*r*	To test the existence of a relationship between two variables	Interval, Ratio	Interval, Ratio
Nonparametric Tests				
Chi-squared test	χ^2	To test the difference in proportions in 2+ independent groups	Nominal	Nominal
Mann-Whitney *U*-test	*U*	To test the difference in ranks of scores on two independent groups	Nominal	Ordinal
Kruskal-Wallis test	*H*	To test the difference in ranks of scores of 3+ independent groups	Nominal	Ordinal
Wilcoxon signed ranks test	*T (Z)*	To test the difference in ranks of scores of two related groups	Nominal	Ordinal
Friedman test	χ^2	To test the difference in ranks of scores of 3+ related groups	Nominal	Ordinal
Phi coefficient	ϕ	To test the magnitude of a relationship between two dichotomous variables	Nominal	Nominal
Spearman's rank order correlation	r_s	To test the existence of a relationship between two variables	Ordinal	Ordinal

*Measurement level of the independent variable (IV) and dependent variable (DV).

◿ MULTIVARIATE STATISTICAL ANALYSIS

Nursing research has become increasingly sophisticated over the past few decades. One of the ways in which this increased sophistication is demonstrated is through the use of complex statistical analyses. This evolution has resulted in increased rigor in nursing studies, but one unfortunate side effect of this evolution is that it is becoming more difficult for novice consumers to understand research reports. Many studies that are reported in the literature now use advanced **multivariate statistics** for data analysis. We use the term *multivariate* here to refer to analyses dealing with at least three—but usually many more—variables simultaneously.

Given the introductory nature of this text and the fact that many of you are not well grounded in even basic statistical procedures, it simply is not possible to describe in any detail the many complex analytic procedures that are appearing in nursing journals. However, we present some basic information that might assist you in reading reports in which three commonly used multivariate statistics are used: Multiple regression, analysis of covariance (ANCOVA), and factor analysis.

Multiple Regression

Correlations enable researchers to make predictions about phenomena. For example, if the correlation between SAT scores and grades in a nursing program were .60, nursing school administrators would be able to make predictions—albeit imperfect predictions—about applicants' future performance. Because the correlation between two variables is rarely perfect, it is often desirable to try to improve one's ability to predict or explain a dependent variable by including more than one independent variable in the analysis. For example, a researcher might predict that an infant's birth weight is related to the amount of prenatal care the mother received. The researcher could collect data on the number of prenatal visits made and on the birth weight of the infant and then compute a correlation coefficient to determine whether a significant relationship between the two variables exists (*i.e.,* whether knowledge of prenatal care could help predict infant birth weights). Birth weight is affected by many other factors, however, such as gestational period, parental height and weight, nutritional practices of the mother during the pregnancy, and the mother's smoking behavior. Increasing numbers of researchers, therefore, are performing an analysis called **multiple regression** (or **multiple correlation**) that allows the researcher to use more than one independent variable to explain or predict a single dependent variable.

In multiple regression, the dependent variable should be an interval- or ratio-level variable. Independent variables should be either interval/ratio-level variables *or* dichotomous nominal level variables. Dichotomous variables are typically coded either 1 or 0 (*e.g.,* smokes = 1, does not smoke = 0).

When multiple independent variables are used to predict a dependent variable, the index of correlation is the **multiple correlation coefficient,** symbolized as **R.** Unlike the bivariate correlation coefficient r, R does not have negative values. R varies only from .00 to 1.00, showing the *strength* of the relationship between several independent variables and a dependent variable, but not *direction*. It would make no sense to indicate direction because one independent variable could be positively correlated with the dependent variable, whereas a second independent variable could be negatively correlated.

There are several ways of evaluating the R statistic. One is to determine, using procedures similar to those described in the preceding section, whether R is statistically significant (*i.e.,* whether the overall relationship between the set of independent variables and the dependent variable is likely to be real or simply the result of chance sampling fluctuations). This is done through the computation of an F statistic that can be compared to tabled F values.

A second way of evaluating a multiple correlation coefficient is to determine whether the addition of new independent variables adds any further predictive power. For example, a researcher might find that the R between infant birth weight on the one hand and maternal weight and prenatal care on the other is .30. By adding a third independent variable—let's say maternal smoking behavior—R might be increased to .36. Is the increased value of R from .30 to .36 statistically significant? In other words, does knowing about whether the mother smoked during her pregnancy really improve our understanding of the birth-weight outcome, or does the increase in the R value simply reflect a relationship that is peculiar to this sample of women? Multiple regression procedures provide a way of answering this question.

The third way of evaluating the R statistic concerns its magnitude. Researchers ideally would like to be able to understand completely and predict perfectly the dependent variables. In the birth-weight example, if it were possible to identify all the factors that lead to differences in infants' weight, the researcher could collect the relevant data and obtain an R value of 1.00. Usually the value of a computed R statistic in a nursing research study is much smaller—seldom higher than .50. An interesting feature of the R statistic is that, when squared, it can be directly interpreted as the proportion of the variability in the dependent variable that is explained or accounted for by the independent variables. If the researcher could identify factors affecting an infant's birth weight that would result in an R of .80 ($R^2 = .64$), then we could say that nearly two thirds (64%) of the variability in the birth weights of the infants in the sample could be accounted for by the independent variables; one third of the variability, however, is caused by factors yet to be identified or measured. Researchers usually report the results of multiple correlation analyses in terms of the value of R^2 rather than R.

Multiple regression analyses typically yield a great deal of information about how each independent variable is related to the dependent variable. Although it is beyond the scope of this text to explain how to read multiple regression tables, you should recognize that what multiple regression analysis attempts to do is indicate whether an independent variable is related to the dependent variable *even when* the other independent variables in the study are controlled or held constant.

Let us assume that our birth-weight researcher used 10 independent variables to predict or explain infant birth weight. If the amount of prenatal care received during pregnancy continued to be significantly related to the birth-weight outcome, this would mean that prenatal care was an important factor in understanding birth weight even with the other nine variables (which might be the extraneous variables) controlled. The example in the next section explains this concept in greater detail.

Analysis of Covariance

Analysis of covariance (ANCOVA) is essentially a combination of ANOVA and multiple regression procedures. ANCOVA is used as a means of providing statistical control for one or more extraneous variables. This approach is especially valuable in certain types of research situations. For example, when random assignment to treatment groups is not feasible, a quasi-experimental design is often adopted. The initial equivalence of the experimental and comparison groups in these studies is always questionable. In this situation, the researcher must consider whether the obtained results were influenced by preexisting group differences. When experimental control through randomization is lacking, ANCOVA offers the possibility of post hoc statistical control.

Because the concept of statistical control may mystify you, we will attempt to explain the underlying principle with a simple illustration. Suppose we were interested in testing the effectiveness of a special physical training program on physical fitness. For this study, we might use intact groups, such as the employees of two companies. The employees of one company would receive the experimental physical fitness intervention, and the employees of the second company would not. As our measure of physical fitness, let us say we have developed a test that involves performance on a number of activities (*e.g.,* running, throwing, weightlifting). The employees' total physical fitness score is the dependent variable in the study. As might be expected, some people in the sample do well on the test, whereas others perform poorly. The research question is: Can some of the individual differences in performance be attributed to the person's participation in the physical fitness program? Physical fitness performance is also related to other, extraneous characteristics of the study participants (*e.g.,* their ages)—characteristics that might differ between the two intact groups.

Figure 11–9 illustrates how ANCOVA can help in this situation. The large circles in this figure may be taken to represent the total variability (*i.e.,* the total extent of individual differences) in scores for both the experimental and comparison groups on the physical fitness measure. A certain amount of that total variability can be explained by differences in the subjects' ages: Younger people will tend to perform better on the test than older ones. This relationship is schematically represented by the overlapping small circle on the left in part A of Figure 11–9. Another part of the variability can be explained by the subjects' participation or nonparticipation in the physical training program, represented here by the overlapping small circle on the right. In part A, the fact that the two small circles (age and

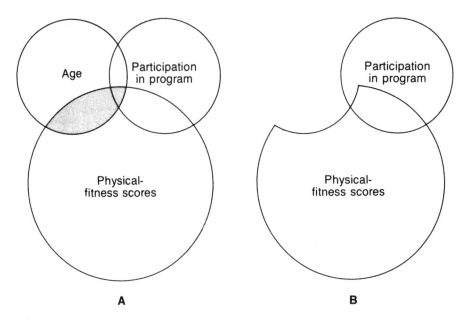

Figure 11-9. Schematic diagram illustrating the principle of analysis of covariance

program participation) overlap indicates that there is a relationship between these two variables. In other words, people in the group receiving the physical training program are, on average, either older or younger than members of the comparison group. Because of this relationship, which could distort the results of the study, age should be controlled.

Analysis of covariance can accomplish this control function by statistically removing the effect of the extraneous variable on the dependent variable. In our illustration, that portion of the physical fitness variability that is attributable to age could be removed through the ANCOVA technique. This is designated in part A of Figure 11-9 by the darkened area of the large circle. Part B illustrates that the final analysis would examine the effect of program participation on fitness scores *after* removing the effect of age (called a **covariate** in ANCOVA) on those scores. With the variability of physical fitness resulting from age removed, we can have a much more precise estimate of the effect of the training program on physical fitness. Note that even after removing the variability resulting from age, there is still individual variability not associated with program participation (the bottom half of the large circle) that is not explained. This means that the precision of the study probably could be further enhanced by controlling additional extraneous variables, such as nutritional habits, gender, and health beliefs. ANCOVA can accommodate multiple extraneous variables.

Analysis of covariance tests the significance of differences between group means after first adjusting the scores on the dependent variable to eliminate the effect of the covariates. This adjustment uses multiple regression procedures. The ANCOVA procedure produces F statistics—one for evaluating the significance of the covariates and another for evaluating the significance of group differences—that can be compared to tabled values of F to determine whether the null hypothesis should be rejected or accepted. ANCOVA, like multiple regression analysis, is an extremely powerful and useful analytic technique for controlling extraneous or confounding influences on dependent measures.

Factor Analysis

Factor analysis is a widely applied procedure that you are likely to find reference to in the research literature, especially in studies seeking to develop, refine, or validate complex instruments. The major purpose of factor analysis is to reduce a large set of variables into a smaller, more manageable set of measures. Factor analysis disentangles complex interrelationships among variables and identifies which variables go together as unified concepts or factors.

As an example, consider a researcher who has prepared 50 Likert statements aimed at measuring women's attitudes toward menopause. Suppose that the research goal is to compare the attitudes of women in different racial and ethnic groups. If the researcher does not combine some of the items to form a scale, it will be necessary to compute 50 chi-squared statistics. The formation of a scale is preferable, but it involves adding together the scores from several individual items. The problem is, which items are to be combined? Would it be meaningful to combine all 50 items? Probably not, because the 50 questions are not all asking exactly the same thing. There are various dimensions, or themes, to women's attitudes toward menopause. One dimension may relate to the issue of aging, whereas another aspect may be concerned with the loss of ability to reproduce. Other questions may touch on the general issue of sexuality, and yet others may concern the release from monthly discomfort or bother. These various dimensions of attitudes toward menopause should serve as the basis for scale construction. Factor analysis offers an objective, empirical method for elucidating the underlying dimensionality of a large number of measures.

Most factor analyses consist of two separate phases. The first step, referred to as **factor extraction,** is to condense the original variables into a smaller number of factors. These factors are derived (almost always by computer) based on the intercorrelations among all the variables. The general goal of this first phase is to seek clusters of highly interrelated variables. In the second phase, called **factor rotation,** the factors are manipulated in such a way that the results can be interpreted by the researcher. The product of this second step is a **factor matrix** that shows how every variable is correlated with the factor. Thus, in our example of the menopause attitudes, the researcher might discover that items 1, 5, 11, 15, 23, 31, 36, 38, 43, and 49 had high correlations with factor 1. By examining the wording of these items, the researcher could attempt to understand what common theme or dimension was being measured. For example, perhaps these 10 questions have to do with the link between menopause and reproductive capacity. These 10 items could then be added together to form a single scale measuring women's attitudes toward the loss of reproductive function that accompanies menopause.

Other Multivariate Techniques

Several other related multivariate techniques increasingly are being used in studies reported in nursing journals. We mention these techniques briefly to acquaint you with terms you might encounter in the research literature.

Discriminant function analysis. In multiple regression analysis, the dependent variable is normally a measure on either the interval or ratio scale. Discriminant function analysis is used to make predictions about membership in categories or groups (*i.e.,* about a dependent variable measured on the nominal scale). For example, a researcher might wish to use several independent variables to predict membership in groups such as: Complying versus noncomplying cancer patients; graduating nursing students versus dropouts; or normal pregnancies versus those terminating in a miscarriage. In discriminant function analysis, as in multiple regression, the independent variables are either interval- or ratio-level measures *or* dichotomous nominal variables (*e.g.,* male versus female, smoker versus nonsmoker).

Multivariate analysis of variance (MANOVA). MANOVA is the extension of ANOVA to more than one dependent variable. This procedure is used primarily to test the significance of differences between the means of two or more groups on two or more dependent variables, considered simultaneously. For instance, if a researcher wanted to examine the effect of two methods of exercise treatment on both diastolic and systolic blood pressure, then a MANOVA would be appropriate. Covariates can also be included, in which case the analysis would be called a **multivariate analysis of covariance (MANCOVA).**

Canonical analysis. Canonical analysis is an extension of multiple regression that is used when there are two or more independent variables *and* two or more dependent variables (*e.g.,* the effect of diet and exercise on heart rate and weight). Canonical analysis determines the nature and extent of the relationship between the two sets of variables. In canonical analysis, composite variables are developed for each set, and the relationship between the sets is expressed by a **canonical correlation coefficient, R_C**.

Logistic regression. Logistic regression (sometimes referred to as **logit analysis**) is a procedure that analyzes the relationships between multiple independent variables and a nominal-level dependent variable. It is thus used in situations similar to discriminant function analysis, but it employs a different statistical estimation procedure that has come to be preferred when the dependent variable involves nominal measurement. Logistic regression transforms the probability of an event occurring (*e.g.,* that a woman will practice breast self-examination or not) into its **odds** (*i.e.,* into the ratio of one event's probability relative to the probability of a second event). After a further transformation, the analysis examines the relationship of the independent variables to the transformed dependent variable. For each predictor, the logistic regression yields an **odds ratio,** which is the factor by which the odds change for a unit change in the predictors.

Causal modeling. Causal modeling involves the development and statistical testing of a hypothesized explanation of the causes of a phenomenon. **Path analysis,** which is based on multiple regression, is the most widely used approach to causal modeling. Alternative methods of testing causal models are also being used by nurse researchers, the most important of which is **linear structural relations analysis,** more widely known as **LISREL.** Both LISREL and path analysis are highly complex statistical techniques whose utility relies on a sound underlying causal theory.

Guide to Multivariate Statistical Analyses

In selecting a multivariate analysis, the researcher must attend to such issues as the number of independent variables, the number of dependent variables, the measurement level of all variables, and the desirability of controlling extraneous variables. Table 11–16 is offered as an aid to help you evaluate the appropriateness of multivariate statistics used in research reports. This chart includes the major multivariate analyses used by nurse researchers.

ASSISTANCE TO CONSUMERS OF NURSING RESEARCH

What to Expect in the Research Literature

The description of statistical analyses is usually the most difficult and intimidating aspect of a quantitative research report for novice research consumers because it includes a lot of numbers, strange-looking symbols, and complex tables. In this section, we present a few tips on what to expect in research reports with regard to statistical information and on how to "read" it.

Tips on Reading Text with Statistical Information
Statistical findings are usually communicated in the results section of a research report and are reported in the text as well as in tables (or, less frequently, figures). This section provides some assistance in reading the text portion.

- There are usually three types of information reported in the results section. First, there are descriptive statistics (such as those shown in Table

Table 11–16. Guide to Widely Used Multivariate Statistical Analyses

Name	Purpose	Measurement Level*			Number of:		
		IV	DV	Cov	IVs	DVs	Covs
Multiple correlation/ regression	To test the relationship between 2+ IVs and 1 DV; to predict a DV from 2+ IVs	N,I,R	I,R		2+	1	
Analysis of covariance (ANCOVA)	To test the difference between the means of 2+ groups, while controlling for 1+ covariate	N	I,R	N,I,R	1+	1	1+
Multivariate analysis of variance (MANOVA)	To test the difference between the means of 2+ groups for 2+ DVs simultaneously	N	I,R		1+	2+	
Multivariate analysis of covariance (MANCOVA)	To test the difference between the means of 2+ groups for 2+ DVs simultaneously, while controlling for 1+ covariate	N	I,R	N,I,R	1+	2+	1+
Canonical analysis	To test the relationship between two sets of variables (variables on the right, variables on the left)	N,I,R	N,I,R		2+	2+	
Factor analysis	To determine the dimensionality/structure of a set of variables						
Discriminant analysis	To test the relationship between 2+ IVs and 1 DV; to predict group membership; to classify cases into groups	N,I,R	N		2+	1	
Logistic regression	To test the relationship between 2+ IVs and 1 DV; to predict the probability of an event; to estimate relative risk (odds ratios)	N,I,R	N		2+	1	

* Measurement level of the independent variable (IV), dependent variable (DV), and covariates (Cov): N = nominal, I = interval, R = ratio.

11–4), which provide the reader with a basic overview of the participants' characteristics and their performance on the dependent variables in the study. Information about the background characteristics of the subjects enables readers to draw conclusions about the groups to which the findings might be generalized. Second, many researchers provide statistical information that enables readers to evaluate the extent of any biases. For example, researchers sometimes compare the characteristics of people who did and did not agree to participate in the study (*e.g.,* using *t*-tests). Or, in a quasi-experimental design, evidence of the preintervention comparability of the experimental and comparison groups might be presented. This information allows the reader to evaluate the internal validity of the study. Finally, statistical information relating directly to the research questions or hypotheses is presented. If the findings are contrary to the researcher's hypotheses, further analyses might be undertaken to help unravel the meaning of the results.

- Inferential statistics are presented in most quantitative studies and are usually more difficult to understand than descriptive statistics. It may help to keep in mind that inferential statistics are just a tool to help us evaluate whether the results obtained in the study are likely to be real and replicable, or simply spurious. As recommended in Chapter 2, you can overcome much of the abstruseness of the results section by translating the basic thrust of the research findings into everyday language.
- The text of research reports normally tells the readers certain facts about the key statistical tests that were performed, including (1) what test was used, (2) the actual value of the calculated statistic, (3) the degrees of freedom, and (4) the level of statistical significance. Examples of how the results of various statistical tests would likely be reported in the text are shown below.

1. *t*-test: $t = 1.68$, $df = 160$, $p = .09$
2. Chi-squared: $\chi^2 = 6.65$, $df = 2$, $p < .05$
3. Pearson's r: $r = .26$, $df = 100$, $p < .01$
4. ANOVA: $F = 0.18$, $df = 1,69$, *NS*

Note that the significance level is sometimes reported as the *actual* computed probability that the null hypothesis is correct, as in example 1. In this case, the observed group differences could be found by chance in 9 out of 100 samples; in other words, this result is *not* statistically significant because the differences have an unacceptably high chance of being spurious. The probability level is sometimes reported simply as having fallen below or above the criterion established by the researcher, as in examples 2 and 3. In both cases, the results are statistically significant because the probability of obtaining such results by chance alone is less than 5 (or 1) in 100. Note that the reader must be careful to read the symbol that follows the **p value** (the probability value) correctly: The symbol, $<$ means *less* *than* and means that the results *are* statistically significant; the symbol > means *greater than* and means that the results are *not* statistically significant. When results do not achieve statistical significance at the desired level, researchers simply may designate that the results were not significant (*NS*), as in example 4.

- The statistical information as just described is normally noted parenthetically following a sentence presenting the findings, as in the following example: The patients in the experimental group had a significantly lower rate of infection than those in the control group ($\chi^2 = 7.99$, $df = 1$, $p < .01$).

- In reading a research report, it is not really important to absorb any numeric information regarding the actual statistical test. For example, the actual value of χ^2 in the preceding example is of no interest in and of itself. What is important is to comprehend whether the statistical tests reveal that the research hypotheses are supported (as indicated by significant results) or not supported (as indicated by nonsignificant results).

Tips on Reading Statistical Tables

Tables are sometimes even more daunting than text and may require considerable scrutiny before all elements in the table are understood. Here are some suggestions that might be useful in reading statistical tables:

- The use of tables for statistical findings allows the researcher to condense a considerable amount of information into a relatively compact space, and space is at a premium in journals. It also prevents a lot of redundancy. Consider, for example, attempting to put the information from a correlation matrix (see Table 11–8) into the text: "The correlation between scores on the Ambiguity and Complexity subscales was .66; the correlation between scores on the Ambiguity and Avoidance subscales was .31. . . ."

- Unfortunately, although tables are efficient, they may be difficult for beginning readers to decipher. Part of the problem is the lack of standardization in table preparation. There is no universally accepted method of presenting *t*-test information, for example. Therefore, each table may present a new challenge to you. Another problem with tables is that some researchers try to include an enormous amount of information in them; we deliberately used tables of relative simplicity and clarity as examples in this chapter. We know of no magic solution for helping you to comprehend tables in research reports. However, we recommend that you (1) read the text and the tables simultaneously because the text may help to unravel what the table is trying to communicate; (2) devote some extra time to making sure you have grasped what the tables are conveying; and (3) for each table, write out a sentence or two that summarizes some of the tabular information in "plain English."

- Before trying to understand the numbers in a table, try to glean as much information as possible from the accompanying words. Table titles and

footnotes often communicate critical pieces of information. The table headings should be carefully reviewed because these indicate what the variables
in the analyses were (often listed in the far left-hand column of the table
as row labels), and what statistical information is included (usually specified
in the top row as the column headings). You may find it helpful to consult
the glossary of symbols in Box 11-2 at the end of this chapter to determine
the meaning of a statistical symbol specified in a report table. (Note that
not all symbols in this appendix were described in this chapter; therefore,
it may be necessary to refer to a statistical textbook, such as that of Polit
(1996), for further information.)
- In tables, the probability levels associated with the significance tests are
  sometimes presented directly, as in Table 11–10. Here, the significance of
  each t-test is indicated in the last column, headed "p." However, researchers
  often indicate the significance of statistical tests in tables through asterisks
  placed right next to the value of the test statistic; by convention, one
  asterisk signifies $p < .05$, two asterisks signify $p < .01$, and three asterisks
  signify $p < .001$ (there is usually a key at the bottom of the table that
  indicates what the asterisks mean). Thus, if this system had been used in
  Table 11–10, the first three ts would have nothing next to them (implying
  nonsignificance), whereas the fourth would be presented as: $-2.40*$.

Critiquing Quantitative Analyses

For novice research consumers, it is often difficult to critique statistical analyses
because they represent the most technical and complex aspects of a report. We
hope this chapter has helped to demystify what statistics are all about, but we also
recognize the limited scope of this presentation. Although it would be unreasonable
to expect you to become adept at evaluating all types of statistical analysis, there
are certain things you should routinely look for in reviewing research reports. Some
specific guidelines are presented in Box 11–1.

The first issue you should consider is whether the data and the research
problem lend themselves to quantitative analysis. Not all information collected in
research projects is in quantitative form, nor should it necessarily be converted to
numbers. In Chapter 12, we discuss how researchers go about analyzing qualitative
information.

Another aspect of the critique should focus on the researcher's decisions about
what analyses to include in the report. Almost invariably, researchers have to be
selective in reporting statistical results; there are generally many more analyses
that the researcher has completed than can be reported in a short journal article.
The reader should determine whether the reported statistical information adequately describes the sample and the important research variables; presents information relating to the internal validity of the study; and reports the results of
statistical tests for all the stated hypotheses. The reader might also wish to consider
if the author included a lot of statistical information that was not really needed, given

---

Box 11-1

Guidelines for Critiquing Quantitative Analyses

1. Does the report include any descriptive statistics? Do these statistics sufficiently describe the major characteristics of the researcher's data set?
2. Were the correct descriptive statistics used? (*e.g.,* were percentages reported when a mean would have been more informative?)
3. Does the report include any inferential statistical tests? If not, should they have been (*e.g.,* were groups compared without information on the statistical significance of group differences)?
4. Was a statistical test performed for each of the hypotheses or research questions?
5. Do the selected statistical tests appear to be appropriate (*e.g.,* are the tests appropriate for the level of measurement of key variables)?
6. Were any multivariate procedures used? If not, should multivariate analyses have been conducted—would the use of a multivariate procedure strengthen the internal validity of the study?
7. Were the results of any statistical tests significant? Nonsignificant? What do the tests tell you about the plausibility of the research hypotheses?
8. Was an appropriate amount of statistical information reported? Were important analyses omitted, or were unimportant analyses included?
9. Were tables used judiciously to summarize statistical information? Is information in the text and tables totally redundant? Are the tables clear, with a good title and carefully labeled headings?
10. Is the researcher sufficiently objective in reporting the results?

---

the stated aims of the study. Another presentational issue concerns the researcher's judicious use of tables to summarize large pieces of statistical information.

A thorough critique also addresses whether the researcher used the appropriate statistical procedures. Tables 11–15 and 11–16 provide useful summaries of the characteristics of the most frequently used statistical tests—although we do not expect that you will readily be able to determine the appropriateness of the tests used in a study without further statistical instruction. The major issues to consider are the number of independent and dependent variables, the levels of measurement of the research variables, the number of groups (if any) being compared, and the appropriateness of using a parametric test. When the researcher has not used a multivariate technique, the reader might well consider whether the use of a bivariate analysis adequately tests the relationship between the independent variable and the dependent variable. For example, if a *t*-test or ANOVA was used, could the internal validity of the study have been enhanced through the statistical control of extraneous variables, using ANCOVA?

Finally, you can be alert to the possibility that the author of a research report is overly subjective in reporting results and insufficiently aware of the tentative nature of research results. The research report should never claim that the data proved, verified, confirmed, or demonstrated that the hypotheses were correct or incorrect. Hypotheses should be described as being *supported* or *not supported*, *accepted* or *rejected.*

The main task for beginning consumers in reading a results section of a research report is to understand the meaning of the statistical tests. What do all the quantitative results indicate about the researcher's hypothesis? How believable are the findings? The answer to such questions form the basis for interpreting the research results, a topic discussed in Chapter 13.

RESEARCH EXAMPLES

The statistical techniques described in this chapter are widely used methods of statistical analysis. Some examples of studies illustrating the use of several of these techniques by nurse researchers are presented in Table 11–17. Three research examples are described in greater detail below. Use the guidelines in Box 11–1 to appraise the analytic decisions made by the researchers, referring to the original studies as needed.

Example of Descriptive Statistics

Gray, Rayome, and Anson (1995), undertook a descriptive study to determine the incidence and characteristics of urinary incontinence among patients with urologic complications caused by spinal injury and managed by clean intermittent catheterization (CIC). A sample of 150 spinal injured patients who had been discharged from a rehabilitation hospital on CIC were questioned about their experiences in the year following their injuries. The data were analyzed through descriptive statistics.

The researchers began by describing their sample. The age range of participants was 6 to 67 years, with a mean age of 30.7 years. The most common (modal) cause of the spinal injury was motor vehicle accident.

The investigators presented a wealth of descriptive information to summarize their findings. For example, the report indicated that only 54% of those patients who performed CIC experienced any incontinent episodes. Of those with any incontinence, 53% reported only episodic incontinence with minimal or moderate leakage. This information was noted in the text and also displayed in graphs.

The investigators found that the use of containment devices was the most commonly used coping strategy among those who experienced incontinence, but 29% of the incontinent patients leaked sufficiently small volumes that no containment device was necessary. However, nearly half (48%) of the 62 incontinent subjects regularly used a condom with a leg bag or a diaper-type device. Pharmacotherapy was the most commonly cited method for preventing leaking, mentioned by 69% of the incontinent patients. The study also revealed that 85% of the sample

Table 11–17. Examples of Statistical Tests
Used by Nurse Reasearchers

Statistical Test	Research Question/Hypothesis	Value of Statistic	p
t-test, independent groups	Pregnant women who self-administer epidural analgesia will use less total fentanyl than women in the control group with nurse-administered boluses (Gordon, Gaines & Hauber, 1994)	$t = -2.96$	$<.001$
t-test, dependent groups	Nonnutritive sucking in intubated infants will reduce the increase in heart rate after onset of cry (Miller & Anderson, 1993)	$t = 9.28$	$<.0005$
ANOVA	Are there differences among underweight, normal weight, and overweight women with regard to gestational weight gain? (Walker, 1996)	$F = 1.30$	$>.05$ (*NS*)
Chi-square test	Rocking infants or giving them a pacifier will reduce bouts of persistent crying following the heelstick procedure (Campos, 1994)	$\chi^2 = 11.87$	$<.01$
Pearson's r	What is the relationship between Parkinson disease patients' physical functioning and their spouse–caregivers' perception of their own health change? (Berry & Murphy, 1995)	$r = .42$	.02
Multiple regression	Which demographic characteristics, social influences, environmental resources, and previous health care experiences predict the number of health care services used by elders with heart disease? (Wallace, Lockhart & Boyle, 1995)	$R^2 = .11$	$<.05$
ANCOVA	What is the efficacy of topical nitroglycerin ointment application on vein size, controlling for pretreatment vein size? (Griffith, James & Cropp, 1994)	$F = 0.96$	.33 (*NS*)
MANOVA	An intervention of intraoperative progress reports for surgical patients' family members will decrease their anxiety scores, mean arterial pressure levels, and heart rates (Leske, 1995)	$F = 12.96$	$<.001$

experienced one or more symptomatic urinary tract infections, and 42% had at least one febrile urinary infection since the commencement of the CIC program.

The authors concluded that the findings provide a basis for nursing management strategies to reduce the incidence and severity of urinary leaking among spinal injured patients managed by CIC.

Example of Bivariate Inferential Statistics: t-Tests and Correlations

Lattavo, Britt, and Dobal (1995) conducted a study designed to compare pulmonary artery (PA), oral, axillary, and two tympanic temperatures. A primary goal of the research was to investigate whether tympanic and core PA temperatures are interchangeable (*i.e.,* whether tympanic temperature is a reliable substitute for pulmonary artery temperature). The research sample consisted of 32 patients from a medical/surgical unit of an urban community hospital. The various temperature measurements were taken in the same order for all patients.

The researchers began by computing correlation coefficients between core PA temperature and all other temperature measures. The correlations ranged from a low of .68 (for axillary temperature) to a high of .84 (for tympanic temperature as measured by the IVAC Core-Check™ tympanic thermometer). All correlations were significant at $p < .01$. However, the researchers reasoned that if the measures are equally reliable in measuring the same phenomenon (body temperature), the r^2s (amount of shared variance) should be at least .80 (*i.e.,* the rs should be about .90 or better). Because none of the measures met this criterion, the authors questioned using alternative temperature measurements as a substitute for core PA temperature.

As a further corroboration, the researchers performed a series of paired *t*-tests. If the PA and tympanic measures were truly comparable, there should be no significant differences between measures made on the same patients. However, most of the *t*-tests *were* statistically significant, indicating true (not spurious) differences between the measures. For example, the mean difference between core PA temperature and IVAC Core-Check™ tympanic temperature was 0.58°F ($t = 3.58$, $df = 31$, $p < .01$). The researchers reached the following conclusion: "Based on these data, the tympanic temperature measurements are not ideal substitutes for the PA temperature measurements" (p. 369).

Example of Multivariate Statistical Analysis: Factor Analysis and Logistic Regression

Kocher and Thomas (1994) used survey data from a random sample of 158 female junior nurse-officers in the Army to examine the factors that might explain the nurses' turnover behavior. The dependent variable in their analysis was nurse retention—whether the nurse remained on active duty 3 years after the survey was completed. The predictor variables available for the analysis included a range of demographic characteristics (*e.g.,* race/ethnicity, age, marital status), as well as 10 items relating to the nurse's satisfaction with various aspects of her job.

For purposes of parsimony, the 10 job satisfaction items were factor analyzed. The analysis indicated that the 10 job satisfaction items could be reduced to four factors. The first factor, which the researchers labeled work/military life, consisted of three items that described various aspects of the nurses' work and working conditions. The second factor, labeled location/assignment stability, involved two items that relate to Army reassignments. The third factor, called advancement opportunities, involved three items (promotions, job training, job security). The fourth factor, called economic benefits, consisted of two items with an economic theme.

Scores on the four factors were then used in a logistic regression analysis designed to predict retention of the Army nurses. The results revealed that two of the satisfaction dimensions (satisfaction with work/military life and satisfaction with location/assignment stability) were significant predictors of retention of nurses in the Army, even when demographic characteristics and characteristics of the external job market were statistically controlled. Marital status and race were also significant predictors. For example, a married nurse who had children had about a one third lower retention likelihood than a nurse who was not married and who had no children.

SUMMARY

There are four major **levels of measurement. Nominal measurement** classifies characteristics of attributes into mutually exclusive categories. **Ordinal measurement** involves the sorting of objects on the basis of their relative standing to each other on a specified attribute. **Interval measurement** indicates not only the rank-ordering of objects on an attribute but also the amount of distance between each object. Distances between numeric values on the interval scale represent equivalent distances in the attribute being measured. **Ratio measurements** are distinguished from interval measurements by virtue of having a rational zero point. Most sophisticated statistical procedures require measures on the interval or ratio scales.

Descriptive statistics enable the researcher to synthesize and summarize quantitative data. A **frequency distribution** is one of the easiest methods of imposing some order on raw data. In a frequency distribution, numeric values are ordered from the lowest to the highest, accompanied by a count of the number (or percentage) of times each value was obtained. **Frequency polygons** are a means of displaying frequency information graphically. A set of data may be completely described in terms of the shape of the distribution, central tendency, and variability. The shape may be symmetric or **skewed,** with one tail longer than the other; it may also be **unimodal** with one peak (*i.e.,* one value of high frequency), or

multimodal with more than one high point. A distribution that is symmetric, unimodal, and not too peaked is a special distribution referred to as a **normal distribution.**

Measures of **central tendency** are indexes that represent the average or typical value of a set of data. The **mode** is the numeric value that occurs most frequently in the distribution. The **median** is that point on a numeric scale above which and below which 50% of the cases fall. The **mean** is the arithmetic average of all the scores in the distribution. In general, the mean is the preferred measure of central tendency because of its stability and its usefulness in other statistical manipulations.

Variability refers to the spread or dispersion of the data. Measures of variability include the range and standard deviation. The **range** is the distance between the highest and lowest score values. The **standard deviation** is an index designed to indicate how much, on average, the scores deviate from the mean.

Bivariate descriptive statistics describe the degree and magnitude of relationships between two variables. A **contingency table** is a two-dimensional frequency distribution in which the frequencies of two nominal- or ordinal-level variables are **cross-tabulated. Correlation coefficients** are statistics designed to describe the direction and magnitude of a relationship between two variables. The values range from -1.00 for a perfect negative correlation, to $.00$ for no relationship, to $+1.00$ for a perfect positive correlation. The most frequently used correlation coefficient is the **product–moment correlation coefficient** (also referred to as **Pearson's *r***), used with variables measured on at least an interval scale.

Inferential statistics, which are based on the **laws of probability,** allow a researcher to make inferences about the characteristics of a population based on data obtained in a sample. Inferential statistics offer the researcher a framework for deciding whether the **sampling error** that results from sampling fluctuation is too high to provide reliable population estimates.

The **sampling distribution of the mean** is a theoretical distribution of the means of many different samples drawn from the same population. The **standard error of the mean**, which is the standard deviation of this theoretical distribution, indicates the degree of average error of a sample mean. The smaller the standard error, the more accurate are the estimates of the population value based on the mean of a sample. Sampling distributions are the basis for inferential statistics.

The testing of hypotheses through statistical procedures enables researchers to make objective decisions about the results of their studies. The **null hypothesis** is a statement that no relationship exists between the variables and that any observed relationship is due to chance or sampling fluctuations. Rejection of the null hypothesis lends support to the research hypothesis. It is possible to fail to reject a null hypothesis when, in fact, it should be rejected; this is a **Type II error.** If a null hypothesis is incorrectly rejected, this is a **Type I error.** Researchers are able to control some of the risk of making a Type I error by establishing a **level of significance** (or **alpha** level), which specifies the probability that such an error will be committed. The .05 level means that in only 5 out of 100 samples would the null hypothesis be rejected when, in fact, it should have been accepted. The results of hypothesis tests are either statistically significant or nonsignificant. The phrase **statistically significant** means that the obtained results are not likely to be due to chance fluctuations at a given probability level (*p* **level**).

Parametric statistical tests involve the estimation of at least one parameter, the use of interval- or ratio-level data, and assumptions of normally distributed variables. **Nonparametric tests** require less stringent assumptions than parametric tests and are used when the level of data is either nominal or ordinal and the normality of the distribution cannot be assumed. Parametric tests are more powerful and are generally preferred.

The most common parametric procedures are the *t*-**test** and **analysis of variance (ANOVA),** both of which can be used to test the significance of the difference between group means. ANOVA is used when there are more than two groups. The nonparametric test that is used most frequently is the **chi-squared test,** which is used in connection with hypotheses relating to differences in proportions. Pearson's *r* can be used to test whether a correlation is significantly different from zero.

Multivariate statistical procedures are increasingly being used in nursing research to untangle complex relationships among three or more variables. **Multiple regression,** or **multiple correlation,** is a method for understanding the effects of two or more independent variables on a dependent variable. The **multiple correlation coefficient,** symbolized by *R*, can be squared to estimate the proportion of the variability of the dependent variable that is explained or accounted for by the independent variables. **Analysis of covariance** (**ANCOVA**) is a procedure that permits the researcher to control statistically extraneous variables (called **covariates**) before determining whether group differences are statistically significant. **Factor analysis** is used to reduce a large set of variables into a smaller set of underlying dimensions. Other multivariate procedures used by nurse researchers include **discriminant function analysis, multivariate analysis of variance (MANOVA), multivariate analysis of covariance (MANCOVA), canonical analysis, logistic regression, path analysis,** and **LISREL.**

◨ STUDY SUGGESTIONS

Chapter 11 of the accompanying *Study Guide to Accompany Essentials of Nursing Research*, 4th edition offers various exercises and study suggestions for reinforcing the concepts presented in this chapter.

Suggested Readings

Methodologic References

Jaccard, J., & Becker, M. A. (1990). *Statistics for the behavioral sciences*. Belmont, CA: Wadsworth.
Jaeger, R. M. (1990). *Statistics: A spectator sport* (2nd ed.). Newbury Park, CA: Sage.

Polit, D. F. (1996). *Data analysis and statistics for nursing research.* Stamford, CT: Appleton & Lange.

Welkowitz, J., Ewen, R. B., and Cohen, J. (1991). *Introductory statistics for the behavioral sciences* (4th ed.). New York: Academic Press.

Substantive References

Anderson, S. E. H. (1995). Personality, appraisal, and adaptational outcomes in HIV seropositive men and women. *Research in Nursing and Health, 18,* 303–312.

Berry, R. A., & Murphy, J. F. (1995). Well-being of caregivers of spouses with Parkinson's disease. *Clinical Nursing Research, 4,* 373–386.

Campos, R. G. (1994). Rocking and pacifiers: Two comforting interventions for heelstick pain. *Research in Nursing and Health, 17,* 321–331.

Gordon, S. C., Gaines, S. K., & Hauber, R. P. (1994). Self-administered versus nurse-administered epidural analgesia after cesarean section. *Journal of Obstetric, Gynecologic, and Neonatal Nursing, 23,* 99–103.

Gray, M., Rayome, R., & Anson, C. (1995). Incontinence and clean intermittent catheterization following spinal cord injury. *Clinical Nursing Research, 4,* 6–21.

Griffith, P., James, B., & Cropp, A. (1994). Evaluation of the safety and efficacy of topical nitroglycerin ointment to facilitate venous cannulation. *Nursing Research, 43,* 203–206.

Groër, M., Mozingo, J., Droppleman, P., Davis, M., Jolly, M. L., Boynton, M., Davis, K., & Kay, S. (1994). Measures of salivary immunoglobin A and state anxiety after a nursing back rub. *Applied Nursing Research, 7,* 2–6.

Kocher, K. M., & Thomas, G. W. (1994). Retaining Army nurses: A longitudinal model. *Research in Nursing and Health, 17,* 59–65.

Koniak-Griffin, D. & Brecht, M. L. (1995). Linkages between sexual risk taking, substance use, and AIDS knowledge among pregnant adolescents and young mothers. *Nursing Research, 44,* 341–345.

Lattavo, K., Britt, J., & Dobal, M. (1995). Agreement between measures of pulmonary artery and tympanic temperatures. *Research in Nursing and Health, 18,* 365–370.

Leske, J. S. (1995). Effects of intraoperative progress reports on anxiety levels of surgical patients' family members. *Applied Nursing Research, 8,* 169–173.

Meeropol, E. (1991). One of the gang: Sexual development of adolescents with physical disabilities. *Journal of Pediatric Nursing, 6,* 243–250.

Miller, H. D., & Anderson, G. C. (1993). Nonnutritive sucking: Effects on crying and heart rate in intubated infants requiring assisted mechanical ventilation. *Nursing Research, 42,* 305–307.

Nelson, J. P. (1991). Perceived health, self-esteem, health habits, and perceived benefits and barriers to exercise in women who have and who have not experienced stage I breast cancer. *Oncology Nursing Forum, 18,* 1191–1197.

Redeker, N. S. (1992). The relationship between uncertainty and coping after coronary bypass surgery. *Western Journal of Nursing Research, 14,* 48–68.

Rudy, S. F., Guckes, A. D., Li, S., McCarthy, G. R., & Brahim, J. S. (1993). Body and orofacial cathexis in edentulous complete-denture-wearing clients. *Clinical Nursing Research, 2,* 296–308.

Sauvé, M. J. (1995). Long-term physical functioning and psychosocial adjustment in survivors of sudden cardiac death. *Heart & Lung, 24,* 133–144.

Walker, L. O. (1996). Predictors of weight gain at 6 months and 18 months after childbirth. *Journal of Obstetric, Gynecologic, and Neonatal Nursing, 25,* 39–48.

Wallace, D. C., Lockhart, J. G., & Boyle, D. K. (1995). Service use by elders with heart disease. *Research in Nursing and Health, 18,* 293–301.

Glossary of Selected Statistical Symbols

This list contains some commonly used symbols in statistics. The list is in approximate alphabetical order, with English and Greek letters intermixed. Nonletter symbols have been placed at the end.

a Regression constant, the intercept

α Greek alpha; significance level in hypothesis testing, probability of Type I error

b Regression coefficient, slope of the line

β Greek beta, probability of a Type II error; also, a standardized regression coefficient (beta weights)

χ^2 Greek chi squared, a test statistic for several nonparametric tests

CI Confidence interval around estimate of a population parameter

df Degrees of freedom

η^2 Greek eta squared, index of variance accounted for in ANOVA context

f Frequency (count) for a score value

F Test statistic used in ANOVA, ANCOVA and other tests

H_0 Null hypothesis

H_1 Alternative hypothesis; research hypothesis

λ Greek lambda, a test statistic used in several multivariate analyses (Wilks' lambda)

μ Greek mu, the population mean

M Sample mean (alternative symbol for $\bar{X}$)

MS Mean square, variance estimate in ANOVA

n Number of cases in a subgroup of the sample

N Total number of cases or sample members

p Probability that observed data are consistent with null hypothesis

r Sample Pearson product-moment correlation coefficient

r_S Spearman's rank order correlation coefficient

R Multiple correlation coefficient

R^2 Coefficient of determination, proportion of variance in Y attributable to Xs

R_C Canonical correlation coefficient

ρ Greek rho, population correlation coefficient

SD Sample standard deviation

SEM Standard error of the mean

σ Greek sigma (lowercase), population standard deviation

Σ Greek sigma (uppercase), sum of

SS Sum of squares

(Continued)

(Continued)

t	Test statistics used in t-tests (sometimes called Student's t)
U	Test statistic for the Mann-Whitney U-test
$\bar{X}$	Sample mean
x	Deviation score
Y'	Predicted value of Y, dependent variable in regression analysis
z	Standard score in a normal distribution
$\mid\ \mid$	Absolute value
$\leq$	Less than or equal to
$\geq$	Greater than or equal to
$\neq$	Not equal to

12

The Analysis of Qualitative Data

Student Objectives

On completion of this chapter, the student will be able to:

- describe some of the challenges that a qualitative analyst faces
- distinguish four prototypical qualitative analysis styles
- describe the four intellectual processes that typically play a role in qualitative analysis
- describe activities that qualitative researchers perform to manage and organize their data, including both manual and computerized approaches
- discuss the procedures used to analyze qualitative data, including both general procedures and those used in the grounded theory approach
- assess the adequacy of the researcher's description of the steps used to analyze the data
- evaluate the steps a qualitative analyst took to validate the understandings gleaned from thematic analysis
- define new terms in the chapter

New Terms

Analytic induction
Axial coding
Basic social process (BSP)
Categorization scheme
Codebook
Conceptual files
Constant comparison
Core category
Editing analysis style
Immersion/crystallization analysis
   style
Level I coding
Level II coding

Level III coding
Manifest content analysis
Memos
Open coding
Qualitative content analysis
Quasi-statistical analysis style
Quasi-statistics
Recontextualization
Selective coding
Template
Template analysis style
Theme

As we have seen in Chapter 9, qualitative data take the form of loosely structured, narrative materials, such as verbatim transcripts of dialogue between an interviewer and a respondent, field notes from participant observation, or personal diaries. These data are generally not amenable to the types of analysis we discussed in the previous chapter. This chapter describes methods for analyzing such qualitative data.

▨ INTRODUCTION TO QUALITATIVE ANALYSIS

Qualitative analysis is a very labor-intensive activity that requires insight, ingenuity, creativity, conceptual sensitivity, and sheer hard work. Qualitative analysis does not proceed in a linear fashion, and is more complex and difficult than quantitative analysis because it is less clear-cut. In this section, we discuss some general considerations relating to qualitative analysis.

Qualitative Analysis: General Considerations

The purpose of data analysis, regardless of the type of data one has and regardless of the tradition that has driven its collection, is to impose some order on a large body of information so that the data can be synthesized, interpreted, and communicated in a research report. Although the overall aim of both qualitative and quantitative analysis is to organize, provide structure to, and elicit meaning from research data, an important difference is that data collection and data analysis usually occur simultaneously in qualitative studies, rather than after all the data are collected. The search for important themes and concepts begins from the moment data collection begins.

The data analysis task is almost always a formidable one, but it is particularly challenging for the qualitative researcher, for three major reasons. First, there are no systematic rules for analyzing and presenting qualitative data. It is at least partly because of this fact that qualitative methods have been described by some critics as "soft." The absence of systematic analytic procedures makes it difficult for the researcher engaged in qualitative analysis to present conclusions in such a way that their validity is patently clear. And, the absence of well-defined and universally accepted procedures makes replication difficult. Some of the procedures described in Chapter 10 (*e.g.,* member checking and investigator triangulation) are extremely important tools for enhancing the trustworthiness of not only the data themselves but also of the analyses and interpretation of those data.

The second aspect of qualitative analysis that makes it challenging is the enormous amount of work that is required. The qualitative analyst must organize and make sense of pages and pages of narrative materials. In a qualitative study directed by one of the authors (Polit), the data consisted of transcribed, unstructured interviews with about 100 women who had recently divorced. The transcriptions ranged from 40 to 80 pages in length, resulting in more than 6000 pages that had to be read and reread and then organized, integrated, and interpreted.

The final challenge comes in reducing the data for reporting purposes. The major results of quantitative research can often be summarized in two or three tables. However, if one compresses qualitative data too much, the very point of maintaining the integrity of narrative materials during the analysis phase becomes lost. If one merely summarizes the conclusions reached without including numerous supporting excerpts directly from the narrative materials, then the richness of the original data disappears. As a consequence, it is sometimes difficult to do a thorough presentation of the results of qualitative research in a format that is compatible with space limitations in professional journals.

Analysis Styles

Crabtree and Miller (1992) observed that there are nearly as many qualitative analysis strategies as there are qualitative researchers. However, they have identified four major analysis styles or patterns that fall along a continuum. At one extreme is a style that is more objective, systematic, and standardized, and at the other extreme is a style that is more intuitive, subjective, and interpretive. The four prototypical styles they described are as follows:

- *Quasi-statistical analysis style.* The researcher using a quasi-statistical style typically begins with some preconceived ideas about the analysis, and then uses those ideas to sort the data. This approach is sometimes referred to as **manifest content analysis**—the researcher reviews the content of the narrative data, searching for particular words or themes that have been specified in advance in a **codebook.** The result of the search is information that can be manipulated statistically—and hence the name **quasi-statistics.** For example, the analyst can count the frequency of occurrence of specific themes, or can cross-tabulate the occurrence of certain words.
- *Template analysis style.* In this style, the researcher develops a **template** or analysis guide to which the narrative data are applied. The units for the template are typically behaviors, events, and linguistic expressions (*e.g.,* words or phrases). A template is more fluid and adaptable than a codebook in the quasi-statistical style. Although the researcher may begin with a rudimentary template before collecting any data, the template undergoes constant revision as more data are gathered. The analysis of the resulting data, once sorted according to the template, is interpretive and not statistical. This type of style is most likely to be adopted by researchers whose research tradition is ethnography, ethology, discourse analysis, and ethnoscience.
- *Editing analysis style.* The researcher using the editing style acts as an interpreter who reads through the data in search of meaningful segments and units. Once these segments are identified and reviewed, the interpreter develops a **categorization scheme** and corresponding codes that can be used to sort and organize the data. The researcher then searches for the patterns and structure that connect the thematic categories. The grounded theory approach typically incorporates this type of style. Researchers whose research tradition is phenomenology, hermeneutics, and ethnomethodology use procedures that fall within the editing analysis pattern.

- ***Immersion/crystallization analysis style.*** This style involves the analyst's total immersion in and reflection of the text materials, resulting in an intuitive crystallization of the data. This highly interpretive and subjective style is exemplified in personal case reports of a semianecdotal nature, and is less frequently encountered in the nursing research literature than the other three styles.

Nurse researchers are especially likely to use an analytic strategy that can best be characterized as an editing style. Most of the remainder of this chapter describes analytic activities that are consistent with that style.

The Qualitative Analysis Process

The analysis of qualitative data typically is an active and interactive process—especially at the interpretive end of the analysis style continuum. Qualitative nurse researchers typically scrutinize their data carefully and deliberatively. Insights and theories cannot spring forth from the data without the researcher becoming completely familiar with those data. Qualitative researchers often read their narrative data over and over in a search for meaning and deeper understandings. Morse and Field (1995) note that qualitative analysis is "a process of fitting data together, of making the invisible obvious, of linking and attributing consequences to antecedents. It is a process of conjecture and verification, of correction and modification, of suggestion and defense" (p. 126).

Several intellectual processes play a role in qualitative analysis. Morse and Field (1995) have identified four such processes:

- *Comprehending.* Early in the analytic process, qualitative researchers strive to make sense of the data and to learn "what is going on." When comprehension is achieved, the researcher is able to prepare a thorough and rich description of the phenomenon under study, and new data do not add much to that description. In other words, comprehension is completed when saturation has been attained.
- *Synthesizing.* Synthesizing involves a "sifting" of the data and putting pieces together. At this stage, the researcher gets a sense of what is "typical" with regard to the phenomenon under study, and what the range and variation are like. At the end of the synthesis process, the researcher can begin to make some generalized statements about the phenomenon and about the study participants.
- *Theorizing.* Another important process in qualitative analysis is theorizing, which involves a systematic sorting of the data. During the theorizing process, the researcher develops alternative explanations of the phenomenon under study, and then holds these explanations up to determine their "fit" with the data. The theorizing process continues to evolve until the best and most parsimonious explanation is obtained.
- *Recontextualizing.* The process of **recontextualization** involves the fur-

ther development of the theory such that its applicability to other settings or groups is explored. In qualitative inquiries whose ultimate goal is theory development, it is the theory that must be recontextualized and generalized.

Although the intellectual processes in qualitative analysis are not linear in the same sense that quantitative analysis is, it is, nevertheless, true that these four processes follow a rough progression over the course of the study. Comprehension occurs primarily while in the field. Synthesis begins in the field but may continue well after the field work has been completed. Theorizing and recontextualizing are processes that are difficult to undertake before synthesis has been completed.

QUALITATIVE DATA MANAGEMENT AND ORGANIZATION

The intellectual processes of qualitative analysis are supported and facilitated by tasks that help to organize and manage the masses of narrative data. Data management tasks involve activities that prepare the data for subsequent analysis. Both manual and computerized techniques for data management are described in this section.

Developing a Categorization Scheme

The first step in analyzing qualitative data is to organize them; without some system of organization, there is only chaos. The main task in organizing qualitative data is developing a method to classify and index the materials. That is, the researcher must design a mechanism for gaining access to parts of the data, without having to repeatedly reread the set of data in its entirety. This phase of data analysis is essentially a reductionistic activity—data must be converted to smaller, more manageable, and more manipulatable units that can easily be retrieved and reviewed.

The most widely used procedure is to develop a categorization scheme and to then code the data according to the categories. Different analysis styles proceed with this task somewhat differently, as previously noted. That is, a categorization system is sometimes prepared (at least in a preliminary version) before data collection. However, in most cases, the qualitative analyst develops categories based on a scrutiny of the actual data.

There are, unfortunately, no straightforward or easy guidelines for this task. The development of a high-quality categorization scheme for qualitative data involves a careful reading of the data, with an eye to identifying underlying concepts and clusters of concepts. Depending on the aims of the study, the nature of the categories may vary in level of detail or specificity, as well as in level of abstraction.

Researchers whose aims are primarily descriptive tend to use categories that are fairly concrete. For example, the category scheme may focus on differentiating various types of actions or events, or different phases in a chronologic unfolding of an experience. The topical coding scheme used in Gagliardi's (1991) study of the family's experience of living with a child with Duchenne muscular dystrophy is presented in Figure 12–1. (Gagliardi's study was described as a research example in Chapter 10). This is an example of a category system that is fairly concrete and descriptive. For example, it allows the coders to code specific relationships among family members, and events occurring in specific locations.

In developing a category scheme, related concepts are often grouped together to facilitate the coding process. As shown in Figure 12–1, Gagliardi's system involved five major clusters of categories. For example, all of the excerpts illustrating how family members feel about living with a child with Duchenne muscular dystrophy are clustered under "Feeling Codes."

Studies designed to develop a theory (*e.g.,* a grounded theory study) are more likely to develop abstract and conceptual categories. In designing conceptual categories, the researcher must break the data into segments, closely examine them, and compare them to other segments for similarities and dissimilarities to determine what type of phenomena are reflected in them, and what the meaning of those phenomena are. (This is part of the process referred to as **constant comparison** by grounded theory researchers.) The researcher asks questions about discrete events, incidents, or thoughts that are indicated in an observation or statement, such as the following:

- What is this?
- What is going on?
- What does it stand for?
- What else is like this?
- What is this distinct from?

Important concepts that emerge from close examination of the data are then given a name or label that form the basis for a categorization scheme. These category names are necessarily abstractions, but the labels are generally sufficiently graphic that the nature of the material to which it refers is clear—and often provocative. Strauss and Corbin (1990), prominent grounded theory methodologists, advise qualitative researchers as follows: "The important thing is to name a category, so that

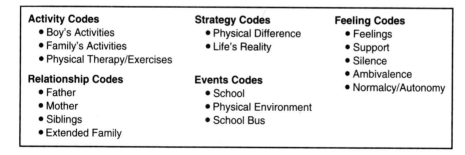

Figure 12–1. Gagliardi's (1991) Coding Scheme of Families' Experiences (Reprinted with permission)

you can remember it, think about it, and most of all begin to develop it analytically" (p. 67–68).

Coding Qualitative Data

Once a categorization scheme has been developed, all of the data are then reviewed for content and coded for correspondence to or exemplification of the identified categories. In a grounded theory study, the entire initial process of breaking down, categorizing, and coding data is often referred to as **open coding.**

The actual codes corresponding to the category system are arbitrary. They can be an abbreviation of the category (*e.g.,* B-ACT for Boy's Activities in Gagliardi's category system), a code corresponding to an outline structure (*e.g.,* Boy's Activities might be A.1 and Family's Activities might be A.2), or some other type of symbolic configuration. When a computer is used to index the data, the software being used often specifies requirements for labeling the codes.

This process of coding qualitative material is seldom an easy one, for several reasons. First, the researcher may have difficulty in deciding which code is most appropriate or may not fully comprehend the underlying meaning of some aspect of the data. It may take a second or third reading of the material to grasp the nuances contained in some portions of the data.

Second, the researcher often discovers in going through the data that the initial category system was incomplete or otherwise inadequate. In many cases, this means going back and starting from scratch. For this reason, it is usually necessary to review a very large portion of the data before an adequate categorization scheme can be developed. It is not unusual for some topics to emerge that were not initially conceptualized. When this happens, it is risky to assume that the topic failed to appear in materials that have already been coded. That is, a concept might not be identified as salient until it has emerged three or four times in the data. In such a case, it would be necessary to reread all previously coded material to have a truly complete grasp of that category.

Another problem stems from the fact that narrative materials are generally not linear. For example, paragraphs from transcribed interviews may contain elements relating to three or four different categories, embedded in a complex fashion. An example of a multitopic segment of an interview from one of the authors' study of divorced women, with codes in the margin, is shown in Figure 12–2.[1]

Manual Methods of Organizing Qualitative Data

A variety of procedures have traditionally been used to organize and manage qualitative data. When the amount of data is small, or when a category system is fairly simple, it may be possible to use color paper clips or color Post-It® Notes to code

[1] Figure 12–2 does not show the categories that the alphanumeric codes in the margin represent. The code categories used in the figure are as follows: 2b—General psychologic state during the divorce; 9—Finances; 5c—Feelings about single parenting; and 1b—Perceived advantages of divorce.

```
Subject 025
June 25, 1980
Page 32

Int:       How did you feel right after the separation?  Will you tell
           me a little more about that?

025:       Well, you know, when I look back...I mean I think anybody
           would have felt hopeless and helpless...because of, you
           know, emotionally...I think maybe it's a little easier if
           you've got more security...more money.  I was really stuck.
           I caught myself thinking..."Oh, if it wasn't for the
           kids..."  I love them both dearly, but...I mean there have
           been times when I've said to myself--I think a lot of women
           go through this too--I really had thought of giving them
           up.  In the beginning I used to think, too, they'd be so
           much better off with somebody that could, you know...When I
           was really struggling--I was on welfare----I used to think,
           "My God, how am I going to educate them?  What are they
           going to have?  I can't make ends meet now."  It's kinda
           projecting the unknown...fear of the unknown.  I think you
           can get mixed up.
```

2b
9
5c
1b.

Figure 12–2. Coded excerpt from an unstructured interview

the content of the narrative materials. For example, if we were analyzing responses to a single unstructured question about women's attitudes toward menopause, we might use blue paper clips for comments relating to the topic of loss of reproductive capacity, red clips for comments relating to physical side effects such as hot flashes, yellow clips for comments relating to aging, and so on. Then the researcher could pull out all of the responses coded with a certain color clip to examine one aspect of menopausal attitudes at a time.

Before the advent of computer programs for managing qualitative data, the most usual procedure was the development of **conceptual files.** In this approach, a physical file is developed for each of the various categories, and all of the materials relating to that topic are cut out and inserted into the file. To create conceptual files, the researcher must first go through all of the data and write the relevant codes in the margins, as in Figure 12–2. Then the researcher cuts up a copy of the material by category area, and places the cut-out excerpt into the file for that category. In this fashion, all of the content on a particular topic can be retrieved by going to the applicable file folder.

The creation of such conceptual files is clearly a cumbersome and labor-intensive task. This is particularly true when segments of the narrative materials have multiple codes, as is true in the excerpt shown in Figure 12–2. In such a situation, there would need to be four copies of the paragraph—one for each file corresponding to the four codes. The researcher must also be sensitive to the need to provide enough context that the cut-up material can be understood. For example, it might be necessary to include material preceding or following the directly relevant materials. Finally, the researcher must usually include pertinent administrative information on each item in the conceptual files. For example, if the data consisted of transcribed interviews, each informant would ordinarily be assigned an identification (ID) number. Each excerpt filed in the conceptual file would also need to include the appropriate ID number so the researcher could, if necessary, obtain additional information from the master copy.

In lieu of conceptual files, some researchers use qualitative sort cards (also known as McBee cards) for indexing their data. These index cards have holes on all sides that can be used for easy retrieval of information on a given topic or concept. That is, the researcher places notches in the holes corresponding to coded topical categories or concepts. Then, when information relating to a particular topic or concept is needed, all of the cards notched for that category can easily be pulled from the deck of index cards. Some researchers directly paste their data on these cards, when the data set is of a manageable size, and then directly code each data segment using the notched holes to indicate a code. Others write an abstract of an entire case (*e.g.,* one interview or one observational session) onto the card, and then indicate on the card the page numbers (*e.g.,* pages of the observational notes or transcribed interview) where different codes may be found.

Computer Programs for Managing Qualitative Data

The traditional manual methods of organizing qualitative data have a long and respected history, but they are becoming increasingly outmoded as a result of the widespread availability of personal computers that can be used to perform the filing and indexing of qualitative material. The early attempts to computerize qualitative data involved numbering all paragraphs of the researcher's field notes or interviews, coding each paragraph for topical codes, and then entering the information into computer files. This is essentially an automated version of the manual indexing/ retrieval systems described previously.

However, sophisticated computer programs for managing qualitative data on personal computers are now available and are becoming widely used. These programs permit the entire data file to be entered onto the computer, each portion of an interview or observational record coded and categorized, and then portions of the text corresponding to specified codes retrieved and printed (or shown on a screen) for analysis. The current generation of programs also has features that go beyond simple indexing and retrieval—they offer possibilities for actual analysis and integration of the data. Among the most widely used programs for qualitative analysis are Ethnograph, GATOR, MARTIN, QUALPRO, Textbase Alpha, Text Analysis Package, and HyperQual.

Computer programs remove the drudgery of cutting and pasting pages and pages of narrative material and are fast becoming indispensable research tools. However, some people argue that beginning researchers should gain at least some experience with manually organizing qualitative data. Part of this argument stems from the sentiment that manual indexing provides a more hands-on type of experience that allows the researcher to get closer to the data. Other concerns have been expressed about the use of computers with qualitative data. For example, one potential pitfall is that the researcher might develop an overly elaborate coding system, resulting from the fact that retrieval of information is vastly simplified with a computer. The advent of sophisticated programs that aid in the analysis of data has also given rise to objections to having a process that is basically cognitive turned into an activity that is mechanical and technical. Despite these concerns, most qualitative researchers have switched to computerized management of their data, and this trend is unlikely to be reversed. Computerized data management frees up the researcher's time so greater attention can be paid to more important conceptual issues. Moreover, a more comprehensive analysis may be possible by using computers, because there is less risk that certain parts of the data set will be overlooked.

Typically, the researcher begins by entering the qualitative data onto a computer file via a word processing program (*e.g.,* WordPerfect, Microsoft Word) and then the data are imported into the analysis program. A few qualitative data management programs (*e.g.,* QUALPRO, HyperQual) do allow text to be entered directly rather than requiring an import file from a word processor.

Next, the researcher marks the boundaries (*i.e.,* the beginning and end) of a segment of data and then codes the data according to the previously developed categorization scheme. *It is important to recognize that, in most cases, the computer does not code the data—the analyst does* (although automatic coding of specific words or phrases can be accomplished by several programs). In some programs, coding can be done directly on the computer screen in a one-step process, but others require two steps. The first step involves the numbering of lines of text and the subsequent printing out of the text with the line numbers appearing in the margins. Then, after coding the paper copy, the researcher tells the computer which codes go with which lines of text. Most (but not all) programs permit overlapping codings and the nesting of segments with different codes within one another.

All of the major qualitative analysis programs permit proofreading and editing. That is, codes can be altered, expanded, or deleted, and the boundaries of segments of text can be changed. Beyond these basic features, the available programs vary considerably in the enhancements they offer the researcher. The following is a nonexhaustive list of features available in some programs, but not in others:

- Compilation of a master list of all codes used
- Selective searches (*i.e.,* restricted to cases with certain characteristics— for example, searching for a code only in interviews with women)
- Retrieval of co-occurring codes (*i.e.,* data segments to which two or more specific codes are attached)
- Retrieval of information on the sequence of coded segments (*i.e.,* on the order of appearance of certain codes)

- Frequency count of the occurrence of codes
- Calculation of code percentages, in relation to other codes
- Calculation of the average size of data segments
- Listing and frequency count of specific words in the data files
- Searches for relationships among coded categories

Several of these enhancements have led to a blurring in the distinction between qualitative data management and data analysis.

ANALYTIC PROCEDURES

Data management tasks in qualitative research are typically reductionist in nature, because they convert large masses of data into smaller, more manageable segments. By contrast, qualitative data analysis tasks are constructionist in nature: they involve putting together segments into a meaningful conceptual pattern. Although different approaches to qualitative data analysis have been advocated, some elements are common to several of them. We provide some general guidelines, followed by a description of the analytic procedures used by grounded theory researchers.

A General Analytic Overview

The analysis of qualitative materials generally begins with a search for **themes** or recurring regularities. In many cases, the thematic analysis begins in the field, as the data are being collected. In other situations, the thematic analysis occurs after the data have been collected, during a reading (or rereading) of the data set.

Themes often develop within categories of data (*i.e.*, within categories of the coding scheme used for indexing materials), but sometimes cut across them. For example, in Gagliardi's study, six themes describing the families' experiences were identified, and these themes were further grouped under three headings corresponding to the stages in the process of adapting to the child's disability. The first theme, disillusionment, embraced content that had been coded under several topical codes (see Figure 12–1), primarily the topics within the feeling category.

The search for themes involves not only the discovery of commonalities across participants, but also a search for natural variation in the data. Themes that emerge from unstructured observations and interviews are never universal. The researcher must attend not only to what themes arise but also to how they are patterned. Does the theme apply only to certain subgroups? In certain types of communities or organizations? In certain contexts? At certain periods? What are the conditions that precede the observed phenomenon, and what are the apparent consequences of it? In other words, the qualitative analyst must be sensitive to *relationships* within the data.

The analyst's search for themes, regularities, and patterns in the data can sometimes be facilitated by charting devices that enable the researcher to summarize the evolution of behaviors, events, and processes. For example, for qualitative studies that focus on dynamic experiences—such as decision making—it is often useful to develop flow charts or time lines that highlight time sequences, major decision points and events, and factors affecting the decisions. An example of such a flow chart from a study of decision making among infertile couples is presented in Figure 12–3. The construction of such flow charts for all subjects would help to highlight any regularities in the subjects' evolving behaviors.

A further step frequently taken involves the validation of the understandings that the thematic exploration has provided. In this phase, the concern is whether the themes inferred are an accurate representation of the perspectives of the people interviewed or observed. Several procedures can be used in this validation step, some of which were discussed in Chapter 10. If more than one researcher is working on the study, debriefing sessions in which the themes are reviewed and specific cases discussed can be highly productive. Multiple perspectives—what we referred to in Chapter 10 as investigator triangulation—cannot ensure the validity of the themes, but it can minimize any idiosyncratic biases. Using an iterative approach is almost always necessary. That is, the researcher derives themes from the narrative materials, goes back to the materials with the themes in mind to see if the materials really do fit, and then refines the themes as necessary. It is generally useful to undertake member checks (*i.e.,* to present the preliminary thematic analysis to some of the subjects or informants, who can be encouraged to offer suggestions that might support or contradict this analysis).

At this point some researchers introduce quasi-statistics—a tabulation of the frequency with which certain themes, relations, or insights are supported by the data. The frequencies cannot be interpreted in the same way as frequencies generated in survey studies, because of imprecision in the sampling of cases and enumeration of the themes. Nevertheless, as Becker (1970) pointed out,

> Quasi-statistics may allow the investigator to dispose of certain troublesome null hypotheses. A simple frequency count of the number of times a given phenomenon appears may make untenable the null hypothesis that the phenomenon is infrequent. A comparison of the number of such instances with the number of negative cases—instances in which some alternative phenomenon that would not be predicted by his theory appears—may make possible a stronger conclusion, especially if the theory was developed early enough in the observational period to allow a systematic search for negative cases. Similarly, an inspection of the range of situations covered by the investigator's data may allow him to negate the hypothesis that his conclusion is restricted to only a few situations, time periods, or types of people in the organization or community. (p. 81)

In the final stage of analysis, the researcher strives to weave the thematic pieces together into an integrated whole. The various themes need to be interrelated in a manner that provides an overall structure (such as a theory or integrated description) to the entire body of data. The integration task is an extremely difficult one, because it demands creativity and intellectual rigor if it is to be successful. A

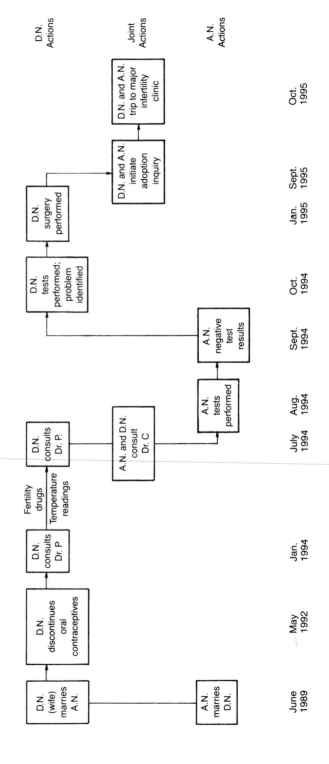

Figure 12–3. Example of a timeline for infertility study

strategy that sometimes helps in this task is to cross-tabulate dimensions that have emerged in the thematic analysis. For example, Barton (1991), in her study of parents' adaptations to their adolescent children's drug abuse problems, found that parental power and parental responsibility were two important dimensions that, when cross-tabulated, reflected important coping patterns among the parents in her sample. Her diagram displaying the cross-tabulated schema is presented in Figure 12–4.

Grounded Theory Analysis

The general procedures and steps previously described provide a general outline of how qualitative researchers make sense of their data and distill from them their understandings of processes and behaviors operating in naturalistic settings. However, some variations in the goals and underlying philosophies of qualitative researchers also lead to variations in how the analytic task is handled. For example, one of the strategies for analyzing qualitative data is referred to as analytic induction. **Analytic induction,** a process that has been used since the 1930s, is a method that involves an iterative approach to testing research hypotheses with qualitative data. Mayo (1992), who conducted an ethnographic study of the processes of managing physical activity among African-American working women, used analytic induction as the method of analyzing her qualitative data.

By far the most widely used analytic approach among nurse researchers is Glaser and Strauss' (1967) grounded theory method of generating theories from data. Because of its popularity, we describe here some of the specific analytic techniques of grounded theory.

	+ POWER **–**	
+ **RESPONSIBILITY** **–**	The parents feel guilty despite professionals' attempts to eliminate guilt Style is "committed"/ "correcting the flaw"	The parents are especially "fused" to the child Style is "stuck"/"secondary gains" or "protection from social responsibility"
	The parents accept not feeling responsible and have power. Style is "successful"/ "mastery"	The parents accept not feeling responsible but let go of power. Style is "letting go"/"new meaning"

Figure 12–4. Barton's (1991) schema describing parental adaptation to adolescent drug abuse (Reprinted with permission)

As we have seen, the first step is the development of a categorization scheme and the substantive coding of data through the preliminary process referred to as open coding (or, sometimes, **level I coding**). Open coding allows the researcher to identify major categories and subcategories, and to describe their major properties and dimensions.

Level II coding (often referred to as **axial coding**) is a reconstructive process that puts the data back together in new ways after open coding is completed by connecting a category and its subcategories. Constant comparison is used again in axial coding to refine theoretical categories. Strauss and Corbin (1990) note that in axial coding the "focus is on specifying a category (*phenomenon*) in terms of the conditions that give rise to it; the *context* (its specific set of properties in which it is embedded; the action/interaction *strategies* by which it is handled, managed, carried out; and the consequences of those strategies" [p. 97]). Axial coding is a complex process involving both inductive and deductive thinking, and is designed to move the coding process to a higher level of abstraction.

Throughout the coding and analysis process, the grounded theory analyst documents his or her ideas, insights, and feelings about the data, themes, and the emerging conceptual scheme in the form of **memos.** Morse and Field (1995) note that the memos serve numerous functions in a grounded theory study. For example, memos help the researcher to identify underlying assumptions. They also preserve ideas that may initially not seem productive but may later prove valuable once further developed. An especially important function is that memos encourage a higher level of abstract thinking by getting the researcher to reflect on and describe themes and patterns in the data, relationships between categories, and emergent conceptualizations.

Once saturation has been achieved and both open coding and axial coding are completed, integration can begin. Here the analyst reviews and sorts the memos to explore theoretical explanations, and searches for the **core category**—the central phenomenon that is used to integrate all other categories. **Level III coding** (also referred to as **selective coding**) is the process of selecting the core category, systematically identifying and integrating relationships between the core category and other categories, and validating those relationships. The integrative process is similar to axial coding, except that it is done at a more highly abstract level of analysis.

Level III coding results in a description of a **basic social process (BSP),** which is the central social process resulting from the data. Because of the activities in which the researcher has engaged, the emergent theory of what this process is and how it works is grounded in the data.

The grounded theory method is concerned with the generation of categories, properties, and hypotheses rather than testing them (as in the case of analytic induction). The product of the typical grounded theory study is a conceptual or theoretical model that endeavors to explain the phenomenon under study. As an example, Figure 12–5 presents the model developed by King and Jensen (1994) in

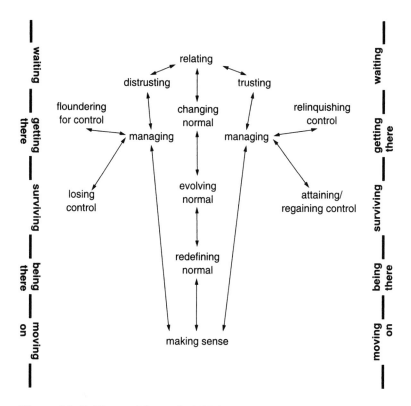

Figure 12–5. King and Jensen's (1994) model of preserving the self during cardiac surgery (Reprinted with permission)

their grounded theory study that conceptualized the process of women's "preserving the self" during cardiac surgery.

 ## ILLUSTRATION OF QUALITATIVE ANALYSIS ACTIVITIES

Qualitative researchers seldom discuss in any detail the ways in which they analyze their data. However, the steps undertaken by one research team have been described and provide a useful illustration of the tasks facing qualitative analysts.

Knafl and Webster (1988) studied how the role of clinical nurse researchers was being defined, enacted, and evaluated. This study involved in-depth telephone interviews with 34 clinical nurse researchers (CNRs) and their corresponding chief nurse executives (CNEs). The data consisted of about 1,000 pages of interview transcripts.

The researchers undertook six major tasks during the data management phase and five major tasks during the data analysis phase. These tasks are as follows:

Phase I: Data Management

1. Independent reading of a sample of interview transcripts by team members; collaborative development of six major descriptive coding categories; development of a codebook to ensure consistent application of final coding categories
2. Independent coding of all interviews in margins of transcripts by two coders; collaborative review of codes and resolution of differences in coding
3. Cut-and-paste transfer of all data onto color-coded 5 × 8 inch index cards, with colors corresponding to the six major categories
4. Identification of subcategories reflecting narrower topical areas within the major categories
5. Coding of the index cards according to the subcategories identified
6. Construction of descriptive summary grids for each subcategory across all subjects, with each cell of the grid containing a brief summary of pertinent content

Phase II: Data Analysis

1. Description of the content of each subcategory, and identification of major themes; preparation of a written analysis summary
2. Description of the content of each major category, constructed from the subcategory summary
3. Description of the CNR group, synthesizing and integrating relevant material
4. Description of the CNE group, synthesizing and integrating relevant material
5. Description of CNR–CNE pairs, contrasting within-pair themes

ASSISTANCE TO CONSUMERS OF NURSING RESEARCH

What to Expect in the Research Literature

Research involving qualitative analyses is increasingly common in the nursing literature, and we can expect this trend to continue. In this section, we present some information designed to help consumers in approaching qualitative analyses.

- Researchers vary considerably in how much information they provide regarding their qualitative analytic procedures. At one extreme, some researchers say little more than that their data were analyzed using qualitative methods; at the other extreme are researchers who explain in detail the steps they took to analyze their data and validate the emerging themes.

Most studies fall between the two extremes, but limited detail is more prevalent than abundant detail.

- In an actual research report, the researcher is unlikely to use terms like *template analysis style* or *editing style;* these terms are post hoc characterizations of prototypical analytic styles that are often adopted. However, if a study was done within a qualitative research tradition such as ethnography or grounded theory, this fact is likely to be reported, thereby providing readers with a sense of the overall analytic strategy.
- A qualitative researcher who has not used a grounded theory or analytic induction approach often says that a content analysis was performed. In most cases, the researcher is not referring to a manifest content analysis involving the quantification of aspects of written materials. **Qualitative content analysis** involves an analysis of the content of narrative data to identify prominent themes and patterns among the themes—primarily using an analysis style that can be characterized as either template analysis or editing analysis. A researcher may use the term content analysis either with a reference to the research tradition (*e.g.,* a phenomenologic study in which the data were content analyzed) or without such a reference.
- Qualitative analyses are often more difficult to *do* than quantitative ones, but qualitative findings are generally much easier to understand than quantitative findings because the stories are more easily told in everyday language. The readability of the qualitative reports is usually enhanced by the inclusion of numerous verbatim excerpts taken directly from the narrative data.
- Despite the readability and comprehensibility of qualitative findings, qualitative analyses are often harder to evaluate critically than quantitative analyses because the person reading the report cannot know first-hand if the researcher adequately captured thematic patterns in the data.

Critiquing Qualitative Analyses

As just noted, the task of evaluating a qualitative analysis is not an easy one, even for researchers with experience in doing qualitative research. The problem stems, in part, from the lack of standardized procedures for data analysis, but the difficulty lies mainly in the fact that readers must accept largely on faith that the researcher exercised good judgment and critical insight in coding the narrative materials, in developing a thematic analysis, and in integrating the materials into a meaningful whole. This is because the researcher is seldom able to include more than a handful of examples of actual data in a research report published in a journal and because the process of inductively abstracting meaning from the data is difficult to describe.

In quantitative analysis, the research can be evaluated in terms of the adequacy of specific analytic decisions (*e.g.,* did the researcher use the appropriate statistical test?). In a critique of qualitative analysis, however, the primary task is usually determining whether the researcher took sufficient steps to validate inferences and

Box 12-1

Guidelines for Critiquing Qualitative Analyses

1. Based on information in the report regarding either the analysis strategy or the research tradition, what type of analysis style appears to have been used?
2. Is the initial categorization scheme described? If so, does the scheme appear logical and complete? Were manual methods used to index and organize the data, or was a computer program used?
3. Is the process described by which an integrated thematic analysis was performed? What major themes emerged? If excerpts from the data are provided, do the themes appear to capture the meaning of the narratives (*i.e.*, does it appear that the researcher adequately interpreted the data and conceptualized the themes)?
4. Is the analysis parsimonious—could two or more themes be collapsed into a broader and perhaps more useful conceptualization?
5. What evidence does the report provide that the researcher's analysis is accurate and replicable?
6. Were data displayed in a manner that allows you to verify the researcher's conclusions? Was a conceptual map, model, or diagram effectively displayed to communicate important processes?
7. Was the context of the phenomenon adequately described? Does the report give you a clear picture of the social or emotional world of the study participants?
8. If the result of the study is an emergent theory or conceptualization, does it seem trivial or obvious? Does the scheme yield a meaningful and insightful picture of the phenomenon under study?

conclusions. A major focus of a critique of qualitative analyses, then, is whether the researcher has adequately documented the analytic process. Some guidelines that may be helpful in evaluating qualitative analyses are presented in Box 12–1.

▨ RESEARCH EXAMPLES

The number of qualitative studies that have been published in nursing journals over the past decade has risen dramatically. Two research examples are described below.

Example of a Grounded Theory Analysis

Bright (1992) studied the birth of a first child as an intergenerational experience with the aim of discovering the basic social process (BSP) associated with this event and generating a theory on normative family process. She collected in-depth interview and observational data over a 15-month period from three families: three first-born infants and their parents and six sets of grandparents. Data collection began during the last trimester of pregnancy and continued until the child's first birthday. The families differed in terms of whether the pregnancy was planned and wanted.

Within each family, the interviews were initially conducted in a group setting, which allowed the researcher to observe family interactional patterns and to learn about family beliefs and customs, as well as expectations about the anticipated birth event. Subsequent interviews were conducted with individual family members, with dyads, and with small groups as deemed needed on the basis of the developing hypotheses. Interviews and observations occurred in parental and grandparental homes, on the hospital maternity ward, and at other locations such as baptismal ceremonies. Telephone interviews were used to clarify data and to check on the validity of the emerging hypotheses.

The analysis of data was done as an ongoing process, integrated with data collection and coding. Interviews were audiotaped, transcribed, and then coded line by line. One three-generation family interaction was videotaped to provide recorded nonverbal as well as verbal data for coding. Coded data were grouped into related categories and then compared with one another and with new data to continually refine or discard emerging hypotheses. Memos were prepared concurrently to record the researcher's theoretical analysis of the data. Several methods were used to validate the themes emerging from the analysis, including review by members of the families.

The analysis resulted in the identification of an evolutionary family process that reflected reorganized interpersonal patterns. "Making place," the central social process that emerged from Bright's analysis, was defined as the family process through which a newborn individual receives recognition as a member of that family. The family made place both physically and socially for the new and expanded relationships created by the child's birth.

Example of an Analysis for an Ethnographic Study

Russell's (1996) ethnographic study focused on the care-seeking process used by elders residing in a continuing-care retirement community. During 8 months of field work in a retirement community, Russell collected data on the elders' process of eliciting care and engaging caregivers in care interactions. Data were collected through in-depth semistructured interviews with 12 elders, participant observation of 34 elders in the facility's adult care center, and a focus group interview with 4 elders. Each of the data collection methods yielded different perspectives about the participants' care seeking. The interviews and focus group sessions were taped and fully transcribed, and the researcher took field notes after observational sessions. Data collection and data analysis were done concurrently. The data were entered into computer files for organization and management.

The first step involved comparing and contrasting data elements from different sources to generate a categorization scheme. The result was the development of a codebook with more than 150 codes and definitions. The codes were organized and reorganized into larger units that enabled the researcher to identify patterns, features, sequences, and relationships in elders' care seeking. Field notes and memos were maintained to document new ideas about the analysis, including both theoretical and methodologic insights.

The basic unit of analysis was a specific care encounter. More than 275 such units were demarcated in the textual database. Each case was characterized in terms of certain structural elements, such as actors, contexts, and behaviors. These cases were used to develop and test an emerging conceptualization of the care-seeking process.

According to Russell's analysis, the care-seeking process comprises two phases, which she labeled "Care Eliciting" and "Care Engaging." Figure 12–6 shows Russell's diagram of the care-seeking process. The Initiating Stage, which began when elders decided that assistance was needed, was shaped by the elders' preferences (*i.e.,* their desires and expectations relating to care) and their beliefs in terms of the appropriateness of a potential caregiver. Stage 2, the Alerting Stage, involved both verbal and nonverbal strategies designed to alert others to their desire for assistance. Stage 3, the Negotiating Stage, began when a caregiver become engaged in an elder's care. The negotiations between the elder and caregiver varied in terms of content, history of the relationship, and "doing"— the extent to which elders did for themselves or worked with caregivers to accomplish their care. Finally, stage 4 was the Evaluation Stage, the periodic appraisal that the elders undertook to make further decisions regarding the caretaking. This stage was characterized by the elders' perceptions about the care settings, caregivers, and the care itself. Russell concluded that the findings support viewing elders' care seeking as an interactional and developmental process.

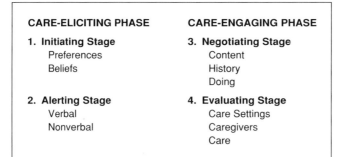

Figure 12–6. Russell's (1996) diagram of sequences in the care-seeking process

▧ SUMMARY

Qualitative analysis is a more challenging and labor-intensive activity than quantitative analysis—and one that is guided by fewer standardized rules. Although there are no universally adopted strategies for analyzing qualitative data, four prototypical styles have been identified that fall on a continuum from objective and systematic to interpretive and subjective: (1) a **quasi-statistical style** that begins with a preestablished **codebook** of themes or words and that lends itself to basic descriptive statistical analysis; (2) a **template analysis style** that involves the development of an analysis guide (**template**) used to sort the data; (3) an **editing analysis style** that involves an interpretation of the data on which a **categorization scheme** is based; and (4) an **immersion/crystallization style** that involves the analyst's total immersion in and reflection of text materials. Most nurse researchers use a strategy that is best characterized as an editing analysis style—a style that typically requires four types of intellectual processes: comprehending, synthesizing, theorizing, and **recontextualizing** (exploration of the developed theory vis-á-vis its applicability to other settings or groups).

The first major step in analyzing qualitative data is to organize the materials according to some plan, so that portions of the data can be readily retrieved. Qualitative researchers usually develop a categorization scheme based on a reading of a portion of the data and then code the content of the data based on this system. Traditionally, researchers have developed **conceptual files** for organizing their data. In using this system, researchers first code their data in the margins of the printed narrative materials (*e.g.*, observational notes or transcripts of interviews); cut out the coded excerpts; and finally place each excerpt into a file corresponding to each of the topics covered in the coding scheme. Then the researcher can retrieve all of the information on a topic by going to a single file. However, the widespread availability of personal computers and appropriate software has lessened the burden of indexing, organizing, and retrieving qualitative materials. There are now a wide variety of programs that perform not only basic indexing functions, but also offer various enhancements that can facilitate analysis of the data.

The actual analysis of data begins with a search for **themes.** The search for themes involves not only the discovery of commonalities across subjects, but also of natural variation in the data. The next step generally involves a validation of the thematic analysis. Some researchers use **quasi-statistics,** which involves a tabulation of the frequency with which certain themes or relations are supported by the data. In a final step, the analyst tries to weave the thematic strands together into an integrated picture of the phenomenon under investigation.

Although this overview summarizes some of the major steps, there are a number of different philosophies underlying qualitative analysis. **Analytic induction** refers to an approach in which the researcher alternates back and forth between tentative definition of emerging hypotheses and tentative explanation, with each iteration making refinements. However, the most widely used approach by nurse researchers is grounded theory. Grounded theory begins with **open coding (level I coding)**—the development of a categorization scheme (using constant comparison) and subsequent initial coding of the data. **Level II coding** (also referred to as **axial coding**) is a reconstructive process that puts data back together in new ways by connecting categories and subcategories. The analyst begins the process of integration by reviewing and sorting the **memos** that have been used to document conceptual ideas throughout the data collection and data analysis process. During **level III coding** (or **selective coding**) the grounded theory analyst searches for the **core category**—the central phenomenon used to integrate all others. This phase results in an emerging theory of a **basic social process (BSP)** that is grounded in the data.

There is no direct correspondence between the underlying qualitative research tradition, which is the basis for certain research questions, and the analytic approach. Some researchers identify neither a specific approach nor a specific research tradition; and some researchers say that they used **qualitative content analysis** as their analytic method.

Suggested Readings

Methodologic References

Becker, H. S. (1970). *Sociological work.* Chicago: Aldine.
Crabtree, B. F., & Miller, W. L., Eds. (1992). *Doing qualitative research.* Newbury Park, CA: Sage.
Glaser, B. G., & Strauss, A. L. (1967). *The discovery of grounded theory: Strategies for qualitative research.* Chicago: Aldine.
Knafl, K. A., & Webster, D. C. (1988). Managing and analyzing qualitative data: A description of tasks, techniques, and materials. *Western Journal of Nursing Research, 10,* 195–218.
Miles, M. B., & Huberman, A. M. (1984). *Qualitative data analysis.* Beverly Hills, CA: Sage.
Morse, J. M., & Field, P. A. (1995). *Qualitative research methods for health professionals* (2nd ed.). Thousand Oaks, CA: Sage.
Strauss, A., & Corbin, J. (1990). *Basics of qualitative research.* Newbury Park, CA: Sage.

Substantive References

Barton, J. A. (1991). Parental adaptation to adolescent drug abuse: An ethnographic study of role formulation in response to courtesy stigma. *Public Health Nursing, 8,* 39–45.
Bright, M. A. (1992). Making place: The first birth in an intergenerational family context. *Qualitative Health Research, 2,* 75–78.
Gagliardi, B. A. (1991). The family's experience of living with a child with Duchenne muscular dystrophy. *Applied Nursing Research, 4,* 159–164.
King, K. M., & Jensen, L. (1994). Preserving the self: Women having cardiac surgery. *Heart & Lung, 23,* 99–105.
Mayo, K. (1992). Physical activity practices among American black working women. *Qualitative Health Research, 2,* 318–333.
Russell, C. K. (1996). Elder care recipients' care-seeking process. *Western Journal of Nursing Research, 18,* 43–62.

Critical Appraisal and Utilization of Nursing Research

PART VI

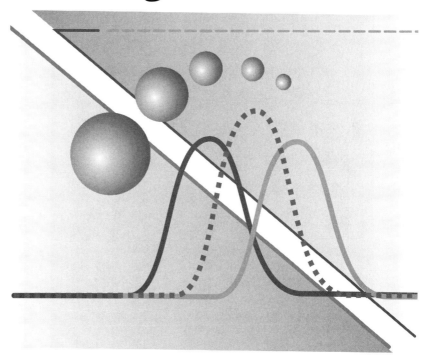

Critiquing Research Reports

Student Objectives

On completion of this chapter, the student will be able to:

- describe five aspects of a study's findings important to consider in developing an interpretation, and distinguish their applicability for quantitative and qualitative studies
- describe strategies for interpreting hypothesized, unhypothesized, or mixed results in quantitative studies
- distinguish practical and statistical significance
- describe the purpose and features of a research critique
- identify the main dimensions along which a reviewer should critique a research report
- evaluate the substantive and theoretical dimensions of a report
- evaluate the methodologic dimensions of a report, with special emphasis on the major methodologic decisions made by researchers
- evaluate the ethical dimensions of a study
- evaluate the stylistic and presentation aspects of a research report
- evaluate a researcher's interpretation of his or her results
- define new terms in the chapter

New Terms

Critique
Interpretation
Methodologic decisions
Mixed results

Replication
Results
Unhypothesized results

Throughout this book, we have provided guidelines for critiquing various aspects of nursing research projects reported in the nursing literature. This chapter describes the purposes of a research critique and offers some further tips on how to evaluate research reports. One important aspect of a research critique involves the reviewer's interpretation of the study findings. Therefore, we begin this chapter by offering some suggestions on interpreting research results.

INTERPRETING STUDY RESULTS

The analysis of research data provides the **results** of the study. These results need to be evaluated and interpreted, which is often a challenging task. The **interpretation** should give due consideration to the overall aims of the project, its theoretical underpinnings, the specific research questions or hypotheses being tested, the existing body of related research knowledge, and the limitations of the adopted research methods.

The interpretive task involves a consideration of various aspects of the study findings, including the following:

- the accuracy and believability of the results
- the meaning of the results
- the importance of the results—the degree to which they make a contribution to knowledge
- the extent to which the results can be generalized or have the potential for utility in other contexts
- the implications of the results for practice, theory, or research

In this section, we review issues relating to these interpretive aspects for quantitative and qualitative research reports.

Interpreting Quantitative Results

Quantitative research results often offer the consumer more interpretive opportunities than qualitative ones—in part because a quantitative report can summarize and display much of the actual data in tables, whereas qualitative reports contain only illustrative examples of the data. Thus, readers of quantitative reports need to think creatively about the possible meaning behind the numbers.

The Accuracy of Quantitative Results

One of the first tasks you will face in interpreting quantitative results is assessing whether they are likely to be accurate and believable. This assessment, in turn, requires a careful analysis of the study's methodologic and conceptual limitations.

A thorough assessment of the accuracy of the results relies on the reviewer's critical thinking skills—and on an understanding of research methods. The assessment of accuracy should be based on an evaluation of evidence, not on personal preferences and "gut feelings." Both external and internal evidence can be brought to bear. External evidence comes primarily from the body of prior research. If the results are inconsistent with prior research, possible reasons for the discrepancy should be sought. What was different about the way the data were collected, the sample was selected, key variables were operationalized, extraneous variables were controlled, and so on?

Internal evidence for the accuracy of the findings comes from an evaluation of the methods used. The validity and meaning of the results depend on the study's strengths and shortcomings. The reviewer needs to evaluate carefully all the major methodologic decisions made in planning and executing the study to determine whether alternative decisions might have yielded different results. This issue is discussed in greater detail later in this chapter.

A critical analysis of the research methods and conceptualization and an examination of various types of external and internal evidence almost inevitably indicates some limitations. These limitations must be taken into account in interpreting the results.

The Meaning of Quantitative Results

In quantitative studies, the results are usually in the form of test statistic values and probability levels, which do not in and of themselves project meaning. The statistical results must be translated into conceptual terms and interpreted. In this section, we discuss the interpretation of various types of research outcomes within a statistical hypothesis testing context.

Interpreting Hypothesized Results. When statistical tests support the researcher's hypotheses, the task of interpreting the results may be straightforward because the rationale for the hypotheses presumably offers an explanation of what the findings mean. However, hypotheses can be correct even when the researcher's explanation of what is going on is not accurate. As a reviewer, you will need to be sure that the researcher does not go beyond the data in interpreting what the results mean. A simple example might help to explain what is meant. Suppose a nurse researcher hypothesizes that a relationship exists between a pregnant woman's level of anxiety about the labor and delivery experience and the number of children she has already borne. The data reveal that a negative relationship between anxiety levels and parity does indeed exist ($r = -.40$, $p < .05$). The researcher, therefore, concludes that increased experience with childbirth causes decreasing amounts of anxiety. Is this conclusion supported by the data? The conclusion appears to be logical, but, in fact, there is nothing within the data that leads directly to this interpretation. An important, indeed critical, research precept is: *correlation does not prove causation.* The finding that two variables are related offers no evidence suggesting which of the two variables—if either—caused the other. Alternative explanations for the findings should always be considered. If competing interpretations can be ruled out on the basis of the data or previous research findings, so much the better, but your initial interpretation should always be given adequate competition. Throughout the interpretation process, you should bear in mind that the support of research hypotheses through statistical testing never constitutes proof of their veracity. Hypothesis testing is probabilistic. There always remains a possibility that any obtained relationships were due to chance.

Interpreting Nonsignificant Results. Failure to reject a null hypothesis is particularly problematic from an interpretive point of view. Standard statistical procedures are geared toward disconfirmation of the null hypothesis. The failure to reject a null hypothesis (*i.e.,* obtaining results suggesting no relationship between the independent variable and dependent variable) could occur for one of two reasons: (1) because the null hypothesis is true (*i.e.,* the nonsignificant result reflects the real absence of relationships among the research variables) or (2) because the null hypothesis is false (*i.e.,* a true relationship among the variables exists but the data failed to reveal it). Neither the researcher nor the reviewer knows which of these situations prevails. In the first situation, the problem is most likely to be in the logical reasoning, the conceptualization, or the theoretical framework that led the researcher to the stated hypotheses. The second situation (retention of a false null hypothesis), by contrast, generally reflects methodologic limitations, such as internal validity problems, the selection of a small or atypical sample, or the use of a weak statistical procedure. Thus, the interpretation must consider both substantive and methodologic reasons for results that fail to confirm the research hypotheses. Whatever the underlying cause, there is never justification for interpreting a retained null hypothesis as proof of a *lack* of relationship among variables. The safest interpretation is that nonsignificant findings represent a lack of evidence for either truth or falsity of the hypothesis.

Interpreting Unhypothesized Significant Results. Although this does not happen frequently, there are situations in which the researcher obtains significant results that are exactly the opposite of the research hypothesis; these are referred to as **unhypothesized results.** For example, a researcher might predict a negative relationship between patient satisfaction with nursing care and the length of stay in hospital, but a significant positive relationship might be found. In such cases, it is less likely, although not impossible, that the methods are flawed than that the reasoning or theory is incorrect. In these cases, the researcher and reviewer should, in attempting to explain the findings, pay particular attention to the results of previous research and alternative theories. It is also useful, however, to consider whether there is anything unusual about the sample that might lead its members to behave or respond in a highly atypical way.

Interpreting Mixed Results. The interpretive process is often confounded by **mixed results:** some hypotheses may be supported by the data, whereas others are not. Or a hypothesis may be accepted when one measure of the dependent variable is used but rejected with a different measure of the same variable. Of all the situations mentioned, mixed results are probably most prevalent. When only some results run counter to a theoretical position or conceptual scheme, the research methods are probably the first aspect of the study deserving critical scrutiny. Differences in the validity and reliability of the various measures may account for such discrepancies, for example. On the other hand, mixed results may be indicative of how a theory needs to be qualified, or of how certain constructs within the theory need to be reconceptualized.

The Importance of Quantitative Results

In quantitative studies, results in support of the researcher's hypotheses are described as being significant. A careful analysis of the results of a study involves an evaluation of whether, in addition to being statistically significant, they are important.

The fact that statistical significance was attained in testing the hypothesis does not necessarily mean the results were of value to the nursing community and their clients. Statistical significance indicates that the results were unlikely to be a function of chance. This means that the observed group differences or observed relationships were probably real but were not necessarily important. With large samples, even modest relationships are statistically significant. For instance, with a sample of 500 subjects, a correlation coefficient of .10 is significant at the .05 level, but a relationship of this magnitude might have little practical value. As a reviewer, therefore, you should pay attention to the numeric values obtained in an analysis in addition to the significance level when assessing the implications of the findings.

The absence of statistically significant results does not mean that the results are unimportant—although because of the difficulty in interpreting nonsignificant results, the case is more complex. Let us suppose that the study involved comparing two alternative procedures for making a clinical assessment (*e.g.,* body temperature). Suppose that a researcher retained the null hypothesis (*i.e.,* found no statistically significant differences between the two methods). If the study involved a small sample, the nonsignificant results would be difficult to interpret. If a very large sample was used, however, a power analysis would likely reveal an extremely low probability of a Type II error. In such a situation, it might reasonably be concluded that the two procedures yield equally accurate assessments. If one of these procedures were more efficient, less painful, or less costly than the other, then the nonsignificant findings could, indeed, be clinically important.

Another criterion for assessing the importance of quantitative research results concerns whether the findings are trivial or obvious. If the findings do little more than confirm common sense or confirm the results from dozens of earlier studies, the contribution they make to knowledge should be questioned.

The Generalizability of Quantitative Results

Another aspect of quantitative results that you should assess when reviewing a report is their generalizability. Researchers are rarely interested in discovering relationships among variables for a specific group of people at a specific point in time. The aim of nursing research is typically to reveal accurate descriptions about phenomena and relationships among them to provide insights that will improve the practice of nursing. For example, if a nursing intervention is found to be successful, others will likely want to adopt it. Therefore, an important interpretive question is whether the intervention will work or whether the relationships will hold in other settings, with other people. Part of the interpretive process involves asking the question: To what groups, environments, and conditions can the results of the study be applied?

The Implications of Quantitative Results

Once you have formed conclusions about the accuracy, meaning, importance, and generalizability of the results, you are ready to draw inferences about the implications of the results. The reviewer should consider the implications of the findings with respect to future research endeavors (What should other researchers working in this area do?), theory development (What are the implications for nursing theory?), and nursing practice (How, if at all, should the results be used by other nurses in their practice?). Research utilization is discussed Chapter 14.

Interpreting Qualitative Results

It is usually more difficult for a reviewer to interpret qualitative findings independently and thoroughly, because the researcher must be selective in the amount and types of data that are included in the report for a reviewer's perusal. Nevertheless, you should strive to consider the same five interpretive dimensions for a qualitative study as for a quantitative one.

The Accuracy of Qualitative Results

As with the case of quantitative reports, qualitative reports must bear a scrutiny of the study's conceptual and methodologic underpinnings. Thus, when reading qualitative reports, you should also begin by questioning whether the results of the inquiry are believable.

It is reasonable to expect the author of qualitative reports to provide evidence of the credibility of the findings, as described in Chapter 10—although this does not always happen. Because readers of qualitative reports are exposed to only a portion of the data, they must rely on the researcher's efforts to corroborate the findings through such mechanisms as peer debriefings and member checks. However, even when such efforts have been undertaken, you should realize that they do not unequivocally establish "proof" that the results are believable. Qualitative reports almost never indicate that the member checks led the researchers to alter their conclusions, and thus it is possible that the member checks are not always effective in illuminating flaws. Perhaps some participants are too polite to disagree with the researcher's interpretations. Or perhaps they become intrigued with a conceptualization they themselves would never have developed on their own—a conceptualization that is not necessarily accurate. Suffice it to say that in thinking about the believability of qualitative results—as with quantitative results—it is advisable to adopt the posture of a person who needs to be persuaded, and to expect the researcher to marshall solid evidence with which to persuade you.

The Meaning of Qualitative Results

In qualitative studies, interpretation and analysis of the data occur virtually simultaneously. That is, the researcher interprets the data as he or she categorizes it, develops a thematic analysis, and integrates the themes into a unified whole. Efforts to validate the qualitative analysis are necessarily efforts to validate the interpretation as well. Thus, in a qualitative study, the meaning of the data flows from the analysis, and it is seldom necessary to puzzle through the findings in search of a deeper meaning. Moreover, the qualitative researcher rarely establishes a priori hypotheses, so the interpretive task does not involve elucidating unhypothesized results or mixed results.

The Importance of Qualitative Results

Qualitative research is especially productive when it is used to explore poorly understood phenomena. But the amount of prior research on a topic is not a sufficient barometer for deciding whether the findings can make a contribution to nursing knowledge. The phenomenon must be one that *merits* rigorous scrutiny. For example, some people prefer the color green and others like red. Color preference may not, however, be a sufficiently important topic for an in-depth inquiry. Thus, you must judge whether the topic under study is important or trivial.

In a critical evaluation of the importance of a study, you should also consider whether the findings themselves are trivial. Perhaps the topic is worthwhile, but you may feel after reading the report that nothing new has been learned. Qualitative researchers often attach catchy labels to their themes and processes, but you should ask yourself whether the labels have really captured an insightful conceptualization that goes beyond common knowledge.

The Transferability of Qualitative Results

Although qualitative researchers do not strive for generalizability, nevertheless the application of the results to other settings and contexts must be considered. If the findings are only relevant to the particular participants in the study, then they cannot be useful to nursing practice. Thus, in interpreting the results of a qualitative study, you should consider how transferable the findings are. In what other types of settings and contexts would you expect the phenomena under study to be manifested in a similar fashion? Of course, to make such an assessment, the author of the report must have described in sufficient detail the context in which the data were collected. Because qualitative studies are context-bound, it is only through a careful analysis of the key parameters of the study context that the transferability of results can be assessed.

The Implications of Qualitative Results

If the findings are judged to be believable and important, and if you are satisfied with your interpretation of the meaning of the results, you can begin to consider what the implications of the findings might be. As with quantitative studies, the implications are often multidimensional. First, you can consider the implications for further research: Should the study be replicated in other settings? Can the study be expanded (or circumscribed) in meaningful or productive ways? Do the results suggest that an important construct has been identified that merits the development of a standardized measuring instrument? Does the emerging theory suggest hypotheses that could be tested through controlled quantitative research? Second, do the findings have implications for nursing practice. For example, could the health-care needs of a subculture (*e.g.,* the homeless) be identified and addressed more effectively as a result of the study? Finally, do the findings shed light on fundamental processes that are incorporated into nursing theory?

RESEARCH CRITIQUE

If nursing practice is to be based on a solid foundation of scientific knowledge, the worth of studies appearing in the nursing literature must be critically appraised. Sometimes consumers mistakenly believe that if a research report was accepted for publication, then the study must be a sound one. Unfortunately, this is not necessarily the case. Indeed, most research has limitations and weaknesses, and, for this reason, no single study can provide unchallengeable answers to research questions. Nevertheless, the methods of disciplined inquiry continue to provide us with the best possible means of answering certain questions. Knowledge is accumulated not by an individual researcher conducting a single, isolated study but rather through the conduct of several studies addressing the same or similar research questions and through the subsequent critical appraisal of these studies by others. Thus, consumers who can thoughtfully critique research reports also play a role in the advancement of nursing knowledge.

Critiquing Research Decisions

Although no single study is infallible, there is a tremendous range in the quality of studies—from nearly worthless to exemplary. The quality of the research is closely tied to the kinds of decisions the researcher makes in conceptualizing, designing, and executing the study and in interpreting and communicating the study results. Each study tends to have its own peculiar flaws because each researcher, in addressing the same or a similar research question, makes somewhat different decisions about how the study should be done. It is not uncommon for researchers who have made different **methodologic decisions** to arrive at different answers to the same research question. It is precisely for this reason that consumers of research must be knowledgeable about the research process. As a consumer, you must be able to evaluate the decisions investigators made so you can determine how much faith should be put in their conclusions. You must ask: What other approaches could have been used to study this research problem? and If another approach had been used, would the results have been more reliable, believable, or replicable? In other words, you must evaluate the impact of the researcher's decisions on the study's ability to reveal the truth.

Much of this book has been designed to acquaint consumers with a range of methodologic options for the conduct of research—options on how to design a study, measure research variables, select a study sample, analyze data, and so on. We hope a familiarity with these options will provide you with the tools to challenge a researcher's decisions when it is appropriate to do so and to suggest alternative methods.

Purpose of a Research Critique

A research **critique** is not just a review or summary of a study but rather a careful, critical appraisal of the strengths and limitations of a piece of research. A written critique should serve as a guide to researchers and practitioners. The critique ideally should suggest possibilities for the design of **replications** (*i.e.,* studies addressing the same research questions using similar methods) and should thus help to advance a particular area of knowledge. The critique should also help those who are practicing nursing to decide how the findings from the study can best be incorporated into their practice, if at all.

The function of critical evaluations of scientific work is not to hunt dogmatically for and expose mistakes. A good critique objectively identifies areas of adequacy and inadequacy, virtues as well as faults. Sometimes the need for this balance is obscured by the terms *critique* and *critical appraisal,* which connote unfavorable observations. The merits of a study are as important as its limitations in coming to conclusions about the worth of its findings. Therefore, the research critique should reflect a thoughtful, objective, and balanced consideration of the study's validity and significance. If the critique is not balanced, it will be of little use to the researcher who conducted the study because it might engender defensiveness, and practicing nurses might erroneously get the impression that the study has no merit at all.

Each chapter in this text has offered guidelines for evaluating various research decisions. Box 13–1 presents some further, more general tips for those preparing a formal research critique.

ELEMENTS OF A RESEARCH CRITIQUE

Each research report has several important dimensions that should be considered in a critical evaluation of the study's worth. The aspects we review here include the substantive and theoretical; methodologic; ethical; interpretive; and presentation and stylistic aspects.

Substantive and Theoretical Dimensions

The reader of a research report needs to determine whether the study was an important one in terms of the significance of the problem studied, the soundness of the conceptualizations, the appropriateness of the theoretical framework, and the creativity and insightfulness of the analysis. The research problem should have obvious relevance to some aspect of the nursing profession. It is not enough that a problem be interesting if it offers no possibility of contributing to nursing knowledge or improving nursing practice. Some topics may be so far afield from the concerns of nurses that they might better be addressed by researchers in other

Box 13–1

Guidelines for the Conduct of a Written Research Critique

1. Be sure to comment on the study's strengths as well as its limitations. The critique should be a balanced consideration of the worth of the research. Each research report has *some* positive features. Be sure to find them and note them.
2. Give specific examples of the study's strengths and limitations. Avoid vague generalizations of praise and fault finding.
3. Try to justify your criticisms. Offer a rationale for how a different approach would have solved a problem that the researcher failed to address.
4. Be as objective as possible. Try to avoid being overly critical of a study because you are not particularly interested in a topic or because you have a world view that is inconsistent with the underlying paradigm.
5. Be sensitive in handling negative comments. Try to put yourself in the shoes of the researcher receiving the critical appraisal. Do not be condescending or sarcastic.
6. Suggest realistic alternatives that the researcher (or future researchers) might want to consider. Don't just identify problems—offer some recommended solutions, making sure that the recommendations are practical ones.
7. Evaluate all aspects of the study—its substantive, theoretical, methodologic, ethical, interpretive, and presentational dimensions.

disciplines. Thus, even before the reader learns how a study was conducted, there should be an evaluation of whether the study should have been conducted in the first place.

The reader's own disciplinary orientation should not intrude in an objective evaluation of the study's significance. A clinical nurse might not be intrigued by a study focusing on the determinants of nursing turnover, but a nursing administrator trying to improve staffing decisions might find such a study highly useful. Similarly, a psychiatric nurse might find little value in a study of the sleep–wake patterns of low-birth-weight infants, but nurses in neonatal intensive care units might not agree. It is important, then, not to adopt a myopic view of the study's relevance to nursing.

Many problems that are relevant to nursing are still not necessarily worthwhile substantively. The reviewer must ask a question such as: Given what we know about this topic, is this research the right next step? Knowledge tends to be incremental. Researchers must consider how to advance knowledge on a topic in the most beneficial way. They should avoid unnecessary replications of a study once a body of research clearly points to an answer, but they also should not leap several steps ahead when there is an insecure foundation. Sometimes replication is exactly what is needed to enhance the believability or generalizability of earlier findings.

Another issue that has both substantive and methodologic implications is the congruence between the study question and the methods used to address it. There must be a good fit between the research problem on the one hand and the overall study design, the method of collecting research data, and the approach to analyzing those data on the other. Questions that deal with poorly understood phenomena, with processes, with the dynamics of a situation, or with in-depth description, for example, are usually best addressed with flexible designs, unstructured methods of data collection, and qualitative analysis. Questions that involve the measurement of well-defined variables, cause-and-effect relationships, or the effectiveness of some specific intervention, however, are usually better suited to more structured, quantitative approaches using designs that offer control over the research situation.

A final issue to consider is whether the researcher has appropriately placed the research problem into a larger theoretical context. As we stressed in Chapter 4, a researcher does little to enhance the value of the study if the connection between the research problem and a conceptual framework is artificial and contrived. But a research problem that is genuinely framed as a part of some larger intellectual problem usually can go much further in advancing knowledge than a problem that ignores its theoretical underpinnings.

Methodologic Dimensions

Researchers make a number of important decisions regarding how to go about answering their research questions or testing their research hypotheses. It is the consumer's job to evaluate critically the consequences of those decisions. In fact, the heart of the research critique lies in the appraisal of the methodologic decisions adopted in addressing the research question.

Although the researcher makes hundreds of decisions about the methods for conducting a study, some are more critical than others. In a quantitative study, the four major decision points on which the consumer should focus critical attention are as follows:

- *Decision 1:* What design will yield the most unambiguous and meaningful (internally valid) results about the relationship between the independent variable and dependent variable, or the most valid descriptions of the concepts under study?
- *Decision 2:* Who should participate in the study? What are the characteristics of the population to which the findings should be generalized? How large should the sample be, from where should participants be recruited, and what sampling approach should be used to select the sample?
- *Decision 3:* How should the research data be gathered? How can the variables be operationalized and reliably and validly measured for each participant in the study?
- *Decision 4:* What statistical analyses will provide the most appropriate tests of the research hypotheses or answers to the research questions?

In a quantitative study, these methodologic decisions are typically made upfront, and the researcher simply executes the prespecified plan. In a qualitative study, by contrast, the researcher makes ongoing methodologic decisions while in the process of collecting and analyzing data—once the very important decision about the research setting has been made. In a qualitative study, the major methodologic decisions you should consider in your critique are as follows:

- *Decision 1:* Where should the study take place? What setting will yield the richest information about the phenomenon under study?
- *Decision 2:* What should the sources of data be and how should the data be gathered? Should multiple sources of data (*e.g.,* unstructured interviews and observations) be used to achieve method triangulation?
- *Decision 3:* Who should participate in the study? How can participants be selected so as to enhance the theoretical richness of the study? How many participants will be needed to achieve data saturation? How much time should be spent in the field to achieve "prolonged engagement"?
- *Decision 4:* What types of evidence can be obtained to support the credibility, transferability, dependability, and confirmability of the data, the analysis, and the interpretation?

Because of practical constraints, research studies almost always involve making some compromises between what is ideal and what is feasible. For example, a quantitative researcher might ideally like to work with a sample of 1000 subjects but because of limited resources must be content to have a sample of 200 subjects. A qualitative researcher might realize that 3 years of field work would yield an especially rich and deep understanding of the culture or group under study, but cannot afford to devote this much time to the effort. The person doing a research critique cannot realistically demand that researchers attain these methodologic ideals but must be prepared to evaluate how much damage has been done by failure to achieve them.

Ethical Dimensions

The person performing a research critique should consider whether there is any evidence that the rights of human subjects were violated during the course of the investigation. If there are any potential ethical problems, the reviewer must consider the impact of those problems on the scientific merit of the study as well as on the subjects' well-being.

There are two main types of ethical transgressions in research studies. The first class consists of inadvertent actions or activities that the researcher did not foresee as creating an ethical dilemma. For example, in one study that examined married couples' experiences with sexually transmitted diseases, the researcher asked the husband and wife to complete privately two self-administered questionnaires. The researcher offered to mail back copies of the questionnaires to couples who wanted an opportunity to review their responses together. This offer was intended as a means of enhancing couple communication and was viewed as a benefit to study participants. However, some subjects may have felt compelled to say, under some spousal pressure, that they wanted to have a copy of their responses returned in the mail, when, in fact, they did not. The use of the mail to return these sensitive completed questionnaires was also questionable. In this case, the ethical problem was inadvertent and could easily be resolved (*e.g.,* the researcher could give out *blank* copies of the questionnaire for the couples to go over together).

In other cases, the researcher is aware of having committed some violation of ethical principles but has made a conscious decision that the violation is relatively minor in relation to the knowledge that could be gained by doing the study in a certain way. For example, the researcher may decide not to obtain informed consent from the parents of minor children attending a family planning clinic because to require such consent would probably dramatically reduce the number of minors willing to participate in the research and would lead to a biased sample of clinic users; it could also violate the minors' right to confidential treatment at the clinic. When the researcher knowingly elects not to follow the ethical principles outlined in Chapter 5, the reviewer must evaluate the decision itself *and* the researcher's rationale.

The reviewer who criticizes the ethical aspects of a study based on a report of completed research obviously is too late to prevent an ethical transgression from occurring. Nevertheless, the critique can bring the ethical problems to the attention of those who might be replicating the research.

Interpretive Dimensions

Research reports almost always conclude with a discussion, conclusions, or implications section. In this final section, the researcher attempts to make sense of the analyses, to understand what the findings mean in relation to the research questions, to consider whether the findings support or fail to support a theoretical framework, and to discuss what the findings might imply for the nursing profession.

As a reviewer, you should be somewhat wary if the discussion section fails to point out the study's limitations. The researcher is in the best position to detect and assess the impact of sampling deficiencies, practical constraints, data quality problems, and so on, and it is a professional responsibility to alert readers to these difficulties. Moreover, when a researcher notes some of the methodologic shortcomings of the study, then readers have some assurance that these limitations were not ignored in the development of the interpretation of the results. As an example, Carty, Bradley, and Winslow (1996) conducted a study of women's perceptions of fatigue during pregnancy and postpartum. Women who were discharged within 3 days of delivery were compared to women who were discharged after 3 days with respect to fatigue levels. The researchers found few differences between the two groups with regard to hours slept, perceptions of tiredness, and impact of tiredness on daily life. However, the researchers included a word of caution in their discussion section:

The following limitations should be considered when interpreting the findings: The women in this study chose their discharge time, those who went home early had significant follow-up by nurses, and the questionnaire developed for this study does not have established reliability. (p. 77)

Of course, researchers are unlikely to note *all* relevant shortcomings of their own work. For instance, in the above example, the authors failed to point out that the absence of significant group differences could have resulted from the use of a relatively small sample. Thus, the inclusion of comments about study limitations in the discussion section, although important, does not relieve you of the responsibility of appraising methodologic decisions.

Your task as reviewer is to contrast your own interpretation with that of the researcher and to challenge conclusions that do not appear to be warranted by the results. If your objective reading of the research methods and study findings leads to an interpretation that is notably different from that endorsed by the researcher, then the interpretive dimension of the study may well be faulty.

In addition to contrasting your interpretation with that of the researchers, your critique should also draw conclusions about the stated implications of the study. Some researchers make rather grandiose claims or offer unfounded recommendations on the basis of modest results. Some guidelines for evaluating the researcher's interpretation and implications are offered in Box 13–2.

Guidelines for Critiquing the Interpretive Dimensions of a Research Report

Box 13–2

1. Does the discussion section offer conclusions or interpretations for all the important results?
2. Are the interpretations consistent with the results? Do the interpretations give due consideration to the limitations of the research methods?
3. What types of evidence in support of the interpretation does the researcher offer? Is that evidence persuasive? Are the results interpreted in light of findings from other studies?
4. Are alternative explanations for the findings mentioned, and is the rationale for their rejection presented?
5. In quantitative studies, does the interpretation distinguish between practical and statistical significance?
6. Are generalizations made that are not warranted on the basis of the sample used?
7. Does the researcher offer implications of the research for nursing practice, nursing theory, and/or nursing research? Are the implications appropriate, given the study's limitations?
8. Are specific recommendations for practice or future studies made? Are the recommendations consistent with the findings and consistent with the body of knowledge on the topic?

Presentation and Stylistic Dimensions

Although the worth of the study is primarily reflected in the dimensions we have reviewed thus far, the manner in which the information is communicated in the research report is also fair game in a comprehensive critical appraisal. Box 13–3 summarizes the major points that should be considered in evaluating the presentation of a research report.

An important consideration is whether the research report has provided sufficient information for a thoughtful critique of the other dimensions. For example, if the report does not describe how participants were selected, then the reviewer cannot comment on the adequacy of the sample, but he or she can criticize the researcher's failure to include information on sampling. When vital pieces of information are missing, the researcher leaves the reader little choice but to assume the worst, because this would lead to the most cautious interpretation of the results.

The writing in a research report, as in any published document, should be clear, grammatical, concise, and well organized. Unnecessary jargon should be kept to a minimum, although colloquialisms generally should also be avoided. Inadequate organization is perhaps the most common presentation flaw in research reports. Continuity and logical thematic development are critical to good communication of scientific information, but these qualities are often difficult to attain.

Styles of writing do differ for qualitative and quantitative reports, and it is

---

Box 13–3

Guidelines for Critiquing the Presentation of a Research Report

1. Does the report include a sufficient amount of detail to permit a thorough critique of the study's purpose, conceptual framework, design and methods, handling of critical ethical issues, analysis of data, and interpretation?
2. Is the report well written and grammatical? Are pretentious words or jargon used when a simpler wording would have been possible?
3. Is the report well organized, or is the presentation confusing? Is there an orderly, logical presentation of ideas? Are transitions smooth, and is the report characterized by continuity of thought and expression?
4. Is the report sufficiently concise, or does the author include a lot of irrelevant detail? Are important details omitted?
5. Does the report suggest overt biases?
6. Is the report written using tentative language as befits the nature of disciplined inquiry, or does the author talk about what the study did or did not "prove"?
7. Is sexist language avoided?
8. Does the title of the report adequately capture the key concepts and the population under investigation? Does the abstract (if any) adequately summarize the research problem, study methods, and important findings?

unreasonable to apply the standards considered appropriate for one paradigm to the other. Quantitative research reports are typically written in a more formal, impersonal fashion, using either the third person or passive voice to connote objectivity. Qualitative studies are likely to be written in a more literary style, using the first or second person and active voice to connote proximity and intimacy with the data and the phenomenon under study. Regardless of style, however, you should, as a reviewer, be alert to indications of overt biases, unwarranted exaggerations, emotionally laden comments, or melodramatic language.

In summary, the research report is meant to be an account of how and why a problem was studied and what results were obtained. The report should be accurate, clearly written, cogent, and concise. It should reflect scholarship, but not pedantry, and it should be written in a manner that piques the reader's interest and curiosity.

RESEARCH EXAMPLES

The appendix offers two research reports—one qualitative and the other quantitative—in their entirety. The guidelines in this chapter and throughout the book can be used to conduct a critical appraisal of these studies. (In addition, there are two complete research reports in the accompanying *Study Guide for Essentials of Nursing Research,* 4th ed., as well as a fictitious research report with a complete critique.)

In this section, we describe two studies by nurse researchers and present excerpts from published written critiques. Note that these comments are not comprehensive—they do not cover all the dimensions of a research critique as described in this chapter. However, the excerpts should provide a flavor for the kinds of things that are noted in a critique. Additionally, we present excerpts from the researchers' responses to the critique.

Example of a Quantitative Report and Critical Comments

Skoner, Thompson, and Caron (1994) conducted a retrospective case-control study to investigate risk factors for stress urinary incontinence (SUI) in women. A sample of 140 women (94 cases and 46 controls), who were recruited from three private physician practices, participated in the study. To be eligible, cases had to have symptoms of SUI, and controls had to have no evidence of SUI. Controls were selected from a list of potential patients without SUI, matched to cases by age within 5-year age intervals. The study was described to cases as an investigation of urinary incontinence in women, whereas it was described as a study of women's health issues to controls.

Telephone interviews were used to obtain data relating to various factors that the research literature suggested were associated with the risk of SUI. The questions covered family history of incontinence, reproductive events and menstrual history, gynecologic-related surgeries and infections, urinary tract infections and procedures, current health behaviors, and medications. No follow-up procedures were instituted for women who were nonrespondents to the telephone survey.

The data were analyzed using logistic regression, which controlled for age and other factors. The results indicated that having a vaginal birth versus having only cesarean sections was associated with a substantially increased risk for SUI. Other significant risk factors included having an episiotomy or tear during delivery, having a mother who had SUI, and having had multiple urinary tract infections.

Knapp and Nickel (1995) prepared a letter to the editor of *Nursing Research,* the journal in which Skoner and colleagues' report appeared, to comment on various aspects of the report. Their first concern related to the matching of the cases and controls:

> The group matching was apparently carried out before the cooperation of cases and controls had been obtained. The original plan called for 123 cases and 198 controls, but with the inevitable attrition and reclassification of some cases as controls, and some controls as cases, the final numbers of 94 and 46 were obtained. The initial matching on age was therefore lost to a considerable degree by the low response rates for both cases and controls and by the reclassifications. No information is provided regarding age distribution and the extent to which the matching was successful within each 5-year interval. (p. 58)

Skoner and Thompson (1995) offered a response to this criticism:

> Regarding age differences, we reported a mean of 51.5 for cases and a mean of 54.3 for controls. In order to control for the possible confounding effects of this modest difference, age was included in the multivariable logistic regression modeling. . . . Control for this and other potential confounding variables did not materially alter the estimates presented in Table 1. (p. 58)

Knapp and Nickel also commented on the operationalization of the dependent variable, namely status as a case with SUI or as a control without SUI. Specifically, they noted that information regarding diagnoses for the controls was not included in the report and wondered why reclassification was based solely on SUI symptoms. The researchers responded that cystourethrograms were a means of expediting the identification of potential cases in only one of the three practices from which participants were recruited. However, for all subjects, the final classification was based on self-report. The researchers acknowledged the limitations of this approach: "Possible selection bias is of concern in any clinic-based case-control study, and we hope that population-based studies of stress urinary incontinence will be undertaken to avoid this potential methodologic problem" (p.58).

Knapp and Nickel also had concerns about the statistical analyses. For example, they noted that, "Given that 35 comparisons were made, some sort of procedure for protection from increased likelihood of Type I errors should have been employed" (p. 58).

Skoner and Thompson (1995) responded as follows:

Finally, regarding the issue of multiple comparisons, we do not feel that some sort of "protection" is warranted. We regard our confidence intervals as approximate indicators of the statistical uncertainty of estimating the odds ratios, and we have not adopted a strict adherence to the qualitative distinction between statistical significance versus non-significance. Of greater interest to us is the overall pattern of findings. . . . (p. 58)

Example of a Qualitative Report and Critical Comments

Vallerand and Ferrell (1995a) performed a secondary analysis of qualitative data to examine issues of control in patients with cancer pain. The original research that generated the data was an in-depth study of pain management at home among cancer patients. Ten patient–caregiver–nurse triads comprised the sample. Participants, who were cancer patients recruited from home health care agencies, had been experiencing cancer-related pain for at least 1 month. All patients had a primary caregiver who was over 18 years of age. Nurses were the primary nurses for the patient and had at least 6 months' experience in home health care.

The data were collected through in-depth interviews, which were tape-recorded and transcribed. The interviews included questions about the patient's illness and pain experience, pain management at home, decision making, and ethical conflicts related to pain. All patient and caregiver interviews were conducted in the patients' homes; the nurses were interviewed at the home health care agencies. Each interview lasted 1 to 2 hours.

For the secondary analysis, Vallerand (who was not involved in the original study) read all the transcripts and coded the data with regard to control; she also coded the data according to a previously developed classification scheme that organized control into five distinct types: processual control, contingency control, cognitive control, behavioral control, and existential control. All data that related directly or indirectly to issues of control were coded, whereas other issues discussed in the interviews were unanalyzed for the purposes of this study. The second author (Ferrell, who was a lead researcher in the original study) independently recoded the data for control-related themes. Agreement between researchers was achieved before analysis.

Using the classification scheme to organize their analysis, the authors found that there were differences in the perception of control by the patient, the caregiver, and the nurse caring for the patient with cancer pain. For the patients, the main focus was their attempt to maintain independence and control of their environment, the management of their pain, and the outcomes of their treatment. Both the primary family caregivers and the home care nurses were confronted with a struggle on a continuum ranging from helplessness to control. The authors concluded their report with some examples of interventions that could be used to increase patient control in the management of pain.

Fowler-Kerry (1995) prepared a commentary that was published in the same journal as this research report. Fowler-Kerry noted the importance of research relating to pain management in cancer patients. However, she expressed a few concerns regarding this research. A main concern was the adequacy of the data set for the conduct of this secondary analysis:

> The authors report that the concept of control emerged as a recurrent theme in the analysis of the primary study transcripts. No in-depth questioning or probing of informants about control occurred in the primary study. . . . The authors provide an explanation of the methodology used in both the primary study and the secondary analysis. There is no discussion of any limitations inherent in the secondary analysis. (pp. 481–482)

In their response to the commentary (Vallerand & Ferrell, 1995b), the researchers noted that, despite the absence of specific in-depth questioning relating to control, control emerged spontaneously as a central topic in the primary study. The absence of prompting, according to the researchers, underscoring the importance of the concept:

> This approach allows for the respondents to select from their own personal experiences those elements that they want to discuss, and therefore the respondents are not biased by the questions of the researcher or early labeling of the concept. Although we have not specifically included the concept of control . . . the participants in these studies consistently discussed the concept of control. (p. 482)

Fowler-Kerry commended the authors for including a detailed list of examples of interventions to increase control in pain management. However, she noted that the researchers did not identify which interventions emerged specifically as a result of the analysis: "Possibly the authors could comment about what novel results emerged from this study that would affect clinical practice or future research questions" (p. 482). The researchers acknowledged that this aspect of their report was not as well developed as might be desired, but noted that there was, indeed, a link between the interventions and their ongoing research on pain management.

▧ SUMMARY

A research **critique** is not simply a review of a study but rather is a careful, critical appraisal of the strengths and limitations of a research report. The critique is meant to provide guidance to the research community and to practitioners who must decide whether and to what extent the results of research findings should be incorporated into nursing practice.

A reviewer should consider five major dimensions of the study: the substantive and theoretical, methodologic, ethical, interpretive, and presentation and stylistic dimensions. Many critiques focus primarily on the methodologic dimension. Researchers designing a study must make a number of important **methodologic decisions** that affect the quality and integrity of the research. Several decisions are especially important in shaping the integrity of the study—although the key methodologic decisions are different for quantitative and qualitative researchers. Consumers preparing a critique must evaluate the decisions the researchers made to determine how much faith can be placed in the results. There is a tremendous range in the quality of the decisions researchers make, but because researchers' decisions are inevitably bound by some practical constraints, virtually every study is subject to some flaws or limitations.

The **interpretation** of research findings, an activity in which both producers and consumers of research engage, basically is a search for the broader meaning and implications of the results of an investigation. The results of the data analysis need to be scrutinized and reflected on with consideration to the conceptual framework, the specific questions that were addressed or the hypotheses that were tested, prior research findings, and the shortcomings of the methods used to answer the research questions. The interpretation typically involves five subtasks: (1) analyzing the accuracy and believability of the results; (2) searching for the underlying meaning of the results; (3) considering the importance of the findings; (4) analyzing the generalizability or transferability of the findings; and (5) assessing the implications of the study in regard to theory, nursing practice, and future research.

▧ STUDY SUGGESTIONS

Chapter 13 of the accompanying *Study Guide to Accompany Essentials of Nursing Research*, 4th edition offers various exercises and study suggestions for reinforcing the concepts presented in this chapter.

Suggested Readings

Methodologic References

Beck, C. T. (1990). The research critique: General criteria for evaluating a research report. *Journal of Obstetric, Gynecologic, and Neonatal Nursing, 19,* 18–22.

Burns, N. (1989). Standards for qualitative research. *Nursing Science Quarterly, 2,* 254–260.

Gehlbach, S. H. (1982). *Interpreting the medical literature.* Lexington, MA: Collamore Press.

Substantive References

Carty, E. M., Bradley, C., & Winslow, W. (1996). Women's perceptions of fatigue during pregnancy and postpartum. *Clinical Nursing Research, 5,* 67–80.

Fowler-Kerry, S. (1995) Commentary on "Issues of control in patients with cancer pain." *Western Journal of Nursing Research, 17,* 481–482.

Knapp, T. R., & Nickel, J. T. (1995). Letter to the editor re "Factors associated with risk of stress urinary incontinence in women." *Nursing Research, 44,* 58.

Skoner, M. M., & Thompson, W. D. (1995). Response to letter to the editor re "Factors associated with risk of stress urinary incontinence in women." *Nursing Research, 44,* 58.

Skoner, M. M., Thompson, W. D., & Caron, V. A. (1994). Factors associated with risk of stress urinary incontinence in women. *Nursing Research, 43,* 301–306.

Vallerand, A. H., & Ferrell, B. R. (1995a). Issues of control in patients with cancer pain. *Western Journal of Nursing Research, 17,* 467–481.

Vallerand, A. H., & Ferrell, B. R. (1995b). Response to commentary by Fowler-Kerry on "Issues of control in patients with cancer pain." *Western Journal of Nursing Research, 17,* 482–483.

14

Utilization of Nursing Research

Student Objectives

On completion of this chapter, the student will be able to:

- describe a continuum along which research utilization can occur
- give examples of how research can be used in the five phases of the nursing process
- discuss the current status of research utilization within nursing
- identify three large-scale nursing research utilization projects
- identify barriers to utilizing nursing research
- propose strategies to improve the utilization of nursing research findings for researchers, practicing nurses, nursing students, and administrators
- describe the general steps in a utilization project
- identify the major criteria that are relevant in a utilization project
- evaluate the extent to which a nurse researcher adequately addresses the issue of utilization in the discussion section of a research report
- define new terms in the chapter

New Terms

Clinical relevance
Collaborative research
Conceptual utilization
Cost–benefit assessment
Decision accretion
Implementation potential

Instrumental utilization
Knowledge creep
Research utilization
Scientific merit
Utilization criteria

Nurse researchers usually are not interested in pursuing knowledge simply for the sake of knowledge itself. In a practicing profession such as nursing, researchers generally want to have their findings incorporated into nursing protocols, nursing decisions, and nursing curricula. In fact, it might be argued that the ultimate worth of a nursing research study is demonstrated by the extent to which its findings eventually are used—alone or in concert with other findings—to improve the delivery of nursing services.

Over the past two decades, a number of changes in nursing education and in nursing research were prompted by the desire to develop a better knowledge base for the practice of nursing. In education, most schools of nursing changed their curricula to include courses on nursing research. Now, almost all baccalaureate and graduate nursing programs offer courses to instill some degree of research competence in their students. In the research arena, as indicated in Chapter 1, there has been a dramatic shift toward a focus on clinical nursing problems. These two changes alone, however, have not been enough to lead to a widespread integration of research findings into the delivery of nursing care. There appears to have been an unwarranted assumption that the production of clinically relevant studies would lead automatically to improved nursing practice—if only there were an audience of practicing nurses who were competent in critically evaluating these studies. Research utilization, as the nursing community has come to recognize, is a complex and nonlinear phenomenon. In this chapter, we discuss various aspects of the utilization of nursing research.

WHAT IS RESEARCH UTILIZATION?

Broadly speaking, **research utilization** refers to the use of some aspect of a study in an application unrelated to the original research. Current conceptions of research utilization recognize a continuum in terms of the specificity or diffuseness of the use to which knowledge is put. At one end of the continuum are discrete, clearly identifiable attempts to base a specific action on the results of research findings. For example, a series of studies in the 1960s and 1970s demonstrated that the optimal placement time of a glass thermometer for accurate oral temperature determination is 9 minutes (Nichols & Verhonick, 1968). When nurses specifically altered their behavior from shorter placement times to the empirically based recommendation of 9 minutes, this constituted an instance of research utilization at this end of the continuum. This type of utilization has been referred to as **instrumental utilization** (Caplan & Rich, 1975). Research utilization projects that have an instrumental goal are most likely to be based on carefully conducted experimental or quasi-experimental studies.

Research also can be utilized more diffusely in a manner that promotes cumulative awareness, understanding, or enlightenment. Caplan and Rich (1975) refer to this end of the utilization continuum as **conceptual utilization.** Thus, practicing nurses may read a research report in which the investigators report that nonnutritive sucking among preterm infants in a neonatal intensive care unit had a beneficial effect on the number of days to the infant's first bottle feeding and on the number of days of hospitalization. Nurses may be reluctant to alter their own behavior or to suggest an intervention based on the results of a single study, but their reading of the research report may make the nurses more observant in their own work with preterm infants and may lead them to watch for the effects of nonnutritive sucking in their own setting. Conceptual utilization, then, refers to situations in which users are influenced in their thinking about an issue based on their knowledge of one or more studies but do not put this knowledge to any specific, documentable use. Qualitative research, because it has the potential to offer rich insights into human needs, behaviors, and experiences, is especially likely to have implications for conceptual utilization.

The middle ground of this continuum involves the partial impact of research findings on nursing activities. This middle ground frequently is the result of a slow evolutionary process that does not reflect a conscious decision to use an innovative procedure but rather reflects what Weiss (1980) has termed knowledge creep and decision accretion. **Knowledge creep** refers to an evolving "percolation" of research ideas and findings. **Decision accretion** refers to the manner in which momentum for a decision builds over a period of time based on accumulated information gained through readings, informal discussions, meetings, and so on.

Research utilization at all points along this continuum appears to be an appropriate goal for nurses.

RESEARCH UTILIZATION IN NURSING

Numerous commentators have noted that progress in utilizing the results of nursing research studies has proceeded slowly—too slowly for many who are anxious to establish a scientific base for nursing actions. In this section, we consider the possibilities for research utilization and evidence of the extent to which utilization has occurred.

Incorporating Research into Practice: The Potential

The nursing process is complex and requires nurses to engage in many decision-making activities. In the course of delivering patient care, nurses collect relevant information, make assessments and diagnoses, develop plans for appropriate nursing actions, initiate interventions, and evaluate the effects of nursing interventions. These activities correspond to the five phases of nursing outlined in the *Standards of Clinical Nursing Practice* established by the American Nurses' Association (1991). Within each of these phases, the findings from research can assist nurses in making more informed decisions and in taking actions that have a solid, scientifically based rationale. Thus, research conducted by nurses can potentially play a pivotal role in improving the quality and efficiency of nursing care, and the process by which the care is delivered.

Assessment Phase
Nurses collect information to assess patient needs from a variety of sources. The information may come from interviews with clients, family members, other nurses, and other types of health professionals as well as from records, charts, and nurses' observations. Each source contributes its unique part to the total assessment. Research can focus on how best to collect the information, what types of information need to be collected, how to integrate various pieces of assessment data, and how

to improve the accuracy of gathering information. Research can also help nurses select alternative methods or forms for particular types of client, settings, and situations. Through research, nurses can determine the extent to which the forms produce comparable information.

Diagnosis Phase

Based on an analysis of the information collected in the assessment phase of the nursing process, nurses are expected to develop nursing diagnoses. Research can play an important role in helping nurses to make more accurate nursing diagnoses by validating the etiology of each diagnosis against the recorded assessment information. In addition, nursing research can help to determine the frequency of occurrence for each defining characteristic or cue associated with each diagnosis. The documentation can be helpful to the nursing profession, which has only recently begun the task of building up its taxonomy of diagnoses. Continued efforts in this area hold promise for the clustering of nursing diagnostic groups and the refinement of accepted nursing diagnoses.

Planning Phase

The planning phase of the nursing process involves decisions concerning *what* nursing actions or interventions are needed; *when* the nursing actions are most appropriately instituted for each nursing diagnosis; *who* the recipients of the nursing interventions should be; and under *what* conditions the interventions are to be implemented. Research findings can fruitfully be used by nurses in planning care by indicating the nursing interventions that are especially effective for particular cultural groups, settings, types of problem, and client characteristics. Research can also help nurses to evaluate the holism of the plan of care and to make more informed decisions about whether the established goals are realistic in a given situation.

Intervention Phase

Ideally, professionally accountable nurses would base as many of their nursing interventions as possible on research findings. Consider, for example, the many decisions made by nurses working the night shift in a nursing home. At what point do they decide that the nursing interventions are no longer producing the desired results for a resident in the process of dying? When is it time to notify the family or physician? What alterations in nursing interventions are available that facilitate, with as much ease as is possible, the transition from a state of life to a state of death? What approach might be used with families? What response might be expected from other residents of the home, and how might their stresses be appropriately alleviated? The systematic documentation of nursing interventions that have been found to be helpful may benefit other nurses facing the same kinds of situations.

Evaluation Phase

The last stage of the nursing process involves the evaluation of the degree to which the behavioral outcomes or goals developed at the planning stage have been met. Research can help document success or failure in achieving the various outcomes.

When success occurs with relative frequency, it may offer other nurses the opportunity to implement the plan in other comparable situations with a fair degree of confidence. When the plan is unsuccessful, then nurses are redirected to examine the accuracy of the assessment, the nursing diagnoses, the plan, and the nursing interventions. Such information, collected systematically, may aid other nurses in avoiding the same dilemmas and lead to improvements in nursing care.

Incorporating Research into Practice: The Record

As suggested above, there is considerable potential for utilizing research throughout the various phases of the nursing process. However, there is considerable concern that nurses have thus far failed to realize fully this potential for using research findings as a basis for making decisions and for developing nursing interventions. This concern is based on some evidence suggesting that nurses are not always aware of research results and do not effectively incorporate these results into their practice.

One of the first pieces of evidence about the gap between research and practice came from a study by Ketefian (1975), who reported on the oral temperature determination practices of 87 registered nurses (RNs). Ketefian's study was designed to learn what "happens to research findings relative to nursing practice after five or ten years of dissemination in the nursing literature" (p. 90). The results of a series of investigations in the late 1960s had clearly demonstrated that the optimal placement time for oral temperature determination using glass thermometers is 9 minutes. In Ketefian's study, only 1 out of 87 nurses reported the correct placement time, suggesting that these practicing nurses were unaware of or ignored the research findings about optimal placement time.

In another study investigating research utilization, Kirchhoff (1982) investigated the discontinuance of coronary precautions in a nationwide sample of 524 intensive care nurses. Several published studies had failed to demonstrate that the practices of restricting ice water and rectal temperature measurement were necessary, yet Kirchhoff's results indicated that these coronary precautions were still widely practiced. Only 24% of the nurses had discontinued ice water restrictions and only 35% had discontinued rectal temperature restrictions.

More recently, Coyle and Sokop (1990) investigated practicing nurses' adoption of 14 nursing innovations that had been reported in the nursing literature, replicating a study by Brett (1987). Brett used the utilization criteria suggested by Haller, Reynolds, and Horsley (1979) in selecting 14 studies. These criteria included scientific merit; significance and usefulness of the research findings to the practice setting; and the suitability of the findings for application to practice. A sample of 113 nurses practicing in 10 hospitals (randomly selected from the medium-sized hospitals in North Carolina) completed questionnaires that measured the nurses' awareness and use of the study findings. The results indicated much variation across the 14 studies. For example, from 34% to 94% of the nurses reported awareness of the various findings. Coyle and Sokop used Brett's original scheme to categorize each study according to its stage of adoption: awareness (indicating knowledge of the innovation); persuasion (indicating the nurses' belief that nurses should use the innovation in practice); occasional use in practice; and regular use in practice. Only 1 of the 14 studies was at the regular-use stage of adoption. Six of the studies were in the persuasion stage, indicating that the nurses knew of the innovation and thought it *should* be incorporated into nursing practice but were not basing their own nursing decisions on it. Table 14–1 describes 4 of the 14 nursing innovations, one for each of the four stages of adoption, according to Coyle and Sokop's results. The results of this study (and the results of Brett's earlier study) are more encouraging than the studies by Ketefian and Kirchhoff in that they suggest that, on average, the practicing nurses were aware of many innovations based on research results, were persuaded that the innovations ought to be used, and were beginning to use them on occasion. Of course, it is possible that the respondents overstated their awareness and use of nursing innovations.

It is clear that a gap exists between knowledge production and knowledge utilization in nursing as well as in other disciplines. Some gap is inevitable and, given the imperfection of scientific research as a means of knowing, even desirable. Moreover, it seems likely that the gap as identified in such studies as those previously described is somewhat overstated, for three reasons. First, the utilization studies do not always take into consideration technologic changes that might make the knowledge irrelevant. Thus, as Downs (1979) has pointed out, electronic thermometers that rapidly replaced glass thermometers in the mid-1970s made the placement time findings obsolete and could account for Ketefian's results. Second, an important factor in research utilization is a cost–benefit analysis, as we will describe later in this chapter. The participants in Kirchhoff's study may have continued using coronary care precautions because the risk of problems that might arise by eliminating them (*e.g.,* if the study results were not correct) outweighed the benefits (such as more efficient use of staff time) that could accrue by keeping them. Third, the studies have focused primarily on utilization at one end of the utilization continuum—the end we have referred to as instrumental utilization. That is, the utilization studies have been interested primarily in the extent to which specific findings are used in specific nursing situations. The studies by Brett (1987) and Coyle and Sokop (1990), which found that half of the innovations were in the persuasion stage, support the notion of a great middle ground in research utilization. No study has investigated conceptual utilization, but we suspect that, with the growing emphasis on nursing research in nursing curricula, there is a much higher level of conceptual utilization throughout the nursing community today than there was 10 years ago. Nurses are becoming enlightened with regard to the value of research by a growing body of research that is challenging traditional ways of practicing nursing.

Table 14-1. Extent of Adoption of Four Nursing Practices*

Stage	Nursing Innovation	Aware (%)	Persuaded (%)	Use Sometimes (%)	Use Always (%)
Awareness	Elimination of lactose from the formulas of tube-feeding diets for adult patients minimizes diarrhea, distention, flatulence, and fullness and reduces patient rejection of feedings (Horsley, Crane, & Haller, 1981)	38	36	13	19
Persuasion	Accurate monitoring of oral temperatures can be achieved on patients receiving oxygen therapy by using an electronic thermometer placed in the sublingual pocket (Lim-Levy, 1982)	68	55	35	29
Occasional use	A formally planned and structured preoperative education program preceding elective surgery results in improved patient outcomes (King & Tarsitano, 1982)	83	81	48	23
Regular use	A closed sterile system of urinary drainage is effective in maintaining the sterility of urine in patients who are catheterized for less than 2 weeks; continuity of the closed drainage system should be maintained during irrigations, sampling procedures, and patient transport (Horsley, Crane, Haller, & Bingle, 1981)	94	91	84	6

* Based on findings reported in Coyle, L. A., & Sokop, A. G. (1990). Innovation adoption behavior among nurses. *Nursing Research, 39,* 176–180. The sample consisted of 113 practicing nurses.

Efforts to Improve Utilization

Much discussion has been generated about the need to reduce the gap between nursing research and nursing practice. Several formal efforts to achieve that goal have been undertaken. In this section, we briefly describe three prominent efforts.

The WICHE Project

One of the earliest research utilization projects was the Western Interstate Commission for Higher Education (WICHE) Regional Program for Nursing Research Development. The 6-year project investigated the feasibility of increasing nursing research activities through regional collaborative activities. According to the final report (Krueger, Nelson, & Wolanin, 1978), the three major project activities were: (1) collaborative, nontargeted research (bringing together nurses from educational and practice settings to design studies based on mutually identified nursing problems); (2) collaborative, targeted research (multiple studies in different settings all designed to investigate the concept of quality of care); and (3) research utilization. The project team visualized research utilization as part of a five-phase resource linkage model. In this model, nurses were conceived as organizational change agents who could provide a link between research and practice. Through a support system (*e.g.,* through workshops, conferences, and consultations), participant nurses were to utilize research results to solve problems identified as occurring in practice.

Nurses who participated in the WICHE project were given the opportunity to identify problems that needed research-based solutions and were then provided with opportunities to develop skills in reading and evaluating research for use in practice. They also developed detailed plans for introducing research innovations into their clinical practice settings. The final report indicated that the project was successful in increasing research utilization, but it also identified a stumbling block. The problem that posed the greatest difficulty was finding scientifically sound, reliable nursing studies with clearly identified implications for nursing care.

The NCAST Project

The Nursing Child Assessment Satellite Training (NCAST) project was a 2-year research dissemination project. Its primary objectives were to determine whether satellite communication technology is an efficient means of disseminating nursing research and whether an interactive communication facility would promote effective application of new health-care assessment techniques (Barnard & Hoehn, 1978). The results of the study supported the use of satellite communication for research dissemination. In terms of research utilization, the project directors proposed a model with four components: (1) recruitment (the identification and recruitment of an appropriate practitioner audience); (2) translation (the transformation of research results into a format and idiom that can easily be understood by nurse practitioners); (3) dissemination (the communication of research findings in an effective and efficient manner); and (4) evaluation (the determination of the impact of the other three processes).

The CURN Project

The best-known nursing research utilization project is the Conduct and Utilization of Research in Nursing (CURN) project, a 5-year development project awarded to the Michigan Nurses Association by the Division of Nursing. The major objective of the CURN project was to increase the use of research findings in the daily practice of RNs by (1) disseminating current research findings; (2) facilitating organizational changes needed for the implementation of innovations; and (3) encouraging the conduct of **collaborative research** that has relevance to nursing practice.

One of the activities of the CURN project was to stimulate the conduct of research in clinical settings. The project resulted in a set of nine volumes on various clinical problems. The titles of these volumes (*e.g., Pain; Preventing Decubitus Ulcers; Structured Preoperative Teaching;* and *Reducing Diarrhea in Tube-Fed Patients*) indicate that a wide range of clinical issues were studied.

The CURN project also focused on helping nurses to utilize research findings in their practice. The CURN project staff saw research utilization primarily as an organizational process (Horsley, Crane, & Bingle, 1978). According to their view, the commitment of organizations that employ practicing nurses to the research utilization process is essential for research to have any impact on nursing practice. The CURN project team concluded that research utilization by practicing nurses is feasible—but only if the research is relevant to practice and if the results are broadly disseminated.

BARRIERS TO UTILIZING NURSING RESEARCH

Typically, several years elapse between the time a researcher conceptualizes and designs a study and the time the results are reported in the research literature. Many more years may elapse between the time the results are reported and the time practicing nurses learn about the results and attempt to incorporate them into practice. Thus, it is not unusual for there to be an interim of a decade or more between the posing of a research problem and the implementation of a solution—if, in fact, there is *ever* an effort to implement. In the next section of this chapter, we discuss some strategies for bridging the gap between nursing research and nursing practice. First, however, we review some of the barriers to research utilization in nursing. These barriers can be broadly grouped into four categories relating to characteristics of the source of the barrier—the research itself, practicing nurses, organizational settings, and the nursing profession.

Research Characteristics

For many nursing problems, the state of the art of research knowledge is at a fairly rudimentary level. Studies reported in the literature often do not warrant the incorporation of their findings into practice. Flaws in research design, sample selection, data collection, or data analysis frequently raise questions about the soundness or generalizability of the study findings. Thus, a major impediment to research utilization by practicing nurses is that, for many problems, an extensive base of valid and trustworthy study results has not been developed.

As we have repeatedly stressed throughout this text, most studies have flaws of one type or another. The study may be flawed conceptually or methodologically, and the flaws may be minor or major; but the fact remains that there are few, if any, perfect studies. If one were to wait for the perfect study before basing clinical decisions and interventions on research findings, one would have a very long wait indeed. It is precisely because of the limits of current research methods that replication becomes essential. When repeated efforts to address a research question in different settings and with different types of participant yields similar results, then there can be greater confidence that the truth has been discovered. Isolated studies can almost never provide an adequate basis for making changes in nursing practice. Therefore, a constraint to research utilization is the dearth of reported replications of studies.

Nurses' Characteristics

Practicing nurses as individuals have characteristics that impede the incorporation of research findings into nursing care. Perhaps the most obvious is the educational preparation of nurses. Most practicing nurses—graduates of diploma or associate degree programs—have not received any formal instruction in research. They may, therefore, lack the skills to judge the merits of scientific projects. Furthermore, because research played a limited role in their training, these nurses may not have developed positive attitudes toward research and may not be aware of the beneficial role it can play in the delivery of nursing care. Champion and Leach (1989) found that nurses' attitudes toward research were strong predictors of the utilization of research findings. Courses on research methodology are now typically offered in baccalaureate nursing programs, but generally insufficient attention is paid to research utilization. The ability to critique a research report is a necessary, but not sufficient, condition for effectively incorporating research results into daily decision making.

Another characteristic of nurses is one that is common to most humans. People are generally resistant to change. Change requires effort, retraining, and restructuring one's work habits. Change may also be perceived as threatening (*e.g.,* proposed changes may be perceived as potentially affecting one's job security). Thus, there is likely to be some opposition to introducing innovations in the practice setting.

Organizational Characteristics

Some of the impediments to research utilization, as the CURN project staff so astutely noted, stem from the organizations that train and employ practicing nurses. Organizations, perhaps to an even greater degree than individuals, resist change, unless there is a strong organizational perception that there is something fundamentally wrong with the status quo. In many settings, the organizational climate is simply not conducive to research utilization. To challenge tradition and accepted practices, a spirit of intellectual curiosity and openness must prevail.

In many practice settings, administrators have established protocols and procedures to reward expertise and competence in nursing practice. Few practice settings, however, have established a reward system for critiquing nursing studies, for utilizing research in practice, or for discussing research findings appropriate to clients. Thus, organizations have failed to motivate or reward nurses to seek ways to implement appropriate findings into their practice. Research review and utilization are often considered appropriate activities only when time is available, but available time is generally limited. Indeed, in a national survey of nearly 1000 clinical nurses, one of the greatest reported barriers to research utilization was "insufficient time on the job to implement new ideas," which was reported as a moderate or great barrier by about 75% of the sample (Funk, Champagne, Wiese, & Tornquist, 1991).

Finally, organizations may be reluctant to expend the necessary resources for attempting utilization projects or for implementing changes to organizational policy. Resources may be required for the use of outside consultants, for staff release time, for administrative review, for evaluating the effects of an innovation, and so on. With the push toward cost containment in health-care settings, resource constraints may pose a barrier to research utilization.

Overall, in the previously cited national survey concerning perceived barriers, those stemming from the organizational setting were viewed by clinical nurses as posing the greatest obstacles to research utilization (Funk et al., 1991).

Characteristics of the Nursing Profession

Some of the impediments that contribute to the gap between research and practice are more global than those previously discussed and can be described as reflecting the state of the nursing profession or, even more broadly, the state of our society.

One issue is that it has sometimes been difficult to encourage clinicians and researchers to interact and collaborate. They generally work in different settings, have different professional concerns, interact with different networks of nurses, and operate according to different philosophical systems. Relatively few systematic attempts have been made to form collaborative arrangements, and, to date, even fewer of these arrangements have been institutionalized as formal, permanent entities. Moreover, attempts to develop such collaboration will not necessarily be welcomed by either group. A deep-seated lack of trust sometimes undermines collaboration between nurse researchers and nurse clinicians.

A related issue is that communication between practitioners and researchers is problematic. Most practicing nurses do not read nursing research journals, nor do they usually attend professional conferences where research results are reported. Many nurses involved in the direct delivery of care are too overwhelmed by the

technical jargon or the statistical analysis contained in research reports to understand fully such reports even when they do read them. Furthermore, nurse researchers may too infrequently attend to the needs of clinical nurses as reported in
specialty journals. For research utilization to happen, there must be two-way communication between the practicing nurse and the nurse researcher. The recent
emergence of two journals—*Applied Nursing Research* and *Clinical Nursing
Research*—represents an important step in this direction.

Phillips (1986) noted two other barriers to bridging the research–practice
gap. One is the shortage of appropriate role models. Phillips comments that "even
if a nurse wants to assume the role of nursing research consumer, there are few
colleagues available to give support for the endeavor and fewer still available to
emulate" (p. 8). The other barrier is the historical "baggage" that has defined nursing
in such a way that practicing nurses may not perceive themselves as independent
professionals capable of recommending changes based on nursing research results.
If practicing nurses believe that their role is to wait for direction from the medical
community, and if they believe they have no power to be self-directed, they will have
difficulty initiating innovations based on nursing research results. In the previously
mentioned national survey, the barrier perceived by the largest percentage of nurses
was the nurse's feeling that he or she did not have "enough authority to change
patient care procedures" (Funk et al., 1991).

SCOPE OF RESPONSIBILITY
FOR RESEARCH UTILIZATION

Where does the responsibility for bridging the gap between research and practice
lie? Should individual practicing nurses pursue research-based nursing innovations?
Should organizations and their administrative staffs take the lead? Or should the
direction come from researchers themselves? In our view, the entire nursing community must be involved in the process of putting research into practice.

Strategies for Researchers

A great deal of the responsibility for research utilization rests in the hands of
researchers. There is little point in pursuing disciplined inquiries if the results do
not get used, so it behooves researchers to take steps to ensure that utilization can
occur. There are a number of strategies that researchers can implement to foster
better adoption of their research results, including the following:

- *Do high-quality research.* A major impediment to utilizing nursing research results, as indicated in the previous section, is that there is often
  an inadequate scientific basis for introducing innovations or for making
  changes.
- *Replicate.* Utilization of research results can almost never be justified on

the basis of a single isolated study, so researchers must make a real commitment to replicating studies and publishing the results of those efforts.

- *Collaborate with practitioners.* Researchers will never succeed in having much of an impact on nursing practice unless they become better attuned to the needs of practicing nurses and the clients they serve, the problems that practicing nurses face in delivering nursing care, and the constraints that operate in practice settings. Researchers should seek opportunities to exchange ideas for research problems with nurse clinicians, to involve clinicians in the actual conduct of research, and to seek their input in the interpretation of study results.
- *Disseminate aggressively.* If a researcher fails to communicate the results of a completed study to other nurses, it is obvious that the results will never be utilized. It is the researcher's responsibility to find some means of communicating research results. It is especially important from a utilization standpoint for researchers to report their results in specialty journals, which are more likely to be read by practicing nurses than the nursing research journals. Researchers should also take steps to disseminate study findings at conferences, colloquia, and workshops that nurse clinicians attend.
- *Communicate clearly.* It is not always possible to present the results of a research project in a way that is readily comprehensible to all nonresearchers. Researchers need to be encouraged, however, to avoid unnecessary jargon whenever possible, to construct tables carefully so that a nonresearcher can get a sense of the findings, and to compose the abstract of the report so that virtually any intelligent reader can understand the research problem, the general approach, and the most salient results.
- *Suggest clinical implications.* In the discussion section of research reports, researchers should suggest how the results of their research can be utilized by practicing nurses. The researcher should be careful to discuss study limitations and to make some assessment of the generalizability of the study findings. If an implications section became a standard feature of research reports, the burden of utilization would be much lighter for the nurse clinician.

Consumers can and should evaluate the extent to which researchers have adopted these strategies to enhance research utilization.

Strategies for Practicing Nurses

Practicing nurses cannot by themselves launch institution-wide utilization projects, but their behaviors and attitudes are, nevertheless, critical to the success of any efforts to base nursing interventions and nursing diagnoses on research findings. Furthermore, individual nurses can clearly engage in and benefit from conceptual utilization. Therefore, every nurse has an important role to play in utilizing nursing research. The following are some strategies in which nurses can engage:

- *Read widely and critically.* Professionally accountable nurses continue their nursing education by keeping abreast of important developments in their field. Nurses ideally should read regularly journals relating to their specialty, including the research reports in them. Research newsletters and columns with research briefs are alternative sources of information on research developments in a field. Brett's study (1987) suggests the importance of reading. Her findings revealed that nurses who spent more time each week reading professional journals were more likely to adopt a research-based innovation than nurses who read infrequently. It is especially important for nurse clinicians to read critical reviews of research on a problem.
- *Attend professional conferences.* Many nursing conferences include presentations of studies that have clinical relevance. It is often more rewarding to hear a research presentation at a conference than to read a research report because conference attenders usually hear of an innovation much sooner than those who wait to read about it in a journal. Furthermore, those attending a conference get an opportunity to meet the researcher and to ask questions about practice implications. Brett's (1987) utilization study revealed a positive relationship between nurses' conference attendance and their degree of adopting a research-based innovation. Nurses should ask their supervisors about the possibility of obtaining stipends to defray the cost of attending such conferences.
- *Learn to expect evidence that a procedure is effective.* Every time nurses or nursing students are told about a standard nursing procedure, they have a right to ask the question: Why? Nurses need to develop expectations that the decisions they make in their clinical practice are based on sound rationales. It is not inappropriate for the nursing student or practitioner to question or challenge the principles and procedures currently in use, although tact is clearly important.
- *Seek environments that support research utilization.* Organizations differ in their openness to research utilization, so nurses interested in basing their practice on research have some control through their employment decisions. If organizations perceive that nurses are basing their employment decisions on such factors as the organization's attitude toward research and research utilization, there will be some pressure to support research utilization.
- *Become involved in a journal club.* Many organizations that employ nurses sponsor journal clubs that meet regularly to review research articles that have potential relevance to practice. Generally, members take turns reviewing and critically appraising a study and presenting the critique to the club's members. If there is no such club in existence, it might be possible to initiate one. Although the bulk of the responsibility for disseminating research results lies with the researcher, this is a responsibility that can be shared by practitioners.

- *Collaborate with a nurse researcher.* Collaboration, which we mentioned as a strategy for nurse researchers, is a two-way street. Practicing nurses who have identified a clinical problem in need of a solution and who lack methodologic skills for the conduct of a study should consider initiating a collaborative relationship with a local nurse researcher. Collaboration with a nurse researcher could also be a useful approach for undertaking formal, institutional utilization projects.

- *Pursue and participate in institutional utilization projects.* Sometimes ideas for utilization projects come from staff nurses. Although large-scale utilization projects require organizational and administrative support, individual nurses or groups of nurses can propose such a project to the nursing department. For example, an idea for such a project may emerge in the context of a journal club. If the idea for a research utilization effort originates from within the administration, individual nurses are still likely to play an important role in carrying out the project. Indeed, a utilization project easily can be undermined by reluctant or uncooperative staff. Although change is not always easy, it is in the interest of the profession to have practicing nurses who are open-minded about the possibility that a new technique or procedure can improve the quality of care that nurses provide. Several studies have found that nurses who are involved in research-related activities (*e.g.,* a utilization project or data collection activities) develop more positive attitudes toward research and better research skills (*e.g.,* Dufault, Bielecki, Collins & Willey, 1995; Bostrom & Suter, 1993).

- *Pursue appropriate personal utilization projects.* Not all findings from research studies require organizational commitment or policy directives. For example, an ethnographic study might reveal that the health beliefs of an immigrant group are different from those of the predominant cultural group, and this may lead a nurse to ask informally several additional questions of clients of that immigrant group during assessment. If the nurse discovers that important and relevant information is gleaned from these additional questions, it may then be appropriate to recommend to the administration a more formal utilization project, which might involve changes to the standard assessment protocols. Of course, not all research findings are amenable to such informal personal utilization projects. If the results of a study or series of studies suggest an action or decision that is contrary to organizational policy or that has *any* potential risk for the clients, nurses should not pursue such projects without supervisory approval. Some criteria for research utilization are discussed in the next section of this chapter.

Strategies for Administrators

According to several models of research utilization, the organizations that employ nurses play a fundamental role in supporting or undermining the nursing profession's efforts to develop a scientific base of practice. In the national survey of clinical nurses, respondents viewed "enhancing administrative support and encouragement" as the single most effective means of facilitating research utilization (Funk et al., 1991). Although the readers of this text are not likely to include a large audience of nursing or hospital administrators, some strategies are described primarily to alert practicing nurses to the kinds of issues facing these groups. To promote research utilization, administrators should engage in the following strategies:

- *Foster a climate of intellectual curiosity.* If there is administrative rigidity and opposition to change, then the staff's interest in research utilization is not likely to become ignited. Open communication is an important ingredient in persuading staff nurses that their experiences and problems are important and that the administration is willing to consider innovative solutions.
- *Offer emotional or moral support.* If nurse administrators are not supportive of research utilization, there is little chance that any utilization efforts will get off the ground. Administrators need to make their support visible by informing staff and prospective staff on an individual basis, by establishing research utilization committees, by helping to develop research journal clubs, and by serving as role models or mentors for the staff nurses.
- *Offer financial or resource support for utilization.* Utilization projects typically require some resources, although resource demands are often modest. If the administration expects nurses to engage in research utilization activities on their own time and at their own expense, the message given is that research utilization is unimportant to those managing the organization.
- *Reward efforts for utilization.* When administrators evaluate nursing performance, they use a number of different criteria. Although research utilization should not be a primary criterion for evaluating a nurse's performance, its inclusion as one of several important criteria is likely to have a large impact on nurses' behaviors.

◩ THE UTILIZATION PROCESS AND CRITERIA FOR UTILIZATION

In this section, we discuss how a research utilization project can be planned and executed. Although the processes described here are most likely to be applicable to an organization or a group of nurses working together on a formal project, many of the steps in the processes are important for individual nurses to consider as they attempt to base their clinical decisions on scientific findings.

Approaches to Research Utilization

Nurses interested in utilizing research findings in their nursing practice generally set about the task in one of two ways. One approach, shown schematically as path A in Figure 14–1, begins with the identification of a clinical problem that needs

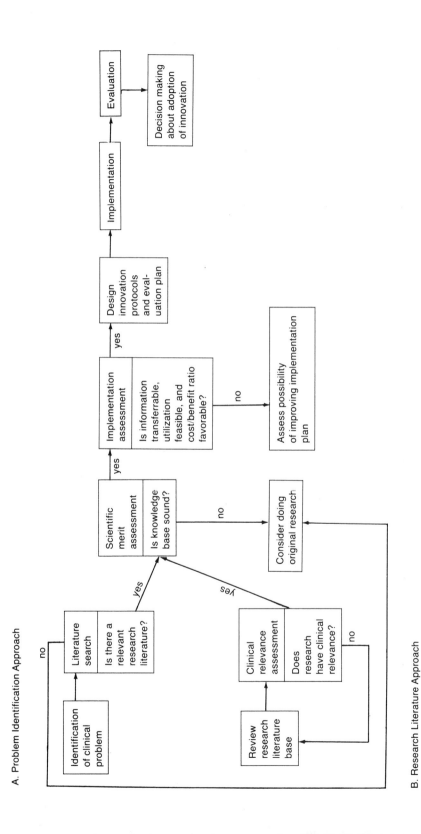

A. Problem Identification Approach

B. Research Literature Approach

Figure 14–1. Two models of research utilization

solution. This problem identification approach is likely to have considerable internal staff support if the selected problem is one that numerous nurses in the practice setting have encountered. This approach to utilization is likely to have a high clinical relevance because a specific clinical situation generated the interest in resolving the problem in the first place.

The next step is a search for relevant literature to determine whether nurse researchers have addressed the problem through scientific research (see Chapter 4). If there is no research base related to the identified problem, there are two choices: to abandon the original problem and perhaps select an alternative one, or to consider initiating an original research project on the topic (*i.e.,* to initiate steps to create a knowledge base). This decision is likely to depend on the research skills of the staff and on the availability of research consultants.

Next, the knowledge base must be critically evaluated. If the knowledge base is sound, then the subsequent step is to conduct an implementation assessment. If, however, the existing knowledge base inspires little confidence that the research could effectively be utilized by nurses, then there remain the two alternatives suggested previously: to go back to the drawing board and select a new problem, or to investigate the possibility of doing original research to improve the knowledge base.

The implementation assessment involves three primary aspects: an assessment of the transferability of the research findings; an assessment of the cost–benefit ratio; and an evaluation of the feasibility of implementing the innovation. These criteria will be discussed in the next section. If all the implementation criteria are met, the team can then proceed to design the protocols for the innovation and its clinical evaluation, implement the innovation in the practice setting, evaluate its effectiveness and costs, and then make a decision about whether the new practice should be institutionalized. If the implementation assessment suggests that there might be problems in testing the innovation within that particular practice setting, the team can either identify a new problem and begin the process anew or consider adopting a plan to improve the implementation potential (*e.g.,* seeking external resources if cost considerations are the inhibiting factor).

The second major approach to conducting a utilization project, shown schematically as path B in Figure 14–1, has many of the same components as the first approach. The major difference, however, is the starting point. Here, the process starts with the research literature. This could occur if, for example, a utilization project emerged as a result of discussions within a journal club. In this approach, the team would proceed through most of the same steps as outlined above, except that a preliminary assessment would need to be made of the clinical relevance of the research findings. If it is determined that the research base is not clinically relevant, then the next step involves further reading and reviewing of the research literature.

Both these approaches involve several types of assessment, the results of which affect the appropriateness of proceeding with the utilization project. Criteria for making these assessments are presented next.

Utilization Criteria

As the two models show in Figure 14–1, there are three broad classes of **utilization criteria** that are important in undertaking a utilization project: (1) clinical relevance, (2) scientific merit, and (3) implementation potential. Each is described below.

Clinical Relevance

Of critical importance is whether the problem and its solution have a high degree of **clinical relevance.** The central issue here is whether a problem of significance to nurses will be solved by making some change or introducing a new intervention. There is little point in undertaking a utilization project if the nursing profession or the clients it serves cannot benefit from the effort. If, under the best of circumstances, there is little potential for solving a nursing problem or helping nurses to make important clinical decisions, then the project probably should not be undertaken.

Five questions relating to clinical relevance, shown in Box 14–1, can be applied to a research report or set of related reports and generally can be answered based on a reading of the introductory sections of the reports. If the answer is yes to any one of the five questions, the next step in the process can be pursued because the innovation has the potential for being useful in practice. If, however, the answers to all the questions are negative, the prospect of clinical relevance is small, and there probably is little point in pursuing the problem area any further.

Scientific Merit

We have discussed the criteria for **scientific merit** throughout this text, and, in each chapter, we presented guidelines for assessing whether the findings and conclusions of a study are accurate, believable, and meaningful. When it comes to

Box 14-1

Criteria for Evaluating the Clinical Relevance of a Body of Research

1. Does the research have the potential to help solve a problem being faced by practicing nurses?
2. Does the research have the potential to help with clinical decision making with regard to (a) making appropriate observations, (b) identifying client risks or complications, or (c) selecting an appropriate intervention?
3. Are clinically relevant theoretical propositions tested by the research?
4. If the research involves an intervention, does the intervention have potential for implementation in real-world clinical settings? Do nurses have control over the implementation of such interventions?
5. Can the data collection measures used in the research be applied to clinical practice?

utilization, however, some additional concerns must be kept in mind. First and foremost is the issue of replication, the repeating of a study in a new setting with a new sample of subjects. It is unwise to base an entire utilization project on a single study that has not been replicated, even if the study is extremely rigorous. Ideally, there would be several replications—each providing similar evidence of the effectiveness of the innovation being considered. At least one and ideally more of the studies should have been conducted in a clinical setting, with real clients.

Replications are seldom exact duplications of an earlier study; usually a replication involves making some changes to some aspects of the research methods, such as the data collection methods, the sampling plan, and so on. It is not essential that the replications be identical to provide a useful basis for pursuing a utilization project. Rather, it is more important that the *problem* being addressed is the same and that the innovations being tested are conceptually similar to each other. For example, several nurse researchers have investigated the effect of infant stimulation on the outcomes of low-birth-weight infants. Although these studies have operationalized stimulation in different ways and have examined different outcomes, it would be reasonable for a utilization project to consider the whole body of research on stimulation strategies for low-birth-weight babies.

Implementation Potential

Even when it has been determined that a problem has clinical significance and when there is a sound knowledge base relating to that clinical problem, it is not necessarily true that a utilization project can be planned and implemented. A number of other issues must be considered when determining implementation potential, which we have grouped under three headings: the transferability of the knowledge, the feasibility of implementation, and the cost–benefit ratio of the innovation. Box 14–2 presents some assessment questions for these categories.

Transferability. The main issue in the transferability of findings question is whether it makes good sense to attempt the selected innovation in the new practice setting. If there is some aspect of the practice setting that is fundamentally incongruent with the innovation—in terms of its philosophy, the types of client it serves, its personnel, or its financial or administrative structure—then it makes little sense to try to transfer the innovation, even if a clinically significant innovation has been shown to be effective in various research contexts.

Feasibility. The feasibility questions address a number of practical concerns about the availability of staff and resources, the organizational climate, the need for and availability of external assistance, and the potential for clinical evaluation. An important issue here is whether nurses will have control over the innovation. When nurses do not have full control over the new procedure being introduced, it is important to recognize the interdependent nature of the utilization project and to proceed as early as possible to establish the necessary cooperative arrangements.

Box 14-2

Criteria for Evaluating the Implementation Potential of an Innovation

Transferability of the Findings

1. Will the innovation "fit" in the proposed new setting?
2. How similar are the target population in the research and that in the new setting?
3. Is the philosophy of care underlying the innovation compatible with the philosophy prevailing in the new setting?
4. Is there a sufficiently large number of clients in the new setting who could benefit from the innovation?

Feasibility

1. Will nurses have the authority to carry out the innovation? Will they have the authority to terminate the innovation if it is considered undesirable?
2. Is there reasonable consensus among staff, administrators, and medical personnel that the innovation should be tested? Are there major pockets of resistance that could undermine efforts to implement and evaluate the innovation fairly?
3. Are the skills needed to carry out the utilization project—both the implementation and the clinical evaluation—available within the nursing staff? If not, how difficult will it be to collaborate with others with the necessary skills?
4. Does the organization have the equipment and facilities necessary for the innovation? If not, is there a way to obtain the needed resources?
5. If nursing staff need to be released from other practice activities to learn about and implement the innovation, what is the likelihood that this will happen?

Cost–Benefit Ratio

1. What are the risks to which clients would be exposed during the implementation of the innovation? What are the potential benefits?
2. What are the risks of maintaining current practices (*i.e.,* the costs of *not* trying the innovation)? What are the benefits?
3. What are the short-term and long-term material costs of implementing the innovation?
4. What are the material costs of *not* implementing the innovation (*i.e.,* could the new procedure result in some efficiencies that could lower the cost of providing care)?
5. What are the potential nonmaterial costs of implementing the innovation to the organization (*e.g.,* lower staff morale, staff turnover, absenteeism)?
6. What are the potential nonmaterial benefits of implementing the innovation (*e.g.,* improved staff morale, improved staff recruitment, positive community publicity)?

Cost–Benefit Ratio. A critical part of any decision to proceed with a utilization project is a careful assessment of the costs and benefits of the innovation. The **cost–benefit assessment** should encompass likely costs and benefits to various groups, including clients, staff, the overall organization, and even the nursing profession as a whole. Clearly, the most important factor is the client. If the degree of risk in introducing a new procedure is high, then the potential benefits must be great. Moreover, if there are risks to client well-being, it is essential that the knowledge base be sound. An innovation that involves client risks should only be implemented when there is a solid body of evidence from several methodologically rigorous studies that the new practice is effective. A cost–benefit assessment should consider the opposite side of the coin as well: the costs and benefits of *not* implementing the innovation. It is sometimes easy to forget that the status quo bears its own risks and that failure to change—especially when such change is based on a firm knowledge base—is costly to clients, to organizations, and to the entire nursing community.

WHAT TO EXPECT IN THE RESEARCH LITERATURE

As indicated throughout this chapter, researchers play a critical role in whether their research findings will be utilized in practice settings. Here are a few things that consumers can expect in the research literature with regard to research utilization.

- Many research reports do not, unfortunately, promote utilization. Even when a study addresses a clinically relevant problem, researchers can undermine utilization when the language they use is unnecessarily complex and full of jargon, when tables are not carefully prepared, and when they fail to help the reader understand the practical implications of the study. Most nursing studies do not carefully lay out how the findings from the study could be used in practice settings and how generalizable those findings are. (Fortunately, a few journals, such as the *Journal of Obstetric, Gynecologic, and Neonatal Nursing,* have specified a format that calls for authors to discuss the implications of the study.)
- Relatively few explicit replications can be found in the research literature. This possibly reflects a bias on the part of researchers, who may prefer to break new ground with their research, or it could reflect a publication bias. Nevertheless, despite the absence of explicit replications, many research topics have been addressed by several nurse researchers and, therefore, are developing a solid knowledge base for nursing practice.
- Unfortunately, relatively few integrative research reviews are published in nursing journals. The availability of thorough critical reviews of the literature on topics of concern to practicing nurses would likely facilitate research utilization. Among the research reviews that are published, there is a trend

toward the conduct of meta-analyses of the literature, which involve the use of statistical procedures to integrate research findings from various studies. Meta-analyses represent an important methodologic tool for advancing scientific knowledge. However, they may be difficult for the typical nurse to comprehend unless the researcher takes pains to translate the results into more clinical terms and to develop recommendations for practice on the basis of the findings.

- Undoubtedly, many utilization projects are being undertaken by nurses in practice settings. Relatively few of these efforts are reported in the nursing literature—although that situation is changing as increased emphasis is being placed on utilization. For example, entire issues of several specialty journals have been devoted to describing utilization efforts in recent years. It should be noted that formal research utilization projects are more likely to be based on quantitative research than on qualitative research. This stems in part from the fact that quantitative researchers are more likely to ask questions about the effectiveness of certain practices or procedures, and in part because quantitative researchers deal with concepts about which there is already a fairly well-defined body of research.

▨ RESEARCH EXAMPLE

Kilpack, Boehm, Smith, and Mudge (1991) undertook a utilization project that focused on efforts to decrease patient falls in their hospital, the Dartmouth-Hitchcock Medical Center. The project began when the hospital's Nursing Quality Assurance Committee noted an increase in patient falls and established a study group to address the problem.

The group began by undertaking a thorough review of the literature to identify nursing interventions that have been documented as being effective in reducing patient falls. After the review, a fall prevention program was implemented in the two units that had especially high rates of inpatient falls. The special program was designed to prevent repeat falls among those who had a fall identified by an incident report.

During the 1-year study period, incident reports were screened, and for each patient who had experienced a fall, the staff nurse caring for the patient completed a form that listed the research-based interventions that had been previously identified in the literature review. The nurse was asked to select those interventions that he or she felt should be incorporated into the plan of care. With this information, the clinical nurse specialist developed a written plan of care using the nursing diagnosis of potential for injury. The staff nurse was asked to implement the plan, and adherence to the plan was monitored. Care plans were adjusted as needed when there was a recurrence of a fall.

The researchers gathered data on falls during the study period and documented their incidence and nature; they also documented the interventions that were utilized. They found that the patient fall rate on the two targeted units decreased (relative to the previous year), whereas the overall rate in the hospital increased. As a result of the project, six major clinical practice recommendations were made to the institution, and all six were implemented.

SUMMARY

In nursing, **research utilization** refers to the use of some aspect of a scientific investigation in a clinical application unrelated to the original research. Research utilization can best be characterized as lying on a continuum, with direct utilization of some specific innovation at one end (**instrumental utilization**) and more diffuse situations in which users are influenced in their thinking about an issue based on some research (**conceptual utilization**) at the other end.

Tremendous potential exists for research utilization at all points along this continuum throughout the nursing process. To date, however, there is little evidence that widespread utilization has occurred—at least not with respect to instrumental utilization. It seems likely, though, that more diffuse forms of utilization have occurred as nurses have increased their research productivity and their awareness of the need for research.

Several major utilization projects have been implemented, the most noteworthy being the WICHE, NCAST, and CURN projects. These utilization projects demonstrated that it is possible to increase research utilization, but they also shed light on some of the barriers to utilization. These barriers include such factors as an inadequate scientific base, nursing staff with little training in research and utilization, resistance to change among nurses and institutions that employ them, unfavorable organizational climates, resource constraints, limited collaboration among practitioners and researchers, poorly developed communication channels among these two groups, and the shortage of appropriate role models.

Responsibility for research utilization should be borne by the entire nursing community. Researchers, practicing nurses, nursing students, and nurse administrators could adopt a number of strategies to improve the extent to which research findings form the basis for nursing practice. In planning a major implementation project, practicing nurses can begin with the identification of an important clinical problem and then proceed to identify and critique the knowledge base and perform an assessment of the implementation potential of the innovation. Under favorable conditions, the nurses could then plan the innovation protocols, implement and evaluate the innovation, and make a rational decision regarding the adoption of the innovation based on the evaluation. Alternatively, nurses can begin with the knowledge base and then perform an evaluation of the clinical relevance of a research area before proceeding through the other steps of the utilization process. Thus, there are three major categories of criteria that must be considered before proceeding with a utilization plan: **clinical relevance, scientific merit,** and **implementation potential.** The last category includes the dimensions of transferability of findings, feasibility of utilization in the particular setting, and the cost–benefit ratio of the innovation.

◩ STUDY SUGGESTIONS

Chapter 14 of the accompanying *Study Guide to Accompany Essentials of Nursing Research*, 4th edition offers various exercises and study suggestions for reinforcing the concepts presented in this chapter.

Suggested Readings

Methodologic References

American Nurses' Association. (1991). *Standards of clinical nursing practice.* Kansas City, MO: ANA.

Barnard, K. E., & Hoehn, R. E. (1978). *Nursing child assessment satellite training: Final report.* Hyattsville, MD: DHEW, Division of Nursing.

Bostrom, J., & Suter, W. N. (1993). Research utilization: Making the link to practice. *Journal of Nursing Staff Development, 9,* 28–34.

Caplan, N., & Rich, R. F. (1975). *The use of social science knowledge in policy decisions at the national level.* Ann Arbor, MI: Institute for Social Research, University of Michigan.

Downs, F. S. (1979). Clinical and theoretical research. In F. S. Downs, & J. W. Fleming (Eds.), *Issues in nursing research.* New York: Appleton-Century-Crofts.

Dufault, M. A., Bielecki, C., Collins, E., & Willey, C. (1995). Changing nurses' pain assessment practice: A collaborative research utilization approach. *Journal of Advanced Nursing, 21,* 634–645.

Funk, S. G., Champagne, M. T., Wiese, R. A., & Tornquist, E. M. (1991). Barriers to using research findings in practice: The clinician's perspective. *Applied Nursing Research, 4,* 90–95.

Haller, D., Reynolds, M., & Horsley, J. (1979). Developing research-based innovation protocols: Process, criteria, and issues. *Research in Nursing and Health, 2,* 45–51.

Horsley, J. A., Crane, J., & Bingle, J. D. (1978). Research utilization as an organizational process. *Journal of Nursing Administration, 8,* 4–6.

Horsley, J., Crane, J., Crabtree, M., & Wood, D. (1983). *Using research to improve nursing practice: A guide.* New York: Grune & Stratton.

Krueger, J. C., Nelson, A. H., & Wolanin, M. O. (1978). *Nursing research: Development, collaboration, and utilization.* Germantown, MD: Aspen Systems Corporation.

O'Sullivan, P. S., & Goodman, P. A. (1990). Involving practicing nurses in research. *Applied Nursing Research, 3,* 169–172.

Pettengill, M. M., Gillies, D. A., & Clark, C. C. (1994). Factors encouraging and discouraging the use of nursing research findings. *Image, 26,* 143–147.

Phillips, L. R. F. (1986). *A clinician's guide to the critique and utilization of nursing research.* Norwalk, CT: Appleton-Century-Crofts.

Stetler, C. B. (1985). Research utilization: Defining the concept. *Image, 17,* 40–44.

Weiss, C. (1980). Knowledge creep and decision accretion. *Knowledge: Creation, Diffusion, Utilization, 1,* 381–404.

Substantive References

Brett, J. L. L. (1987). Use of nursing practice research findings. *Nursing Research, 36,* 344–349.

Champion, V. L., & Leach, A. (1989). Variables related to research utilization in nursing. *Journal of Advanced Nursing, 14,* 705–710.

Coyle, L. A., & Sokop, A. G. (1990). Innovation adoption behavior among nurses. *Nursing Research, 39,* 176–180.

Horsley, K., Crane, J., & Haller, J. (1981). *Reducing diarrhea in tube-fed patients (CURN Project).* New York: Grune & Stratton.

Horsley, K., Crane, J., Haller, D., & Bingle, J. (1981). *Closed urinary drainage system (CURN Project).* New York: Grune & Stratton.

Ketefian, S. (1975). Application of selected nursing research findings into nursing practice. *Nursing Research, 24,* 89–92.

Kilpack, V., Boehm, J., Smith, N., & Mudge, B. (1991). Using research-based interventions to decrease patient falls. *Applied Nursing Research, 4,* 50–56.

King, I., & Tarsitano, E. (1982). The effect of structured and unstructured preoperative teaching: A replication. *Nursing Research, 31,* 324–329.

Kirchhoff, K. T. (1982). A diffusion survey of coronary precautions. *Nursing Research, 31,* 196–201.

Lim-Levy, F. (1982). The effect of oxygen inhalation on oral temperature. *Nursing Research, 31,* 150–152.

Nichols, G. A., & Verhonick, P. J. (1968). Placement times for oral temperatures: A nursing study replication. *Nursing Research, 17,* 159–161.

Glossary

abstract A brief description of a completed or proposed research investigation; in research journals, usually located at the beginning of a research report.

accessible population The population of people available for a particular study; often a nonrandom subset of the target population.

accidental sampling Selection of the most readily available persons (or units) as participants in a study; also known as *convenience sampling.*

acquiescence response set A bias in self-report instruments, especially in social psychological scales, created when study participants characteristically agree with statements ("yea-say") independent of their content.

after-only design An experimental design in which data are collected from subjects only after the experimental intervention has been introduced.

alpha (α) (1) In tests of statistical significance, the level designating the accepted probability of committing a Type I error; (2) in estimates of internal consistency, a reliability coefficient, as in Cronbach's alpha.

analysis A method of organizing data in such a way that research questions can be answered.

analysis of covariance (ANCOVA) A statistical procedure used to test mean differences among groups on a dependent variable, while controlling for one or more extraneous variables (covariates).

analysis of variance (ANOVA) A statistical procedure for testing mean differences among three or more groups by comparing the variability between groups to the variability within groups.

analytic induction A method of analyzing qualitative data that involves an iterative approach to testing research hypotheses.

anonymity Protection of the participant in a study such that even the researcher cannot link him or her with the information provided.

applied research Research that concentrates on finding a solution to an immediate practical problem.

assumptions Basic principles that are accepted as being true on the basis of logic or reason, without proof or verification.

asymmetric distribution A distribution of values that is skewed (*i.e.*, has two halves that are not mirror images of each other).

attribute variables Preexisting characteristics of the study participants, which the researcher simply observes or measures.

attrition The loss of participants during the course of a study, which can introduce bias by changing the composition of the sample initially drawn—particularly if more participants are lost from one group than another; can thereby be a threat to the internal validity of a study.

audit trail The systematic collection and documentation of material that allows an independent auditor (in an inquiry audit of qualitative data) to draw conclusions about the data.

axial coding The second level of coding in a grounded theory study, involving the process of categorizing, recategorizing, and condensing all first level codes by connecting a category and its subcategories.

basic research Research designed to extend the base of knowledge in a discipline for the sake of knowledge production or theory construction, rather than for solving an immediate problem.

before–after design An experimental design in which data are collected from research subjects both before and after the introduction of the experimental intervention.

beneficence A fundamental ethical principle that seeks to prevent harm and exploitation of, and maximize benefits for, human subjects.

between-subjects design A research design in which there are separate groups of people being compared (*e.g.*, smokers and nonsmokers).

bias Any influence that produces a distortion in the results of a study.

bimodal distribution A distribution of values with two peaks (high frequencies).

bivariate statistics Statistics derived from the analysis of two variables simultaneously for the purpose of assessing the empirical relationship between them.

"blind" review The review of a manuscript or proposal such that neither the author nor the reviewer is identified to the other party.

borrowed theory A theory borrowed from another discipline or field to guide nursing practice or research.

bracketing In phenomenologic inquiries, the process of identifying and holding in abeyance any preconceived beliefs and opinions one has about the phenomena under study.

canonical analysis A statistical procedure for examining the relationship between two or more independent variables *and* two or more dependent variables.

case-control study A research design, typically found in retrospective ex post facto research, that involves the comparison of a "case" (*i.e.*, a person with the condition under scrutiny, such as lung cancer) and a pair-matched control (*i.e.*, a person without the condition).

categorical variable A variable with discrete values rather than incremental placement along a continuum (*e.g.*, a person's marital status).

category system In observational studies, the prespecified plan for organizing and recording the behaviors and events under observation.

causal modeling The development and statistical testing of an explanatory model of hypothesized causal relationships among phenomena.

causal relationship A relationship between two variables such that the presence or absence of one variable (the "cause") determines the presence or absence, or value, of the other (the "effect").

cell (1) The intersection of a row and column in a table with two or more dimensions; (2) in an experimental design, a cell is the representation of an experimental condition in a schematic diagram.

central tendency A statistical index of the "typicalness" of a set of scores that comes from the center of the distribution of scores; the three most common indices of central tendency are the mode, the median, and the mean.

chi-squared test A nonparametric test of statistical significance used to assess whether a relationship exists between two nominal-level variables. Symbolized as χ^2.

clinical relevance The degree to which a study addresses a problem of significance to the practice of nursing; a major criterion for research utilization.

clinical research Research designed to generate knowledge to guide nursing practice.

clinical trial An experiment involving a test of the effectiveness of a clinical treatment, generally involving a large and heterogeneous sample of subjects.

closed-ended question A question that offers respondents a set of mutually exclusive and jointly exhaustive alternative replies, from which the one that most closely approximates the "correct" answer must be chosen.

cluster sampling A form of multistage sampling in which large groupings ("clusters") are selected first (*e.g.,* nursing schools), with successive subsampling of smaller units (*e.g.,* nursing students).

code of ethics The fundamental ethical principles established by a discipline or institution to guide researchers' conduct in research with living beings.

codebook A record that documents the researcher's categorization and coding decisions.

coding The process of transforming raw data into standardized form for data processing and analysis; in quantitative research, the process of attaching numbers to categories; in qualitative research, the process of identifying and labeling recurring words, themes, or concepts within the data.

coefficient alpha (Cronbach's alpha) A reliability index that estimates the internal consistency or homogeneity of a measure composed of several items or subparts.

coercion In a research context, the explicit or implicit use of threats (or excessive rewards) to get people to agree to participate in a study.

comparison group A group of subjects whose scores on a dependent variable are used as a basis for evaluating the scores of the group of primary interest (*e.g.,* nonsmokers as a comparison group for smokers); term used in lieu of control group when the investigation does not involve a true experimental design.

concealment A tactic involving the unobtrusive collection of research data without the participants' knowledge or consent, used as a means of obtaining an accurate view of naturalistic behavior when the known presence of an observer would distort the behavior of interest.

concept An abstraction based on observations of certain behaviors or characteristics (*e.g.,* stress, pain).

conceptual model Interrelated concepts or abstractions that are assembled together in some rational scheme by virtue of their relevance to a common theme; sometimes referred to as *conceptual framework*.

conceptual utilization The use of research findings in a general, conceptual way to broaden one's thinking about an issue, although the knowledge is not put to any specific, documentable use.

concurrent validity The degree to which scores on an instrument are correlated with some external criterion, measured at the same time.

confidentiality Protection of participants in a study such that their individual identities will not be linked to the information they provide and will never be publicly divulged.

confirmability A criterion for evaluating data quality with qualitative data, referring to the objectivity or neutrality of the data.

consent form A written agreement signed by a study participant and a researcher concerning the terms and conditions of a study participant's voluntary participation in a study.

constant comparison A procedure often used in a grounded theory analysis wherein newly collected data are compared in an ongoing fashion with data obtained earlier, to refine theoretically relevant categories.

construct An abstraction or concept that is deliberately invented (constructed) by researchers for a scientific purpose (*e.g.,* health locus of control).

construct validity The degree to which an instrument measures the construct under investigation.

consumer An individual who reads, reviews, and critiques research findings and who attempts to use and apply the findings in practice.

content analysis The process of organizing and integrating narrative, qualitative information according to emerging themes and concepts; also refers to a procedure for analyzing written or verbal communications in a systematic and objective fashion, typically with the goal of quantitatively measuring variables—sometimes referred to as *manifest content analysis.*

content validity The degree to which the items in an instrument adequately represent the universe of content.

contingency table A two-dimensional table that permits a cross-tabulation of the frequencies of two categorical variables.

continuous variable A variable that can take on a large range of values representing a continuum (*e.g.,* height).

control The process of holding constant possible influences on the dependent variable under investigation.

control group Subjects in an experiment who do not receive the experimental treatment and whose performance provides a baseline against which the effects of the treatment can be measured (see also *comparison group*).

convenience sampling Selection of the most readily available persons (or units) as participants in a study; also known as *accidental sampling.*

core category In a grounded theory study, the central phenomenon that is used to integrate all categories of the data.

correlation A tendency for variation in one variable to be related to variation in another variable.

correlation coefficient An index that summarizes the degree of relationship between two variables. Correlation coefficients typically range from +1.00 (for a perfect positive relationship) through .00 (for no relationship) to −1.00 (for a perfect negative relationship).

correlation matrix A two-dimensional display showing the correlation coefficients between all combinations of variables of interest.

correlational research Research that explores the interrelationships among variables of interest, without any active intervention on the part of the researcher.

cost–benefit analysis An evaluation of the financial costs of a program or intervention relative to the financial gains attributable to it.

cost–benefit assessment The assessment of relative costs and benefits, to individuals, organizations, and society, of implementing an innovation.

counterbalancing The process of systematically varying the order of presentation of stimuli, treatments, or items in a scale to control for ordering effects, as in counterbalancing the order of treatments in a repeated measures design.

covariate A variable that is statistically controlled (held constant) in analysis of covariance. The covariate is typically an extraneous, confounding influence on the dependent variable or a pre-intervention measure of the dependent variable.

covert data collection The collection of information in a study without the participant's knowledge.

credibility A criterion for evaluating the data quality of qualitative data, referring to confidence in the truth of the data.

criterion variable The quality or attribute used to measure the effect of an independent variable; sometimes used instead of *dependent variable.*

criterion-related validity The degree to which scores on an instrument are correlated with some external criterion.

critical incidents technique A method of obtaining data from study participants by in-depth exploration of specific incidents and behaviors related to the matter under investigation.

critique An objective, critical, and balanced appraisal of a research report's various dimensions (*e.g.,* conceptual, methodologic, ethical).

Cronbach's alpha A widely used reliability index that estimates the internal consistency or homogeneity of a measure composed of several subparts; also referred to as *coefficient alpha.*

crossover design See *repeated measures design.*

cross-sectional study A study based on observations of different age groups or developmental groups at a single point in time for the purpose of inferring time-related changes.

cross-tabulation A determination of the number of cases occurring when simultaneous consideration is given to the values of two or more variables (*e.g.,* gender—male/female—cross-tabulated with smoking status—smoker/nonsmoker). The results are typically presented in a table with rows and columns divided according to the categories of the variables.

data The pieces of information obtained in the course of a study (singular is *datum*).

data analysis The systematic organization and synthesis of research data, and the testing of research hypotheses using those data.

data collection The gathering of information needed to address a research problem.

data saturation See *saturation.*

debriefing Communication with study participants, generally after their participation has been completed, regarding various aspects of the study.

deception The deliberate withholding of information, or the provision of false information, to study participants; usually used to reduce potential biases.

deductive reasoning The process of developing specific predictions from general principles (see also *inductive reasoning*).

degrees of freedom (*df*) A concept used in tests of statistical significance, referring to the number of sample values that cannot be calculated from knowledge of other values and a calculated statistic (*e.g.,* by knowing a sample mean, all but one value would be free to vary); degrees of freedom is often $N - 1$, but different formulas are relevant for different tests.

dependability A criterion for evaluating data quality in qualitative data, referring to the stability of data over time and over conditions.

dependent variable The outcome variable of interest; the variable that is hypothesized to depend on or be caused by another variable (called the *independent variable*).

descriptive research Research studies that have as their main objective the accurate portrayal of the characteristics of persons, situations, or groups, and/or the frequency with which certain phenomena occur.

descriptive statistics Statistics used to describe and summarize data (*e.g.,* mean, standard deviation).

descriptive theory A broad characterization that thoroughly accounts for a single phenomenon.

determinism The belief that phenomena are not haphazard or random, but rather have antecedent causes; an assumption within the positivist paradigm.

dichotomous variable A variable having only two values or categories (*e.g.,* gender).

directional hypothesis A hypothesis that makes a specific prediction about the direction and nature of the relationship between two variables.

discriminant function analysis A statistical procedure used to predict group membership or status on a categorical (nominal level) variable on the basis of two or more independent variables.

disproportionate sample A sample that results when the researcher samples differing proportions of subjects from different strata in the population to ensure adequate representation of subjects from strata that are comparatively smaller.

double-blind experiment An experiment in which neither the subjects nor those who administer the treatment know who is in the experimental or control group.

electronic database Bibliographic files that can be accessed by computer for the purpose of conducting a literature search.

element The most basic unit of a population, from which a sample will be drawn; in nursing research, the element is typically humans.

eligibility criteria The criteria used by a researcher to designate the specific attributes of the target population, and to select participants for a study.

emergent design A design that unfolds in the course of a qualitative study as the researcher makes ongoing design decisions reflecting what has already been learned.

emic perspective A term used by ethnographers to refer to the way members of a culture themselves view their world; the "insider's view."

empirical evidence Evidence that is rooted in objective reality and that is gathered through the collection of data using one's senses; used as the basis for generating knowledge through the scientific approach.

equivalence The degree of similarity between alternate forms of a measuring instrument.

error of measurement The difference between true scores and obtained scores when measuring a characteristic.

ethics A system of moral values that is concerned with the degree to which research procedures adhere to professional, legal, and social obligations to the study participants.

ethnography A branch of human inquiry, associated with the field of anthropology, that focuses on a culture (or subculture) of a group of people, with an effort to understand the world view of those under study.

ethnomethodology A branch of human inquiry, associated with sociology, that focuses on the way in which people make sense of their everyday activities and come to behave in socially acceptable ways.

ethnonursing research The study of human cultures, with a focus on a group's beliefs and practices relating to nursing care and related health behaviors.

etic perspective A term used by ethnographers to refer to the "outsider's" view of the experiences of a cultural group.

evaluation research Research that investigates how well a program, practice, or policy is working.

event sampling In observational studies, a sampling plan that involves the selection of integral behaviors or events.

ex post facto research Research conducted after the variations in the independent variable have occurred in the natural course of events; a form of nonexperimental research in which causal explanations are inferred "after the fact."

experiment A research study in which the investigator controls (manipulates) the independent variable and randomly assigns subjects to different conditions.

experimental group The subjects who receive the experimental treatment or intervention.

experimental intervention (experimental treatment) See *intervention; treatment.*

exploratory research A study designed to explore the dimensions of a phenomenon or to develop or refine hypotheses about the relationships between phenomena.

external validity The degree to which the results of a study can be generalized to settings or samples other than the ones studied.

extraneous variable A variable that confounds the relationship between the independent and dependent variables and that needs to be controlled either in the research design or through statistical procedures.

extreme response set A bias in self-report instruments, especially in social psychological scales, created when participants characteristically express their opinions in terms of extreme response alternatives (*e.g.,* "strongly agree") independent of the question's content.

face validity The extent to which a measuring instrument looks as though it is measuring what it purports to measure.

factor analysis A statistical procedure for reducing a large set of variables into a smaller set of variables with common characteristics or underlying dimensions.

factorial design An experimental design in which two or more independent variables are simultaneously manipulated; this design permits an analysis of the main effects of the independent variables separately, plus the interaction effects of those variables.

field notes The notes taken by researchers describing the unstructured observations they have made in the field, and their interpretation of those observations.

field research Research in which the data are collected "in the field" from individuals in their normal roles, with the aim of understanding the practices, behaviors, and beliefs of individuals or groups as they normally function in real life.

findings The results of the analyses of the research data; in quantitative studies, the results of the hypothesis tests.

fixed alternative question A question that offers respondents a set of prespecified responses, from which the respondent must choose the alternative that most closely approximates the correct response.

focus group interview An interview with a group of individuals assembled discuss a given topic.

focused interview A loosely structured interview in which the interviewer guides the respondent through a set of questions using a topic guide.

follow-up study A study undertaken to determine the subsequent development of individuals with a specified condition or who have received a specified treatment.

framework The conceptual underpinnings of a study; often referred to as a *theoretical framework* in studies based on a theory, or as a *conceptual framework* in studies that have roots in a specific conceptual model.

***F* ratio** The statistic obtained in several statistical tests (*e.g.,* ANOVA) in which variation attributable to different sources (*e.g.,* between groups and within groups) is compared.

frequency distribution A systematic array of numeric values from the lowest to the highest, together with a count of the number of times each value was obtained.

frequency polygon Graphic display of a frequency distribution, in which dots connected by a straight line indicate the number of times a score value occurs in a set of data.

Friedman test A nonparametric analog of ANOVA, used when the researcher is working with paired groups or a repeated measures situation.

full disclosure The communication of complete information to potential research participants regarding the nature of the study, the person's right to refuse participation, and the likely risks and benefits that would be incurred.

functional relationship A relationship or association between two variables wherein it cannot be assumed that one variable caused the other; however, it can be said that the variable X changes values as a function of changes in variable Y.

gaining entrée The process of gaining access to study participants in in-depth qualitative studies through the cooperation of key actors in the selected community or site.

generalizability The degree to which the research procedures justify the inference that the findings represent something beyond the specific observations on which they are based; in particular, the inference that the findings can be generalized from the sample to the entire population.

grand theory A broad theory aimed at describing large segments of the physical, social, or behavioral world; also referred to as a *macro-theory.*

grand tour question A broad question asked in an unstructured interview to gain a general overview of a phenomenon, on the basis of which more focused questions are subsequently asked.

grounded theory An approach to collecting and analyzing qualitative data with the aim of developing theories and theoretical propositions grounded in real-world observations.

Hawthorne effect The effect on the dependent variable caused by subjects' awareness that they are participants under study.

hermeneutics A qualitative research tradition, closely related to phenomenology, that uses the lived experiences of humans as a tool for better understanding the social, cultural, political, and/or historical context in which those experiences occur.

heterogeneity The degree to which objects are dissimilar (*i.e.,* characterized by high variability) with respect to some attribute.

historical research Systematic studies designed to establish facts and relationships concerning past events.

history threat A threat to the internal validity of a study; refers to the occurrence of events external to the intervention but concurrent with it that can affect the dependent variable.

homogeneity (1) In terms of the reliability of an instrument, the degree to which the subparts are internally consistent (*i.e.,* are measuring the same critical attribute). (2) More generally, the degree to which objects are similar (*i.e.,* characterized by low variability).

hypothesis A statement of predicted relationships between the variables under investigation.

impact analysis An evaluation of the effects of a program or intervention on some outcomes of interest, net of other factors influencing those outcomes.

implementation analysis An evaluation that describes the process by which a program or intervention was implemented in practice.

implementation potential The extent to which an innovation is amenable to implementation in a new setting, an assessment of which is usually made in a research utilization project; includes the criteria of transferability, feasibility, and the cost–benefit of the innovation.

independent variable The variable that is believed to cause or influence the dependent variable; in experimental research, the manipulated (treatment) variable.

inductive reasoning The process of reasoning from specific observations to more general rules (see also *deductive reasoning*).

inferential statistics Statistics that permit inferences on whether relationships observed in a sample are likely to occur in a larger population of concern.

informant Individuals who provide information to researchers about a phenomenon under study; term often used in qualitative studies.

informed consent An ethical principle that requires researchers to obtain the voluntary participation of subjects, after informing them of possible risks and benefits.

inquiry audit An independent scrutiny of qualitative data and relevant supporting documents by an external reviewer, a method used to determine the dependability and confirmability of qualitative data.

Institutional Review Board (IRB) A group of individuals who convene to review proposed and ongoing studies with respect to ethical considerations.

instrument The device or technique that a researcher uses to collect data (*e.g.*, questionnaires, tests, observation schedules, and so forth).

instrumental utilization Clearly identifiable attempts to base some specific action or intervention on the results of research findings.

interaction effect The effect on a dependent variable of two or more independent variables acting in combination (interactively) rather than as unconnected factors.

internal consistency A form of reliability, referring to the degree to which the subparts of an instrument are all measuring the same attribute or dimension.

internal validity The degree to which it can be inferred that the experimental treatment (independent variable), rather than uncontrolled, extraneous factors, is responsible for observed effects.

interrater (interobserver) reliability The degree to which two raters or observers, operating independently, assign the same ratings or values for an attribute being measured.

interval measurement A level of measurement in which an attribute is rank ordered on a scale that has equal distances between points on that scale (*e.g.*, Fahrenheit degrees).

intervention In experimental research, the experimental treatment or manipulation.

interview A method of data collection in which one person (an interviewer) asks questions of another person (a respondent); interviews are conducted either face to face or by telephone.

interview schedule The formal instrument, used in structured self-report studies, that specifies the wording of all questions to be asked of respondents.

inverse relationship A negative correlation between two variables (*i.e.*, a relationship characterized by the tendency of high values on one variable to be associated with low values on a second variable).

item A single question on a test or questionnaire, or a single statement on an attitude or other scale (*e.g.,* a final examination might consist of 100 items).

journal club A group that meets regularly (often in clinical settings) to discuss and critique research reports appearing in research journals, often with the goal of assessing the utilization potential of the findings.

judgmental sampling A type of nonprobability sampling method in which the researcher selects participants for the study on the basis of personal judgment about which ones will be most representative or productive; also referred to as *purposive sampling.*

key informant A person well versed in the phenomenon of research interest and who is willing to share the information and insight with the researcher; key informants are often used in needs assessments.

known-groups technique A technique for estimating the construct validity of an instrument through an analysis of the degree to which the instrument separates groups that are predicted to differ on the basis of some theory or known characteristic.

Kruskal-Wallis test A nonparametric test used to analyze the differences among three or more independent groups, based on ranked scores.

level of measurement A system of classifying measurements according to the nature of the measurement and the type of mathematical operations to which they are amenable; the four levels are nominal, ordinal, interval, and ratio.

level of significance The risk of making a Type I error, established by the researcher before the statistical analysis (*e.g.,* the .05 level).

life history A narrative self-report about a person's life experiences vis-à-vis some theme of interest to the researcher.

Likert scale A type of composite measure of attitudes that involves summation of scores on a set of items (statements) to which respondents are asked to indicate their degree of agreement or disagreement.

LISREL The widely used acronym for linear structural relation analysis, typically used for testing causal models.

literature review A critical summary of research on a topic of interest, often prepared to put a research problem in context or as the basis for an implementation project.

log In participant observation studies, the observer's daily record of events and conversations that took place.

logical positivism The philosophy underlying the traditional scientific approach; see also *positivist paradigm.*

logistic regression A multivariate regression procedure that analyzes relationships between multiple independent variables and categorical dependent variables; also referred to as *logit analysis.*

longitudinal study A study designed to collect data at more than one point in time, in contrast to a cross-sectional study.

macro-theory A broad theory aimed at describing large segments of the physical, social, or behavioral world; also referred to as a *grand theory.*

main effect In a study with multiple independent variables, the effect of a single independent variable on the dependent variable.

manifest content analysis See *content analysis.*

manipulation An intervention or treatment introduced by the researcher in an experimental or quasi-experimental study; the researcher manipulates the independent variable to assess its impact on the dependent variable.

Mann-Whitney U test A nonparametric test used to test the difference between two independent groups, based on ranked scores.

MANOVA See *multivariate analysis of variance.*

matching The pairing of subjects in one group with those in another group based on their similarity on one or more dimension, done to enhance the overall comparability of groups.

maturation threat A threat to the internal validity of a study that occurs when changes to the outcome measure (dependent variable) result from the passage of time.

mean A descriptive statistic that is a measure of central tendency, computed by summing all scores and dividing by the number of subjects.

measurement The assignment of numbers to objects according to specified rules to characterize quantities of some attribute.

median A descriptive statistic that is a measure of central tendency, representing the exact middle score or value in a distribution of scores; the median is the value above and below which 50 percent of the scores lie.

mediating variable A variable that mediates or acts like a "go-between" in a chain linking two other variables (*e.g.,* coping skills may be said to mediate the relationship between stressful events and anxiety).

member check A method of validating the credibility of qualitative data through debriefings and discussions with informants.

meta-analysis A technique for quantitatively combining and thus integrating the results of multiple studies on a given topic.

methodologic notes In observational field studies, the notes kept by the researcher regarding the methods used in collecting the data.

methodologic research Research designed to develop or refine procedures for obtaining, organizing, or analyzing data.

methods (research) The steps, procedures, and strategies for gathering and analyzing the data in a research investigation.

middle range theory A theory that focuses on only a piece of reality or human experience, involving a selected number of concepts (*e.g.,* theories of stress).

minimal risk Anticipated risks that are no greater than those ordinarily encountered in daily life or during the performance of routine tests or procedures.

mode A descriptive statistic that is a measure of central tendency; the score or value that occurs most frequently in a distribution of scores.

model A symbolic representation of concepts or variables, and interrelationships among them.

mortality threat A threat to the internal validity of a study, referring to the differential loss of participants (attrition) from different groups.

multimethod research Generally, research in which multiple approaches are used to address the research problem; often used to designate research in which both qualitative and quantitative data are collected and analyzed.

multimodal distribution A distribution of values with more than one peak (high frequency).

multiple comparison procedures Statistical tests, normally applied after an ANOVA indicates statistically significant group differences, that compare different pairs of groups; also referred to as *post hoc tests.*

multiple correlation coefficient An index that summarizes the degree of relationship between two or more independent variables and a dependent variable; symbolized as *R*.

multiple regression analysis A statistical procedure for understanding the simultaneous effects of two or more independent (predictor) variables on a dependent variable.

multistage sampling A sampling strategy that proceeds through a set of stages from larger to smaller sampling units (*e.g.,* from states, to nursing schools, to faculty members).

multivariate analysis of variance (MANOVA) A statistical procedure used to test the significance of differences between the means of two or more groups on two or more dependent variables, considered simultaneously.

multivariate statistics Statistical procedures designed to analyze the relationships among three or more variables; commonly used multivariate statistics include multiple regression, analysis of covariance, and factor analysis.

N Often used to designate the total number of study participants (*e.g.,* "the total *N* was 500").

n Often used to designate the number of participants in a subgroup or in a cell of a study (*e.g.,* "each of the four groups had an *n* of 125, for a total *N* of 500").

naturalistic paradigm An alternative paradigm to the traditional positivist paradigm that holds that there are multiple interpretations of reality, and that the goal of research is to understand how individuals construct reality within their context; often associated with qualitative research.

naturalistic setting A setting for the collection of research data that is natural to those being studied (*e.g.,* homes, places of work, and so on).

needs assessment A study in which a researcher collects data for estimating the needs of a group, community, or organization; usually used as a guide to policy planning and resource allocation.

negative case analysis A method of refining a hypothesis or theory in a qualitative study that involves the inclusion of cases that appear to disconfirm earlier hypotheses.

negative relationship A relationship between two variables in which there is a tendency for higher values on one variable to be associated with lower values on the other (*e.g.,* as temperature increases, people's productivity may decrease); also referred to as an *inverse relationship.*

negative results Research results that fail to support the researcher's hypotheses.

negatively skewed distribution An asymmetric distribution of values such that a disproportionately high number of cases have high values (*i.e.,* fall at the upper end of the distribution); when displayed graphically, the tail points to the left.

network sampling The sampling of participants based on referrals from others already in the sample, sometimes referred to as *snowball sampling.*

nominal measurement The lowest level of measurement that involves the assignment of characteristics into categories (*e.g.,* males, category 1; females, category 2).

nondirectional hypothesis A research hypothesis that does not stipulate in advance the direction and nature of the relationship between variables.

nonequivalent control group design A quasi-experimental design involving a comparison group that was not developed on the basis of random assignment, but from whom preintervention data are obtained to assess the initial equivalence of the groups.

nonexperimental research Studies in which the researcher collects data without introducing any new treatments or changes.

nonparametric statistics A general class of inferential statistics that does not involve rigorous assumptions about the distribution of the critical variables; most often used when the data are measured on the nominal or ordinal scales.

nonprobability sampling The selection of participants or sampling units from a population using nonrandom procedures; examples include convenience, judgmental, and quota sampling.

nonresponse bias A bias that can result when a nonrandom subset of people invited to participate in a study fail to participate.

nonsignificant result The result of a statistical test that indicates that the result could have occurred as a result of chance, given the researcher's level of significance; sometimes abbreviated as *NS* in research journals.

normal distribution A theoretical distribution that is bell-shaped and symmetric; also referred to as a *normal curve* or *bell-shaped curve*.

null hypothesis The hypothesis that states there is no relationship between the variables under study; used primarily in connection with tests of statistical significance as the hypothesis to be rejected.

objectivity The extent to which two independent researchers would arrive at similar judgments or conclusions (*i.e.,* judgments not biased by personal values or beliefs); considered a desirable attribute within the positivist paradigm.

observational notes In field studies, the observer's descriptions about observed behaviors, events, and conversations.

observational research Studies in which the data are collected by means of observing and recording behaviors or activities of interest.

obtained (observed) score The actual score or numeric value assigned to a person on a measure.

open coding The first level of coding in a grounded theory study, referring to the basic descriptive coding of the content of narrative materials.

open-ended question A question in an interview or questionnaire that does not restrict the respondents' answers to preestablished alternatives.

operational definition The definition of a concept or variable in terms of the operations or procedures by which it is to be measured.

operationalization The process of translating research concepts into measurable phenomena.

ordinal measurement A level of measurement that yields rank orders of a variable along some dimension.

outcome analysis An evaluation of what transpires with respect to outcomes of interest after implementing a program or intervention, without use of an experimental design to assess net effects; see also *impact analysis.*

outcome variable A term sometimes used to refer to the dependent variable in experimental research (*i.e.,* the measure that captures the outcome of the experimental intervention).

***p* value** In statistical testing, the probability that the obtained results are due to chance alone; the probability of committing a Type I error.

pair matching See *matching.*

panel study A type of longitudinal study in which the same people are used to provide data at two or more points in time.

paradigm A way of looking at natural phenomena that encompasses a set of philosophical assumptions and that guides one's approach to inquiry.

parameter A characteristic of a population (*e.g.,* the mean age of all US citizens).

parametric statistics A class of inferential statistics that involves (a) assumptions about the distribution of the variables, (b) the estimation of a parameter, and (c) the use of interval measures.

participant See *study participant.*

participant observation A method of collecting data through the observation of a group or organization in which the researcher participates as a member.

path analysis A regression-based procedure for testing causal models, typically using nonexperimental data.

Pearson's *r* The most widely used correlation coefficient, designating the magnitude and direction of relationship between two variables measured on at least an interval scale; also referred to as the *product–moment correlation.*

peer reviewer A person who reviews and critiques a research report or research proposal, who himself/herself is a researcher (usually working on similar types of research problems as those in the research report under review), and who makes a recommendation about publishing or funding the research.

perfect relationship A relationship or correlation between two variables such that the values of one variable permit perfect prediction of the values of the other; designated as 1.00 or −1.00.

personal interview An interview that occurs between an interviewer and a respondent in a face-to-face situation.

personal notes In field studies, written comments about the observer's own feelings during the research process.

phenomenology A qualitative research tradition, with roots in philosophy and psychology, that focuses on the lived experience of humans.

phenomenon The abstract entity or concept under investigation in a study, most often used by qualitative researchers in lieu of the term "variable."

phi coefficient An index describing the magnitude of relationship between two dichotomous variables.

pilot study A small-scale study, or trial run, done in preparation for a major study.

population The entire set of individuals (or objects) having some common characteristic(s) (*e.g.,* all RNs in the state of California); sometimes referred to as *universe.*

positive relationship A relationship between two variables in which there is a tendency for high values on one variable to be associated with high values on the other (*e.g.,* as physical activity increases, pulse rate also increases).

positive results Research results that are consistent with the researcher's hypotheses.

positively skewed distribution An asymmetric distribution of values such that a disproportionately high number of cases have low values (*i.e.,* fall at the lower end of the distribution); when displayed graphically, the tail points to the right.

positivist paradigm The traditional paradigm underlying the scientific approach, which assumes that there is a fixed, orderly reality that can be objectively studied; often associated with quantitative research.

post hoc test A test for comparing all possible pairs of groups following a significant test of overall group differences (*e.g.,* in an ANOVA).

posttest The collection of data after the introduction of an experimental intervention.

posttest-only design An experimental design in which data are collected from subjects only after the experimental intervention has been introduced; also referred to as an *after-only design.*

power analysis A procedure for estimating either the likelihood of committing a Type II error or sample size requirements.

prediction One of the aims of the scientific approach; the use of empirical evidence to make forecasts about how variables of interest will behave in a new setting and with different individuals.

predictive validity The degree to which an instrument can predict some criterion observed at a future time.

preexperimental design A research design that does not include controls to compensate for the absence of either randomization or a control group.

pretest (1) The collection of data before the experimental intervention; sometimes referred to as *baseline data*. (2) The trial administration of a newly developed instrument to identify flaws or assess time requirements.

pretest–posttest design An experimental design in which data are collected from research subjects both before and after the introduction of the experimental intervention; also referred to as a *before–after design*.

primary source First-hand reports of facts, findings or events; in terms of research, the primary source is the original research report as prepared by the investigator who conducted the study.

principal investigator The person who is the lead researcher and who will have primary responsibility for overseeing the project.

probability sampling The selection of participants or sampling units from a population using random procedures; examples include simple random sampling, cluster sampling, and systematic sampling.

probing Eliciting more useful or detailed information from a respondent in an interview than was volunteered in the first reply.

problem statement The statement of the research problem, often phrased in the form of a research question.

process analysis An evaluation focusing on the process by which a program or intervention gets implemented and used in practice.

process consent In a qualitative study, an ongoing, transactional process of negotiating consent with study participants, allowing them to play a collaborative role in the decision making regarding their ongoing participation.

product moment correlation coefficient (r) The most widely used correlation coefficient, designating the magnitude of relationship between two variables measured on at least an interval scale; also referred to as *Pearson's r*.

projective techniques Methods for measuring psychological attributes (values, attitudes, personality) by providing respondents with unstructured stimuli to which to respond.

prolonged engagement In qualitative research, the investment of sufficient time in the collection of data to have an in-depth understanding of the group under study; a mechanism for achieving data credibility.

proportionate sample A sample that results when the researcher samples from different strata of the population in direct proportion to their representation in the population.

proposal A document specifying what the researcher proposes to study; it communicates the research problem, its significance, planned procedures for solving the problem, and, when funding is sought, how much the research will cost.

prospective study A study that begins with an examination of presumed causes (*e.g.,* cigarette smoking) and then goes forward in time to observe presumed effects (*e.g.,* lung cancer).

psychometric evaluation An assessment of the quality of an instrument, based primarily on evidence of its reliability and validity.

purposive (purposeful) sampling A type of nonprobability sampling method in which the researcher selects participants for the study on the basis of personal judgment about which ones will be most representative or productive; also referred to as *judgmental sampling.*

Q sort A method of scaling in which the participant sorts statements into a number of piles (usually 9 or 11) according to some bipolar dimension (*e.g.,* most like me/least like me; most useful/least useful).

qualitative analysis The organization and interpretation of nonnumeric data for the purpose of discovering important underlying dimensions and patterns of relationships.

qualitative data Information collected in the course of a study that is in narrative (nonnumeric) form, such as the transcript of an unstructured interview.

qualitative research The investigation of phenomena, typically in an in-depth and holistic fashion, through the collection of rich narrative materials using a flexible research design.

quantitative analysis The manipulation of numeric data through statistical procedures for the purpose of describing phenomena or assessing the magnitude and reliability of relationships among them.

quantitative data Information collected in the course of a study that is in a quantified (numeric) form.

quantitative research The investigation of phenomena that lend themselves to precise measurement and quantification, and often involving a rigorous and controlled design.

quasi-experiment A study in which subjects cannot be randomly assigned to treatment conditions, although the researcher does manipulate the independent variable and exercises certain controls to enhance the internal validity of the results.

quasi-statistics An "accounting" system used to assess the validity of conclusions derived from qualitative analysis.

questionnaire A method of gathering self-report information from respondents through self-administration of questions in a paper-and-pencil format.

quota sampling The nonrandom selection of participants in which the researcher prespecifies characteristics of the sample to increase its representativeness.

r The symbol typically used to designate a bivariate correlation coefficient, summarizing the magnitude and direction of a relationship between two variables.

R The symbol used to designate the multiple correlation coefficient, indicating the magnitude (but not direction) of the relationship between the dependent variable and multiple independent variables, taken together.

R^2 The squared multiple correlation coefficient, indicating the proportion of variance in the dependent variable accounted for or explained by a group of independent variables.

random assignment The assignment of subjects to treatment conditions in a random manner (*i.e.,* in a manner determined by chance alone); also known as *randomization.*

random number table A table displaying hundreds of digits (from 0 to 9) set up in such a way that each number is equally likely to follow any other; used in randomization and random sampling.

random sampling The selection of a sample such that each member of a population (or subpopulation) has an equal probability of being included.

randomization The assignment of subjects to treatment conditions in a random manner (*i.e.,* in a manner determined by chance alone); also known as *random assignment.*

range A measure of variability, consisting of the difference between the highest and lowest values in a distribution of scores.

ratio measurement A level of measurement in which there are equal distances between score units and which has a true meaningful zero point (*e.g.*, weight); the highest level of measurement.

reactivity A measurement distortion arising from the study participant's awareness of being observed, or, more generally, from the effect of the measurement procedure itself.

regression A statistical procedure for predicting values of a dependent variable based on the values of one or more independent variables.

relationship A bond or a connection between two or more variables.

reliability The degree of consistency or dependability with which an instrument measures the attribute it is designed to measure.

reliability coefficient A quantitative index, usually ranging in value from .00 to 1.00, that provides an estimate of how reliable an instrument is; computed through such procedures as Cronbach's alpha technique, the split-half technique, test–retest approach, and interrater approaches.

repeated-measures design An experimental design in which one group of subjects is exposed to more than one condition or treatment in random order; sometimes referred to as a *cross-over design*.

replication The deliberate repetition of research procedures in a second investigation for the purpose of determining if earlier results can be repeated.

representative sample A sample whose characteristics are highly similar to those of the population from which it is drawn.

research Systematic inquiry that uses orderly, disciplined methods to answer questions or solve problems.

research control See *control*.

research design The overall plan for addressing a research question, including specifications for enhancing the integrity of the study.

research problem A situation involving an enigmatic, perplexing, or conflictful condition that can be investigated through disciplined inquiry.

research proposal See *proposal*.

research question A statement of the specific query the researcher wants to answer to address a research problem.

research report A document that summarizes the main features of a study, including the research question, the methods used to address it, the findings, and the interpretation and implications of the findings.

research utilization The use of some aspect of a scientific investigation in an application unrelated to the original research.

respondent In a self-report study, the research participant who responds to questions posed by the researcher.

response rate The rate of participation in a study, calculated by dividing the number of persons participating by the number of persons invited to participate.

response set bias The measurement error introduced by the tendency of some individuals to respond to items in characteristic ways (*e.g.*, always agreeing), independently of the item's content.

results The answers to research questions, obtained through an analysis of the collected data; in a quantitative study, the information obtained through statistical tests.

retrospective study A study that begins with the manifestation of the dependent variable in the present (*e.g.*, lung cancer) and then links this effect to some presumed cause occurring in the past (*e.g.*, cigarette smoking).

risk/benefit ratio The relative costs and benefits, to an individual participant and to society at large, of participation in a scientific study; also, the relative costs and benefits of implementing an innovation.

rival hypothesis An alternative explanation, competing with the researcher's hypothesis, for understanding the results of a study.

sample A subset of a population selected to participate in a research study.

sampling The process of selecting a portion of the population to represent the entire population.

sampling bias Distortions that arise from the selection of a sample that is not representative of the population from which it was drawn.

sampling distribution A theoretical distribution of a statistic using the values of the statistic computed from an infinite number of samples as the data points in the distribution.

sampling error The fluctuation of the value of a statistic from one sample to another drawn from the same population.

sampling frame A list of all the elements in the population, from which the sample is drawn.

saturation The process of collecting data in a grounded theory study to the point where a sense of closure is attained because new data yield only redundant information.

scale A composite measure of an attribute, consisting of several items that have a logical or empirical relationship to each other; involves the assignment of a score to place people on a continuum with respect to the attribute.

scientific approach A set of orderly, systematic, controlled procedures for acquiring dependable, empirical—and typically quantitative—information; the methodologic approach associated with the positivist paradigm.

scientific merit The degree to which a study is methodologically and conceptually sound; a major criterion for research utilization.

secondary analysis A form of research in which the data collected by one researcher are reanalyzed by another investigator, to answer new research questions.

secondary source Second-hand accounts of events or facts; in a research context, a description of a study or studies prepared by someone other than the original researcher.

selection threat (self-selection) A threat to the internal validity of the study resulting from preexisting differences between the groups under study; the differences affect the dependent variable in ways extraneous to the effect of the independent variable.

selective coding The third level of coding in a grounded theory study that involves the process of selecting the core category, systematically integrating relationships between the core category and other categories, and validating those relationships.

self-determination A person's ability to voluntarily decide whether to participate in a study.

self-report Any procedure for collecting data that involves a direct verbal report by the person who is being studied (*e.g.*, by interview or questionnaire).

semantic differential A technique used to measure attitudes that asks respondents to rate a concept of interest on a series of bipolar rating scales.

setting The physical location and conditions in which data collection takes place in a study.

significance level The probability that an observed relationship could be caused by chance (*i.e.*, as a result of sampling error); significance at the .05 level indicates the probability that a relationship of the observed magnitude would be found by chance only 5 times out of 100.

simple random sampling The most basic type of probability sampling, wherein a sampling frame is created by enumerating all members of a population of interest, and then selecting a sample from the sampling frame through completely random procedures.

skewed distribution The asymmetric distribution of a set of scores around a central point.

snowball sampling The selection of participants by means of nominations or referrals from earlier participants; also referred to as *network sampling.*

social desirability response set A bias in self-report instruments created when participants have a tendency to misrepresent their opinions in the direction of answers consistent with prevailing social norms.

Spearman's rank-order correlation (Spearman's rho) A correlation coefficient indicating the magnitude of a relationship between variables measured on the ordinal scale.

split-half technique A method for estimating the internal consistency reliability of an instrument by correlating scores on half of the measure with scores on the other half.

standard deviation The most frequently used statistic for measuring the degree of variability in a set of scores.

standard error The standard deviation of a sampling distribution, such as the sampling distribution of means.

statement of purpose A broad declarative statement of the overall goals of a research project.

statistic An estimate of a parameter, calculated from sample data.

statistical analysis The organization and analysis of quantitative data using statistical procedures, including both descriptive and inferential statistics.

statistical inference The process of inferring attributes about the population based on information from a sample, using laws of probability.

statistical significance A term indicating that the results obtained in an analysis of sample data are unlikely to have been caused by chance, at some specified level of probability.

statistical test An analytic procedure that allows a researcher to determine the probability that obtained results from a sample reflect true population results.

stipend A monetary payment to individuals participating in a study to serve as an incentive for participation and/or to compensate for time and expenses.

strata Subdivisions of the population according to some characteristic (*e.g.,* males and females); singular is *stratum.*

stratified random sampling The random selection of subjects from two or more strata of the population independently.

structured data collection An approach to collecting information from participants, either through self-report or observations, wherein the researcher determines in advance the categories of interest.

study participant An individual who participates and provides information in a qualitative or quantitative research investigation.

subject An individual who participates and provides data in a study; term used primarily in quantitative research.

summated rating scale See *Likert scale.*

survey research Nonexperimental research that focusses on obtaining information regarding the activities, beliefs, preferences, and attitudes of people via direct questioning of a sample of respondents.

symmetric distribution A distribution of values that has two halves that are mirror images of each other; a distribution that is not skewed.

systematic sampling The selection of study participants such that every kth (*e.g.,* every tenth) person (or element) in a sampling frame or list is chosen.

table of random numbers See *random number table.*

target population The entire population in which the researcher is interested and to which he or she would like to generalize the results of a study.

test statistic A statistic used to test for the statistical significance of relationships between variables; the sampling distributions of test statistics are known for circumstances in which the null hypothesis is true; examples include chi-square, F-ratio, t, and Pearson's r.

test–retest reliability Assessment of the stability of an instrument by correlating the scores obtained on repeated administrations.

theme A recurring regularity emerging from an analysis of qualitative data.

theoretical notes In field studies, notes detailing the researcher's interpretations of observed behavior.

theoretical sampling In qualitative studies, the selection of sample members based on emerging findings as the study progresses, to ensure adequate representation of important themes.

theory An abstract generalization that presents a systematic explanation about the relationships among phenomena.

thick description A rich and thorough description of the research context in a qualitative study.

time sampling In observational research, the selection of time periods during which observations will take place.

time series design A quasi-experimental design that involves the collection of information over an extended period of time, with multiple data collection points both before and after the introduction of a treatment.

topic guide A list of broad question areas to be covered in a semistructured interview or focus group interview.

transferability (1) A criterion for evaluating the quality of qualitative data, referring to the extent to which the findings from the data can be transferred to other settings or groups—analogous to generalizability; (2) also, a criterion used in an implementation assessment of a utilization project.

treatment The experimental intervention under study; the condition being manipulated.

treatment group The group receiving the intervention being tested; the experimental group.

trend study A form of longitudinal study in which different samples from a population are studied over time with respect to some phenomenon (*e.g.,* annual Gallup polls on abortion attitudes).

triangulation The use of multiple methods or perspectives to collect and interpret data about some phenomenon, in order to converge on an accurate representation of reality.

true score A hypothetical score that would be obtained if a measure were infallible; it is the portion of the observed score not due to random error or measurement bias.

trustworthiness A term used in the evaluation of qualitative data, assessed via the criteria of credibility, transferability, dependability, and confirmability.

t-**test** A parametric statistical test used for analyzing the difference between two means.

Type I error An error created by rejecting the null hypothesis when it is true (*i.e.,* the researcher concludes that a relationship exists when, in fact, it does not).

Type II error An error created by accepting the null hypothesis when it is false (*i.e.,* the researcher concludes that *no* relationship exists when, in fact, it does).

unimodal distribution A distribution of values with one peak (high frequency).

univariate descriptive study A study that gathers information on the occurrence, frequency of occurrence, or average value of the variables of interest, one variable at a time, without focusing on interrelationships among variables.

univariate statistics Statistical procedures for analyzing a single variable for purposes of description.

unstructured interview An oral self-report in which the researcher asks a respondent questions without having a predetermined plan regarding the specific content or flow of information to be gathered.

unstructured observation The collection of descriptive information through direct observation, whereby the observer is guided by some general research questions but does not follow a prespecified plan for observing, enumerating, or recording the information.

utilization See *research utilization.*

utilization criteria The criteria that are brought to bear in considering whether a tested innovation is amenable to utilization in a practice setting; includes the criteria of clinical relevance, scientific merit, and implementation potential.

validity The degree to which an instrument measures what it is intended to measure.

validity coefficient A quantitative index, usually ranging in value from .00 to 1.00, that provides an estimate of how valid an instrument is; often computed in conjunction with the criterion-related approach to validating an instrument.

variability The degree to which values on a set of scores are widely different or dispersed.

variable A characteristic or attribute of a person or object that varies (*i.e.,* takes on different values) within the population under study (*e.g.,* body temperature, age, heart rate).

variance A measure of variability or dispersion, equal to the square of the standard deviation.

vignette A brief description of an event, person, or situation to which respondents are asked to react and to describe their reactions.

visual analog scale A scaling procedure used to measure a variety of clinical symptoms (*e.g.,* pain, fatigue) by having people indicate on a straight line the intensity of the attribute being measured.

vulnerable subjects Special groups of people whose rights in research studies need special protection because of their inability to provide meaningful informed consent or because their circumstances place them at higher-than-average risk of adverse effects; examples include young children, the mentally retarded, and unconscious patients.

weighting A correction procedure used to arrive at population values when a disproportionate sampling design has been used.

Wilcoxon signed ranks test A nonparametric statistical test for comparing two paired groups, based on the relative ranking of values between the pairs.

within-subjects design A research design in which a single group of subjects is compared under different conditions or at different points in time (*e.g.,* before and after surgery).

Appendix: Research Reports

Patient Outcomes for The Chronically Critically Ill: Special Care Unit Versus Intensive Care Unit

ELLEN B. RUDY, BARBARA J. DALY, SARA DOUGLAS, HUGO D. MONTENEGRO, RHAYUN SONG, MARY ANN DYER

The purpose of this study was to compare the effects of a low-technology environment of care and a nurse case management case delivery system (special care unit, SCU) with the traditional high-technology environment (ICU) and primary nursing care delivery system on the patient outcomes of length of stay, mortality, readmission, complications, satisfaction, and cost. A sample of 220 chronically critically ill patients were randomly assigned to either the SCU (n = 145) or the ICU (n = 75). Few significant differences were found between the two groups in length of stay, mortality, or complications. However, the findings showed significant cost savings in the SCU group in the charges accrued during the study period and in the charges and costs to produce a survivor. The average total cost of delivering care was $5,000 less per patient in the SCU than in the traditional ICU. In addition, the cost to produce a survivor was $19,000 less in the SCU. Results from this 4-year clinical trial demonstrate that nurse case managers in a SCU setting can produce patient outcomes equal to or better than those in the traditional ICU care environment for long-term critically ill patients.

The original purpose of intensive care units (ICUs) was to locate groups of patients together who had similar needs for specialized monitoring and care so that highly trained health care personnel would be available to meet these specialized needs. As the success of ICUs has grown and expanded, the assumption that a typical ICU patient will require only a short length of stay in the unit during the most acute phase of an illness has given way to the recognition that stays of more than 1 month are not uncommon (Berenson, 1984; Daly, Rudy, Thompson, & Happ, 1991).

These long-stay ICU patients represent a challenge to the current system, not only because of costs, but also because of concern for patient outcomes. These patients are often elderly, have underlying chronic conditions that complicate or exacerbate their acute illness, and often require sustained ventilatory and nutritional support. A prime example of these types of patients are those referred to as "ventilator dependent," found to varying degrees in nearly every ICU in the country (American Association for Respiratory Care, 1991).

The term "chronically critically ill" has been previously used (Daly et al., 1991) to describe patients who have extended stays in the ICU. These patients have become the most burdensome to nurses and physicians, who see their progress as slow and frustrating, to hospital administrators because of the extended bed occupancy in times of high demand, and to hospital financial officers because of costs that usually exceed the diagnosis-related group (DRG) cost allocation. Patients who have ICU length of stays greater than 21 days account for approximately 3% of the total number of patients admitted to the ICUs, yet they account for approximately 25% to 38% of the patient days (Daly et al.).

While ample evidence confirms that this subpopulation of ICU patients represents a drain on hospital resources, few studies have attempted to evaluate the effects of a care delivery system outside the ICU setting on patient outcomes, costs, and nurse outcomes. The majority of studies that have examined ICU patient outcomes have been limited primarily to mortality and length of stay (Bersenson, 1984; Borlase et al., 1991; Madoff, Sharpe, Fath, Simons, & Cerra, 1985). More recently, attention has been given to cost in terms of risk-adjusted ICU length of stays, cost and utility of diagnostic and laboratory tests, and time on mechanical ventilation (Gundlach & Faulkner, 1991; Kappstein et al., 1992; Roberts et al., 1993; Schapira, Studnicki, Bradham, Wolff, & Jarrett, 1993; Zimmerman et al., 1993).

In studies limited to mechanically ventilated patients, comparisons on length of stay and costs have been examined in "a before-and-after" design following initiation of a ventilatory management team (Cohen et al., 1991), on overall costs for mechanically ventilated patients cared for in an ICU versus a noninvasive respiratory care unit (Elpern, Silver, Rosen, & Bone, 1991), and on hospital charges and life expectancy for elderly mechanically ventilated ICU patients (Cohen, Lambrinos, & Fein, 1993). The lack of randomized trials comparing care delivery systems for these high-cost patients is noteworthy, as well as the limitation of outcome measurements to mortality and cost.

The purpose of the current study was to compare the effects of a low-technology environment of care based on a nurse-managed care delivery system [special care unit (SCU) environment] with the traditional high-technology ICU environment based on a primary nursing care delivery system. The two groups were compared on the outcomes of length of stay, mortality, readmission to the hospital, complications, patient and family satisfaction, and cost. The complications were defined as number and type of infections, number and type of respiratory complications, and number and type of life-threatening complications.

◧ **METHOD**

Sample: A total of 276 subjects were eligible for the study. Table 1 lists eligibility criteria. Only four refused to participate; of the remaining 272 subjects, 220 (81%) were able to be randomized. Of the 52 subjects who were not randomly assigned to a treatment group, the majority (n = 37, 71%) were due to bed availability, with only 13 (25%) due to physician refusal to allow randomization to treatment assignment, and 2 (4%) because of family unwillingness to allow treatment assignment.

The final sample for analysis consisted of 145 subjects cared for in the SCU environment and 75 subjects in the ICU environment. The sample was nearly equally divided between males and females, was predominantly white (70%), with an average age of 64 years (range 16 to 90 years). The groups were equivalent on gender, age, and race, on the prior ICU length of stay (M = 16 days, SD = 13.3), and on the general medical diagnosis of patients. Significant differences were found in the type of ICU where patients received their care prior to the study and in source of payment for care. A higher percentage of no payment source and private insurance was found in the ICU group, with a higher percentage of public (Medicare and Medicaid) insurance in the SCU group.

To ensure similarity in acuity of illness between the two groups of subjects, a variety of variables were compared. No significant difference between the groups was noted on the Acute Physiological and Chronic Health Evaluation II (APACHE II) on admission to the ICU or at time of eligibility for the study, the Therapeutic Intervention Scoring System (TISS) at the time of eligibility for the study, and the number of infections prior to admission to the study. In terms of these known risk predictors, then, the experimental and control groups were equivalent. There were, however, significantly ($p \le .03$) more respiratory complications prior to the study

Table 1. Eligibility Criteria for Patients in the Study

Length of stay (LOS) in ICU >5 days[a]
Non currently receiving IV vasopressor (exception: low-level maintenance drip)
No pulmonary artery monitor required
No acute event (arrest, unstable event) in past 3 days
APACHE II 18 or less
TISS class II or III (10 to 39 points)
Unable to be cared for on a general nursing unit

NOTE. APACHE, Acute physiological and chronic health evaluation; TISS, Therapeutic intervention scoring system.
[a] First 2 years of study LOS in ICU was >7 days, but with experience the LOS was shortened to ≥5 days.

in the patients admitted to the SCU. While statistically significant, in practical terms, the means of the two groups varied by only 0.5, with a very similar range and standard deviation. Furthermore, the higher risk from prior respiratory complications was in the SCU sample, so claims that patients in the ICU were sicker can be refuted.

Setting: The environments of care were conceptualized according to the socio-technical theory of work, which proposes that both the physical environment in which work occurs, the procedures and processes of work, and the way workers interact with one another and with the environment will influence the way in which the work is accomplished and ultimately the output of the work (Happ, 1993; Pasmore, 1988, Pasmore & Sherwood, 1978).

The SCU environment of care was designed to decrease technology and ensure privacy in order to promote sleep and rest, allow for more freedom for interaction with family and friends, ensure continuity of care by nurse case managers working with medical protocols, and create an opportunity for a self-directed governance model. The significant contrasting features of the SCU versus the ICU were the physical environment, the nursing practice model, and the nursing management model.

The SCU environment was a 7-bed unit with only private rooms. Technology was limited to electrocardiographic monitors, ventilators, and occasional arterial pressure monitoring. Family involvement was encouraged through unlimited visiting and overnight accommodations. The care delivery system was case management, with the nurse case manager accountable clinically and financially for each patient's outcomes. Interns and residents were not in the unit. Each patient's plan of care was established, coordinated, and evaluated by the case manager working in close collaboration with the unit's attending physician. Case managers participated in an 8-week training program for the SCU and, with the medical director of the unit, developed protocols that addressed such activities as ventilator weaning, nutrition, pain management, and sedation. In addition, the SCU initiated a shared governance management model, which vested the authority and responsibility for managing the work environment in the staff nurses.

The ICU environments included primarily a 12-bed medical intensive care unit and an 18-bed surgical intensive care unit. A small percentage of subjects (19%) who met the study criteria came from the neurosurgical intensive care unit or the coronary intensive care unit. The majority (80%) of bed spaces were open or curtained off from a central nursing station. Visitor lounges were outside the units, family visiting was controlled, and overnight stays were not accommodated. Technology and physiological monitoring devices were not limited, and lighting and noise from the overall unit was difficult to exclude from the patient bed spaces. A primary nursing model of care was used in all of the ICUs, with total nursing care the responsibility of the primary nurse. Interns and residents delivered most of the medical care, as is the standard practice in academic medical centers. A bureaucratic management model was used with centralized decision making at the head nurse level, and organizational responsibility and authority descending within each unit through a distinct chain of command.

Procedure: Rounds were made every other day in all ICUs to assess patient eligibility. Using a coin toss, eligible patients were assigned to either the experimental or control group. Consent to participate was then obtained from both the primary physician and the patient. If the patient was unable to consent, the next of kin was asked for permission. If the patients and their physicians consented, patients were then enrolled and, if in the experimental group, transferred to the SCU. This procedure for consent and group assignment was approved by the hospital's Institutional Review Board.

Every effort was made to randomize subject assignment to groups, but because of the practical need to keep the 7-bed SCU occupied, a distribution of approximately 2:1 was needed to meet this obligation. Based on various options for randomization of subject assignment in the clinical trials literature (Efron, 1971; Hjelm-Karlsson, 1991; Meinert & Tonasicia, 1986), a biased-coin format was used in which two out of every three eligible subjects were assigned to the experimental group (SCU), and one was assigned to the control (Rudy, Vaska, Daly, Happ, & Shiao, 1993). While this design helped to ensure a more steady occupancy of the SCU, the disadvantage was that at certain times the investigator knew ahead of time where the next eligible patient would be assigned. Efforts were made to overcome this bias. First, the date on which a patient became eligible for the study was used to determine who was next in line for assignment, and this was outside the direct control of the investigators. Second, caregivers in both the SCU and ICU were not involved in determining patient eligibility or patient assignments. Furthermore, patients transferred to SCU because of a low census in the SCU rather than through the randomized assignment were not part of the study sample. Even with these disadvantages, this assignment procedure was far superior to a simple comparative design without a randomization procedure, allowing real comparisons to occur within the limitations of a clinical setting.

Following group assignment and transfer of experimental subjects to the SCU, data collection was done prospectively. Patient records were reviewed at least every other day until the patient was discharged from the hospital or died.

Instruments: The ACUTE PHYSIOLOGICAL AND CHRONIC HEALTH EVALUATION II (APACHE II) was used to establish the similarity of severity of illness between the experimental and control groups and as a measure of severity of illness at entry to the study. This instrument, a refinement of the original APACHE (Knaus, Draper, Wagner, & Zimmerman, 1986), is a severity of disease classification system that predicts risk of death. It is based on the assumption that the severity of disease can be quantified by the degree of abnormality of physiologic variables in combination with age and the presence of chronic disease. The range of possible scores is 0 to 71. Accuracy in predicting death was found to be 86% in a study of 5,815 patients (Knaus et al.). This is consistent with earlier studies in which regression analysis was used to validate mortality prediction using the acute physiology portion of the tool (Wagner, Knaus, & Draper, 1983). In a multihospital study of critically ill patients that used the APACHE classification, an interrater agreement of .95 was maintained (Knaus et al.).

The THERAPEUTIC INTERVENTION SCORING SYSTEM (TISS) (Keene & Cullen, 1983) was designed to classify intensive care patients according to intensity of resource utilization. The TISS score is obtained by recording the number of weighted interventions actually used on the patient from a list of 76. The range of total scores is 0 to 181. TISS has been used since 1974 in multiple studies to assess severity of illness, outcomes of critical care, and utilization of ICU beds (Byrick, Mindorff, McKee, & Mudge, 1980; Schwartz & Cullen, 1981), and recently to examine the relationship between charges and reimbursement in different patient populations (Bekes, Fleming, & Scott, 1988; Teres et al., 1988). It was used in this study to compare utilization of resources in groups matched for severity of illness by APACHE. Validity is based on the initial study by Cullen, Civetta, Briggs, & Ferrara (1974) who recorded all interventions according to critically ill subjects and subsequently divided these into classes to be used to describe resource utilization: Class I = 0 to 9, Class II = 10 to 19, Class III = 20 to 39, Class IV $\geq$ 40. Experts in critical care validated the list of interventions as adequately and accurately reflecting critical care patient management (Byrick et al.; Schwartz & Cullen). Four experienced ICU nurses were trained in the use of TISS and 20 critically ill patients were evaluated at the start of this study, each by two nurses within 1 hour of each other. The correlation coefficient for this interrater reliability was $r = .96$.

The LAMONICA-OBERST PATIENT SATISFACTION SCALE measures satisfaction with care, defined as the degree of congruence between patients' expectations of nursing care and their perceptions of care actually received (LaMonica, Oberst, Madea, & Wolf, 1986). Three dimensions of nursing care are measured: technical-professional, trusting relationship, and education relationship. The scale was based on the Risser scale (1975) and was modified to be appropriate for the acute care setting. Internal consistency of the three subscales in separate studies ranged from .80 to .90. The LaMonica-Oberst instrument consisted of 41 statements about nursing care to which the patient indicated agreement or disagreement using a Likert scale.

After preliminary use in this study, it became apparent that the instrument was too difficult for patients who were recovering from a critical illness to complete. Following a factor analysis, the scale was shortened to 15 items by removing items that demonstrated redundancy. Post-hoc analysis identified three factors. The alpha coefficient for the revised Patient Satisfaction scale has averaged .92 ($n = 93$). Construct validity is supported in that the identified factors are the same as those identified in LaMonica's original work.

A similar analysis was performed on the Family Satisfaction scale. This instrument was developed from the LaMonica-Oberst Patient Satisfaction scale by changing the wording of items to reflect the family member's satisfaction with the care received by the patient. This scale was shortened from the original 41 items to 29 items.

The RESPIRATORY COMPLICATIONS INDEX (RCI) was developed by the investigators. It is a checklist that is easily administered and scored. It includes the categories of respiratory complications evident in critical care areas. The range of total possible scores is 0 to 10. The criteria used to determine the presence of a pulmonary complication include: radiologic reports of atelectasis, consolidation, or collapse; fever; arterial blood gas results; positive sputum cultures; and clinical signs as documented in progress notes. While this checklist was constructed specifically for the study, these criteria are routinely used by other investigators in studying frequency of pulmonary complications (Ali, Serrette, Wood, & Anthomisen, 1985; Kirilloff, Owens, Rogers, & Mazzocco, 1985; Morran et al., 1983). Some association between occurrences of individual complications can be expected. For example, respiratory infections may commonly be associated with increased likelihood of hypoxia or failure to wean. The construct validity of the instrument is supported by the data obtained from both preliminary studies and the special care unit. Rules for use of the tool were established in these preliminary studies and average interrater reliability of .94 was maintained.

The INFECTION COMPLICATIONS INDEX (ICI) is an investigator-developed checklist. It includes the specific sites of infections commonly found in critical care areas, as well as general indicators of infection. The checklist identifies critical indicators from the respiratory and urinary tracks, blood, and wound, as well as general indicators of present infections. The general criteria are considered to be positive critical indicators of infection of unknown source only when other noninfectious causes are absent. While this checklist was constructed specifically for the study, these criteria are routinely used by other investigators studying nosocomial infections (Bartlett, O'Keefe, Tally, Louie, & Gorbach, 1986; Garner & Favero, 1986; Parkhurst, Blaser, Laxson, & Wang, 1985).

Construct validity was established by testing the relationship between the total number of infections and length of hospital stay ($r = .78$) and ICU length of stay ($r = .88$). Interrater reliability was maintained at $\leq 90\%$ throughout the study.

The LIFE-THREATENING COMPLICATION INDEX (LTCI) was developed in the second year of the study when it became evident that the occurrence of such complications as seizures, ventricular fibrillation, and gastrointestinal bleeding were frequent enough that the rate of occurrence could serve as additional outcome measures. The LTCI includes 15 life-threatening events or episodes. To be counted as life threatening, the event must have required medical treatment.

The LTCI is scored by giving one point for each event. Scores range from 0 to 15. Construct validity is supported by the positive correlation between the LTCI and hospital mortality ($r = .24$), hospital length of stay ($r = .32$), and critical care days ($r = .40$). The interrater reliability averaged .97 over the 4 years of the study. Data for the LTCI were obtained retrospectively for those patients who had entered the study prior to the design of the instrument; for all other patients, the data were collected prospectively with the other outcome measures.

Since each instrument is dependent on accurate abstraction of data from the patient record, interrater agreement was carefully monitored. Each member of the research team who participated in data collection was trained by the project director and had to achieve a 90% agreement on each measurement before independent data were collected. In addition, a detailed rule book was kept so that reliability could be maintained. Interrater reliability was checked on a random selection of 10% of records and maintained at 90% agreement between coders. Whenever agreement dropped below 90%, differences in scoring were analyzed and resolved, usually through the construction of additional coding rules.

COST. Two sources of financial information were used in this study: charge data from actual patient bills and cost data from the hospital's cost management information system (CMIS). The CMIS uses product- or service-specific cost data provided by each hospital department. In most cases, the costs per product or per service delivered were derived by calculating the actual cost of material and labor, such as a CAT scan or physical therapy session, projecting the estimated volume of all services, and then adding a weighted portion of that department's indirect cost to each product or service. Room costs included only direct cost of nursing salaries, including benefits, and unit specific costs such as equipment depreciation and supplies. While questions of accuracy always arise, the method of calculating specific costs at the level of individual products or services delivered is generally acceptable and is as close to "true" costs as possible at this setting. A variety of analyses were performed on these data and a fuller description is provided in another publication (Douglas, Daly, Rudy, Song, & Dyer, in press). The comparisons between DRG weight, total charges for the entire hospitalization, total costs, total payment or reimbursement from any payor, the margin, study period charges, and charges and costs to produce a survivor are described in this report.

DRG weight is the adjustment for variance of complexity used by the federal government for diagnosis-related groups. The margin is the difference between the cost of each patient's care and the reimbursement or payment actually received. Charges accruing after the patient entered the study were also obtained by subtracting the prestudy period charges from the total hospitalization charges. The cost and charge to produce a survivor in each of the study environments was also calculated by adding the charges (or costs) for every study patient in each unit and then dividing this total by the number of survivors in that unit.

▨ RESULTS

The results are presented according to each patient outcome that was compared (see Table 2). When data were in interval level, ANOVA was used with significance set at $p \leq .05$. When nominal level data were compared, a chi-square statistic was used with significance set at $p \leq .05$.

Mortality: Although a higher percentage of patients cared for in the ICUs died in the hospital (41.3% versus 30.3% for the SCU), this difference was not statistically significant. While a higher percentage of patients from the SCU were discharged home ($n = 45; 31\%$) or to a rehabilitation facility ($n = 21; 14.5\%$), these differences were also not significant.

Table 2. Comparison of Patient Outcomes Between ICU Patients and SCU Patients[a]

Variable	Special Care Unit $n = 145$	Intensive Care Unit $n = 75$	Stat	p Value	Effect Size	Power
Mortality			$\chi^2 = .66$	.103	.05	.36
Died	44 (30.3%)	31 (41.3%)				
Lived	101 (69.7%)	44 (58.7%)				
Discharge disposition from hospital:			$\chi^2 = 4.55$	.473	.14	.33
Died	44 (30.3%)	31 (41.3%)				
Other hospital	3 (2.1%)	0 (0%)				
Long-term care	31 (21.4%)	14 (18.7%)				
Rehabilitation	21 (14.5%)	11 (14.7%)				
Home	45 (31.0%)	19 (25.3%)				
Home ventilator	1 (0.7%)	0				
Length of hospital stay (days)	48.6 ± 29.5 (9 to 160)	50.6 ± 33.4 (8 to 176)	$F = 0.20$	.655	.03	.07
Readmit[b]			$\chi^2 = 4.65$	.031	.18	.48
Yes	8 (8%)	9 (20%)				
No	93 (92%)	35 (80%)				
Total number of infections	1.6 ± 2.3 (0 to 10)	1.7 ± 2.3 (0 to 10)	$F = 0.27$	.870	.02	.05
Total number of respiratory complications	2.14 ± 1.9 (0 to 7)	2.25 ± 1.9 (0 to 7)	$F = 0.10$	.688	.03	.06
Life-threatening complications	1.12 ± 1.4 (0 to 8)	.88 ± 1.2 (0 to 5)	$F = 2.16$	.1917	.09	.26

[a] Continuous variables reported as $M \pm SD$, with range noted below;
[b] The n used for this calculation included only patients who survived to discharge ($n = 145$).

481

Length of Stay: The hospital length of stay (LOS) for the total sample ranged from 8 to 176 days, with an overall mean of 49.3 days. There was a large standard deviation in both groups of patients. While the mean LOS for the SCU patients was 2 days less than the ICU patients, this difference was not significant.

Readmission: A total of 17 patients were readmitted to the hospital after discharge. The SCU percentage at 8% is significantly ($p \leq .03$) lower than the ICU's at 20%.

Infections: The total number of infections ranged from 0 to 10 for both groups with an overall mean of 1.6 ($SD = 2.3$) and with no difference between the groups. Approximately one third of the patients in both groups had respiratory infections and one third had urinary track infections. Only 9% ($n = 13$) of the SCU patients had sepsis (blood infections) compared to 16% ($n = 12$) of ICU patients. None of the differences noted between the groups was significant.

Respiratory Complications: In both groups, the number of respiratory complications ranged from 0 to 7, with an overall mean of 2.17 ($SD = 1.9$) per patient and with no significant difference between groups. Only 1% ($n = 2$) of SCU patients had adult respiratory distress syndrome (ARDS) versus 5% ($n = 4$) of ICU patients.

Life-Threatening Complications: There was no difference between the groups in the number of life-threatening complications, with an average of about one life-threatening complication per patient. However, the SCU patients had significantly more documented episodes of bradycardia (pulse < 40 BPM), 14.5% vs. 3% in the ICUs ($p \leq .006$), and more episodes of a decrease in neurological status (SCU 13% vs. ICUs 4%, $p \leq .033$).

Patient and Family Satisfaction: No difference was noted between the groups on either patient or family satisfaction. The overall patient satisfaction scores ranged from 43 to 105 ($M = 90.1$), and the family satisfaction scores ranged from 125 to 210 ($M = 186.5$). Satisfaction scores were all skewed to the high end of the scale with minimal variability for nearly all patients and family members. Because of this, data collection on this variable was discontinued after 2 years.

Cost: Comparisons of financial data associated with the two study environments are shown in Table 3. Although the differences in total charges, costs, and margin were not significantly different, both charges and costs were lower for patients in the SCU by 6% to 7%. Combined with the lower mortality rate in the SCU, this resulted in both significantly lower costs and charges to produce a survivor. The actual cost savings were $5,000 less per patient in the SCU, and the cost to produce a survivor was $19,000 less in the SCU versus the ICU. SCU charges were also significantly lower when the prestudy period (prior to the point at which the patient became eligible for the study and experimental patients were transferred into the SCU) was excluded.

◧ DISCUSSION

While the original expectation of ICUs was for short-term stays during a vulnerable period of an acute illness, patients today may require life-support technology with

Table 3. Comparison of Finance Data Between ICU Patients and SCU Patients[a]

Variable	Special Care Unit $n = 145$	Intensive Care Unit $n = 70$	F	p Value	Effect Size	Power
Charges	$151,226 ± $92,621 (29,388 to 586,139)	$162,718 ± 107,818 (26,621 to 548,829)	.6792	.4107	.05	.12
Payment	$65,709 ± $46,391 (0 to 212,452)	$66,364 ± $55,452 (0 to 305,362)	.0084	.9272	.01	.04
Cost	$76,077 ± $45,101 (13,853 to 231,125)	$81,212 ± $50,186 (9,436 to 251,000)	.5832	.4459	.05	.11
Margin	$−10,899 ± $39,241 (−153,795 to 103,184)	$−14,694 ± $48,083 (−138,015 to 131,297)	.3806	.5379	.04	.09
DRG weight	8,230 ± 5,708 (.451 to 16,986)	8,579 ± 6,039 (.5123 to 16,986)	.1783	.6733	.00	.04
Study period charge	$69,132 ± $53,222 (9,330 to 277,239)	$94,045 ± $85,915 (7,474 to 472,470)	5.3394	.022*	.17	.69
Charge per survivor	$215,351 ± $85,303 (98,690 to 482,733)	$279,870 ± $110,407 (139,522 to 661,730)	14.5741	.0002*	.30	.95
Cost per survivor[b]	$109,220 ± $45,117 (48,007 to 265,279)	$138,434 ± $44,736 (66,467 to 234,619)	12.684	.0005*	.30	.95

[a] Continuous variables reported as $M ± SD$, with range noted below.
[b] The n used for this calculation included only survivors; SCU $n = 101$. ICU $n = 41$.
* Significant at $p \leq .05$ level.

intensive monitoring and care for extended periods. These chronically critically ill represent a subgroup of patients whose outcomes of care have not been carefully examined and whose care may be equally effective outside the traditional ICU setting.

The similarity in outcomes is striking considering the differences in the two environments. The special care unit environment was purposely planned to have less technology, be more open to visitors, have less ambient noise and distraction through the use of private rooms, and patient care managed by nurse case managers. The lack of differences between the groups including mortality and length of stay indicate that chronically critically ill patients can be cared for outside the standard ICU setting when their care is managed by skilled nurse case managers. The study confirms that care managed by nurses working with collaboratively derived medical protocols produces outcomes that are equal to or that exceed those of patients whose care is managed by residents and interns in the routine ICU setting. While a significantly lower percentage of SCU patients required readmission, the effect size and power were low, indicating a need for a larger sample size.

The average LOS for all patients was extremely long, and therefore costly in terms of intensive care resources. Because of the wide variability in length of stay (8 to 176 days), those patients at the extreme end of the spectrum should be examined. Patients who require intensive care services up to 3 months are obviously a major financial and personnel burden to hospitals. This calls for an examination of such patients beyond simple mortality statistics to questions of functional status, quality of life, and family response to an extended critical illness. Patients such as the chronically critically ill survive one complication only to develop another. Thoughts regarding the futility of care in some cases of elderly patients with multiple complications, setbacks, and prolonged lengths of stay need to be addressed by the entire health care team before health care providers are forced into making decisions solely on the basis of cost. To provide a fuller picture of the differences between the two groups, post-hoc effect size and power were calculated for each of the fiscal variables (Borenstein & Cohen, 1988; SOLO Power Analysis, 1992). The differences in the fiscal aspects of care associated with the SCU environment were marked. It is important to note that these differences do not represent savings associated only with reduced nursing care or lower nurse-patient ratios. In fact, the nurse-patient ratio for each patient was nearly identical to that found in ICUs, with the exception of the night shift when the ratio in the SCU was occasionally 1:3 rather than 1:2 or 1:1 in the ICUs. Use of cost data, rather than charge data, confirms the conclusion that the differences between the study units was not just a reflection of charging different rates for the SCU.

The primary source of savings in the SCU stems from a different philosophy and approach to the care of these very ill patients. Most ICUs, quite appropriately, are founded on the assumption that the goal of care is to preserve life at all costs. Every precaution is taken to identify and prevent complications; the rule of thumb is to err on the side of aggressive intervention. This approach is appropriate for the typical ICU patient who experiences a very brief and very acute episode of a life-threatening, but survivable illness. It is less appropriate and less effective for chronically critically ill patients whose problems are not short-term, whose illness may not be reversible, and whose course is not improved by the use of therapies, each of which carries with it the possibility of iatrogenic harm. By segregating these patients in the current study, it was possible to change the norms underlying the approach to care, to question what gains were to be made by aggressive pursuit of every abnormal diagnostic test, to reduce the use of daily laboratory testing surveillance, and to tailor care to the specific needs and goals of each patient. This resulted directly in reduced use of X rays, blood tests, and some therapies. The management of the patients in the SCU by expert nurses undoubtedly contributed to the success of this conservative approach to care.

The results of this study demonstrate that carefully selected patients can be cared for outside of the ICU setting under the care of well-trained nurse case managers, with no threat to patient outcomes and with significant cost savings. This finding has major implications for the care of long-term critically ill patients. It would seem prudent for those institutions that have such patients to explore the potential for creating a special care unit with trained nurse case managers.

To replicate these results, it is necessary to recognize the sociotechnical theory that underpins the SCU environment of care (Daly et al., 1991; Happ, 1993), thereby creating a work environment that encompasses both a carefully designed physical space for these patients, as well as an expanded case management role for nurses who work in and contribute to the environment of care. A medical director of the unit who not only understands the medical care of critically ill patients but who supports the collaborative development of treatment protocols and the need for consistency of care provided by case managers is an essential part of the model. Thus, the evidence strongly suggests that the use of a special environment for chronically critically ill patients headed by nurse case managers, as reported in this study, offers health care facilities a viable, cost-effective alternative to traditional ICU units, without sacrificing quality of care.   NR

Accepted for publication September 22, 1995.
This study was funded in part by a grant from the National Institute of Nursing Research, Grant number R01-NR02248.

Ellen B. Rudy, PhD, FAAN, is dean and professor, University of Pittsburgh, School of Nursing, Pittsburgh, PA.

Barbara J. Daly, PhD, FAAN, is an assistant professor, Case Western Reserve University, School of Nursing, Cleveland, OH.

Sara Douglas, PhD, RN, is an assistant professor, Case Western Reserve University, School of Nursing, Cleveland, OH.

Hugo D. Montenegro, MD, is an associate professor, School of Medicine, Case Western Reserve University, Cleveland, OH.

Rhayun Song, PhD, RN, was project director during the time of the study at Case Western Reserve University, School of Nursing, Cleveland, OH.

Mary Ann Dyer, MSN, RN, is project staff, Case Western Reserve University, School of Nursing, Cleveland, OH.

REFERENCES

Ali, J., Serrette, C., Wood, L. D. H., & Anthomisen, N. R. (1985). Effect of postoperative intermittent positive pressure breathing on lung function. *Chest, 85,* 192–196.

American Association for Respiratory Care. (1991). A study of chronic ventilator patients in the hospital. Dallas: Author.

Bartlett, J. G., O'Keefe, P., Tally, F. P., Louie, T. J., & Gorbach, S. L. (1986). Bacteriology of hospital-acquired pneumonia. *Archives of Internal Medicine, 146,* 868–871.

Bekes, C., Fleming, J., & Scott, W. E. (1988). Reimbursement for intensive care services under diagnosis-related groups. *Critical Care Medicine, 16,* 470–481.

Berenson, R. A. (1984). Intensive care units: Clinical outcomes, costs, and decision making. Health Technology Case Study 28 (OTA-28). Office of Technology Assessment. Washington DC: U.S. Government Printing Office.

Borenstein & Cohen, J. (1988). Statistical power analysis: A computer program. New Jersey: Lawrence Erlbaum.

Borlase, B. C., Baxter, J. T., Benotti, P. N., Stone, M., Wood, E., Forse, R. A., Blackburn, G. L., & Steele, G. Jr. (1991). Surgical intensive care unit resource use in a specialty referral hospital: I. Predictors of early death and cost implications. *Surgery, 109,* 687–693.

Byrick, R. J., Mindorff, C., McKee, L., & Mudge, B. (1980). Cost-effectiveness of intensive care for respiratory failure patients. *Critical Care Medicine, 8,* 332–337.

Cohen, I. L., Bari, N., Strosberg, M. A., Weinberg, P. F., Waskswan, R. M., Millstein, B. H., & Fein, I. A. (1991). Reduction of duration and cost of mechanical ventilation in an intensive care unit by use of a ventilatory management team. *Critical Care Medicine, 19,* 1278–1281.

Cohen, I. L., Lambrinos, J., & Fein, I. A. (1993). Mechanical ventilation for the elderly patient in intensive care. Incremented changes and benefits. *JAMA,* 269f–1029.

Cullen, D. J., Civetta, J. M., Briggs, B. A., & Ferrara, L. C. (1974). Therapeutic intervention scoring system: A method for quantitative comparison of patient care. *Critical Care Medicine, 2,* 57–62.

Daly, B. J., Rudy, E. R., Thompson, K. S., & Happ, M. B. (1991). Development of a special care unit for chronically critically ill patients. *Heart and Lung, 20,* 45–51.

Douglas, S., Daly, B., Rudy, E., Song, R., & Dyer, M. A. (in press). Cost effectiveness of a special care unit to care for the chronically critically ill. *Journal of Nursing Administration.*

Efron, B. (1971). Forcing a sequential experiment to be balanced. *Biometrika, 58,* 403–417.

Elpern, E. H., Silver, M. R., Rosen, R. L., & Bone, R. C. (1991). The non-invasive respiratory care unit. Patterns of use and financial implications. *Chest,* 990–208.

Garner, J. S., & Favero, M. S. (1986). CDC guidelines for handwashing and hospital environmental control, 1985. *Infection Control, 7,* 231–243.

Gundlach, C. A., & Faulkner, T. P. (1991). Charge and reimbursement analysis for intensive care unit patients in a large tertiary teaching hospital. *DICP, 25,* 1231–1235.

Happ, M. B. (1993). Sociotechnical system's theory: Analysis and application for nursing administration (tables/charts). *Journal of Nursing Administration, 23*–54.

Hjelm-Karlsson, K. (1991). Using the biased coin design for randomization in health care research. *Western Journal of Nursing Research, 13,* 284–288.

Kappstein, I., Schulgen, G., Beyer, U., Geiger, K., Schumacher, M., & Daschner, F. D. (1992). Prolongation of hospital stay and extra costs due to ventilator-associated pneumonia in an intensive care unit. *European Journal of Clinical Microbiology and Infectious Diseases, 11,* 504–508.

Keene, A. R., & Cullen, D. J. (1983). Therapeutic intervention scoring system: Update, 1983. *Critical Care medicine, 11,* 1–4.

Kirilloff, L. H., Owens, G. R., Rogers, R. M., & Mazzocco, M. C. (1985). Does chest physical therapy work: A review. *Chest, 88,* 436–444.

Knaus, W. A., Draper, E. A., Wagner, D. P., & Zimmerman, J. E. (1986). An evaluation of outcome from intensive care in major medical centers. *Annals of Internal Medicine, 104,* 410–418.

LaMonica, E. L., Oberst, M. T., Madea, A. R., & Wolf, R. M. (1986). Development of a patient satisfaction scale. *Research in Nursing and Health, 9,* 43–50.

Madoff, R. D., Sharpe, S. M., Fath, J. J., Simons, R. L., & Cerra, F. B. (1985). Prolonged surgical intensive care. *Archives of Surgery, 120,* 698–702.

Meinert, C. L., & Tonasicia, S. (1986). *Clinical trials, design, conduct and analysis.* New York: Oxford University Press, pp. 90–112.

Morran, C. G., Finlay, I. G., Mathieson, M., McKay, A. J., Wilson, N., & McArdle, C. S. (1983). Randomized controlled trial of physiotherapy for postoperative pulmonary complications. *British Journal of Anesthesia, 55,* 1113–1116.

Parkhurst, S. M., Blaser, M. J., Laxson, L., & Wang, W. (1985). Surveillance for the detection of nosocomial infections and the potential for nosocomial outbreaks: Development of a laboratory-based system, part 2. *American Journal of Infection Control, 13*(1), 7–15.

Pasmore, W. (1988). *Designing effective organizations: The sociotechnical systems perspective.* New York: John Wiley.

Pasmore, W., & Sherwood, J. (1978). *Sociotechnical systems: A source-book.* San Diego, CA: University Associates, Inc.

Risser, N. (1975). Development of an instrument to measure patient satisfaction with nurses and nursing care in primary care settings. *Nursing Research, 24,* 45–52.

Roberts, D. E., Bell, D. D., Ostryzniuk, T., Dobson, K., Oppenheimer, L., Marten, D., Honcharik, N., Cramp, H., Loewen, E., Bodnar, S., Guenther, A., Pronger, L., Roberts, E., & McEwen, T. (1993). Eliminating needless testing in intensive care—an information-based team management approach. *Critical Care Medicine, 21,* 1452–1458.

Rudy, E. B., Vaska, P., Daly, B., Happ, M. B., & Shiao, P. (1993). Permuted block design for randomization in a nursing clinical trial. *Nursing Research, 42,* 287–289.

Schapira, D. V., Studnicki, J., Bradham, D. D., Wolff, P., & Jarrett, A. (1993). Intensive care, survival, and expense of treating critically ill cancer patients. *Journal of the American Medical Association, 269,* 783–786.

Schwartz, S., & Cullen, D. J. (1981). How many intensive care beds does your hospital need? *Critical Care Medicine, 9,* 625–630.

SOLO Power Analysis (1992). Los Angeles, CA: BMDP Statistical Software.

Teres, D., Rapaport, J., Lemeshow, S., Haber, R., Gage, R. W., & Avrunin, J. S. (1988). Using a severity of illness measurement with critically ill patients to explain cost validity within diagnostic-related groups (abstract). *Critical Care Medicine, 16,* 406.

Wagner, D. P., Knaus, W. A., & Draper, E. A. (1983). Statistical validation of a severity of illness measure . . . Acute physiology score of APACHE. *American Journal of Public Health, 73,* 878–884.

Zimmerman, J. E., Shortell, S. M., Knaus, W. A., Rousseau, D. M., Wagner, D. P., Gilles, R. R., Draper, E. A., & Devers, K. (1993). Value and cost of teaching hospitals: A prospective, multicenter, inception cohort study. *Critical Care Medicine, 21,* 1432–1442.

Family Members' Experiences Living With Members With Depression[1]

TERRY A. BADGER

Using interview data from 11 family members and grounded theory methods, this study describes family members' experiences in living with a member with depression. Findings suggest that this process can be described as family transformations. In the first stage of this process—acknowledging the strangers within—family members described observing the metamorphosis of the person and other family members, finding socially acceptable explanations, living two lives, searching for reasons and solutions, and hoping for what was. In the second stage—fighting the battle—family members alternated between the strategies of holding our ground (protective) and of moving forward (coercive) to counteract the metamorphosis, and the strategy of working the system to get help for their ill member. In the third and final stage, family members described gaining a new perspective and identified preserving oneself, refocusing on others, redesigning the relationship, and becoming hopeful as strategies used in this stage.

Depression is a public health problem affecting approximately 25 million Americans and their families. The prevalence estimates for lifetime major depression is 17.1%; there is a higher prevalence for women, young adults, and people with less than a college education (Blazer, Kessler, McGonagle, & Swartz, 1994). Most people suffering from depression live with their families, usually their spouses and children. Recent studies of families with members with depression[2] have focused more on the biological causes and treatment of depression and less on its interpersonal context (Beach, Sandeen, & O'Leary, 1990; Coyne, 1990; Keitner, Miller, & Ryan, 1993). Yet the interpersonal nature of depression suggests families have a critical role in both understanding and treating depression.

The majority of recent studies of families with members with depression have used primarily inpatient samples, have focused on depressed women as the identified patient, have been from the patient perspective, have often excluded parents of children with depression, and are quantitative in methodology (Keitner, Miller,

Epstein, & Bishop, 1990; Schwab, Stephenson, & Ice, 1993). This study extends previous work by including the perspectives of seven women whose husbands were depressed, two men whose wives were depressed, and two parents whose children were depressed. The purpose of this study was to describe family members' experiences in living with a member with depression.

◪ RELATED LITERATURE

Families with members with depression experience difficulties with communication, marital adjustment and dissatisfaction, expressed emotion, problem solving, and family functioning (Biglan et al., 1985; Keitner, Miller, Epstein, Bishop, & Fruzzetti, 1987; Schwab et al., 1993). Communication between members with depression and their spouses is characterized by high levels of tension, negative expressions, self-preoccupation, and diminished nonverbal patterns of support. The strain of the poor communication in the couples' relationships often continues after recovery. Couples that include one partner with depression consistently rate higher than control couples on marital difficulties and dissatisfaction (Beach et al., 1990).

Although the cause-and-effect relationships of expressed emotion remain unclear, expressed emotion has been found to be significantly associated with increased symptom levels and relapse (Hooley, Orley, & Teasdale, 1986). People with depression are more likely to be criticized by their spouses than other family members. Couples with greater spousal criticism have shown consistently higher relapse rates than control couples (Beach et al., 1990). Further, divorce rates for these couples have been reported as nine times higher than the national average.

It should not be surprising that depression has its most negative impact on families during acute depressive episodes. Negative symptoms such as a lack of interest in social life, fatigue, constant worrying, irritability, and hopelessness were the most disturbing aspects of living with ill family members and caused greater disruption in family functioning and greater burden for family members than did other symptoms (Coyne et al., 1987; Fadden, Bebbington, & Kuipers, 1987; Miller et al., 1992). In their studies of families with members with depression, Keitner et al. (1990) found that these families showed greater impairment in family functioning than families who contained members with alcohol dependence, adjustment disorders, schizophrenia, or bipolar disorders.

Fortunately, negative symptoms decrease in the approximately 75% of people with depression who respond to treatment (Depression Guideline Panel, 1993). However, studies have consistently found that families with a member with depression continue to experience more difficulties at remission than matched control families. These families continue to experience problems with social functioning 1 year after initial treatment (Billings & Moos, 1985). Families with remitted members failed to reach the level of social resources (friends, supportive family interactions) observed for control families. Similarly, Keitner et al. (1987) found that 46% of their clinical families reported impairment in their overall functioning at remission in contrast to only 18% of control families.

Families with members with depression report greater health problems than families with other types of illness (Hinrichsen, Hernandez, & Pollack, 1992; Pruchno, Kleban, Michaels, & Dempsey, 1990; Wells et al., 1989). Coyne et al. (1987) found that over 40% of adults living with family members with depressive episodes were distressed themselves to the point of needing therapeutic intervention. The detrimental effect on children living with a parent with depression has also been well documented (Buckwalter, Kerfoot, & Stolley, 1988; Merikangas, Weissman, & Prusoff, 1990). Children of parents with depression exhibit greater symptomatology and impairment than control children, and their risk of developing an affective disorder has been reported as high as 45%. Billings and Moos (1985) had similar findings. The children of parents with depression were still functioning more poorly than control group children 1 year after remission of parental illness.

METHOD

Sample

Purposeful sampling was used to recruit 11 English-speaking family members who were living or who had recently lived with someone with depression. A combination of advertising at a local mental health clinic and network/snowball sampling in which initial informants referred others to the study was used. Of the family members, 9 were women, and 10 were white. A total of 7 family members were wives of men with depression, 2 were husbands of women with depression, and 2 were parents of children (1 son, 1 daughter) with depression. The mean age of the family members was 46 years (ranging from 32 to 61 years). Of the family members, 8 were married, and the mean number of years married was 18.8. A total of 8 had at least a baccalaureate education, and annual incomes ranged from below the poverty level to above $50,000. All people who are termed *members with depression* in this study met standard diagnostic criteria as determined by a psychiatrist or psychologist (American Psychiatric Association, 1994). Members with depression included those currently in acute episodes, in recovery, and at remission. Although half had been hospitalized, not one was hospitalized at the time of the interview.

Data Collection

After screening to ensure family members met study criteria, consent forms were signed. Open-ended interviews were usually conducted in the researcher's office because most family members preferred the office over the home setting. These audiotaped interviews lasted between 1 and 2 hours. The following broad data-generating question was used to begin the interview: "Tell me what it has been like living with your [husband, wife, child] who [is/was] depressed." Informants responded with full descriptions to this question, and few subsequent probes or clarifiers were required.

Data Analysis

Interviews were conducted simultaneously with data analysis (Chenitz & Swanson, 1986; Glaser, 1978; Hutchinson, 1986). Interviews were professionally transcribed and checked by the researcher for accuracy. Each interview was coded and guided the selection of subsequent informants. Open coding was used for the initial analysis of the transcribed data, and initial categories were adjusted with subsequent interviews. Categories were refined by merging categories into smaller sets of higher level concepts to fit the emerging theory. Concurrent coding and analysis continued until unique categories no longer appeared in the data, and no additional informants were obtained after data saturation (Glaser & Strauss, 1967). Verification of the categories occurred as similar patterns from previous interviews appeared over time. A central or core category that best explained the process of living with a person with depression was identified as *family transformations.*

Lincoln and Guba (1985) suggested that four factors can be used to assess the rigor of the qualitative study: credibility, transferability, dependability, and confirmability. Credibility refers to having confidence in the truth of the findings. Methods used to check credibility included peer debriefing, exposure of the investigator's thinking to consultants with expertise in both grounded theory and family members' experiences of living with members with other chronic illnesses, discussion with clinicians who work with people with depression and their families, and member checks with some family members who were asked to verify the emerging constructions. Transferability is concerned with providing sufficient data to enable others to make judgments about the degree of similarity between contexts. The sample included adult family members who provided thick descriptions from their perspectives as husbands, wives, parents, and so forth. Dependability refers to the stability and tracking of the data over time. The researcher used a systematic data management system to track the data by hand using detailed memos. Equivalence checks were also conducted within the interviews by asking similar questions and evaluating consistency of the informants' answers (Brink, 1991). Confirmability was supported by gathering information from a variety of sources, and alternative explanations were explored with both family members and professionals. Colleagues experienced in grounded theory methods functioned as inquiry auditors. Transcribed consultations with these colleagues were used to reexamine, recode, or recategorize portions of the data. Further, initial codings, comparative memos and process and personal notes were reevaluated, enabling changes in earlier data formulations.

▨ FINDINGS

The basic social psychological process of family transformations was identified from the data (see Figure 1). The process refers to the cognitive and behavioral changes that occur within the family from the time the member begins to exhibit symptoms

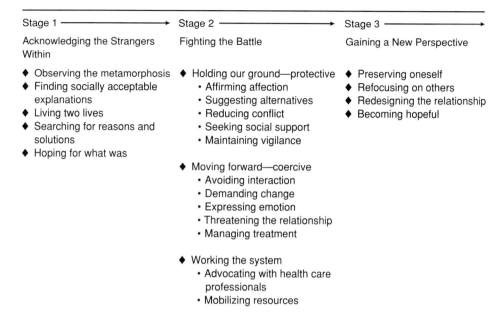

Figure 1. Family transformations: stages of living with a member with depression.

of depression through recovery and at remission. As family members move through the three stages of family transformations, all family members are transformed, and family functioning is changed.

Stage 1: Acknowledging the Strangers Within

Acknowledging the strangers within was described as the stage when family members first acknowledged the profound changes in the member with depression, other family members, and family functioning. Family members described *observing the metamorphosis, finding socially acceptable explanations, living two lives, searching for reasons and solutions,* and *hoping for what was.* The length of this stage varied among family members from months to years, and for some, it was primarily a retrospective process occurring after intervention by a third party.

Family members described observing the metamorphosis of the member with depression. Family members described their member with depression as becoming a completely different person, but they did not associate the metamorphosis with a diagnosis of depression until much later. The following examples illustrate the metamorphosis of the member with depression:[3]

> You are not living with the same person that you've known all these years. He used to be a very patient, very easy-going, very kind, caring person. He's not

anybody I recognize at this point. He is very testy, he is very tense . . . there is no hope. (Ida)

I think the biggest thing for [me], was hard for me to deal with because of my personality and with her, like that she'd be negative. It would just be, and I know it wasn't her and that would make me more angry. (Eddie)

It's like day and night, Jekyll and Hyde, he's this totally different person. But I see glimmers of him in there . . . it's so discouraging. (Fran)

The depressive symptoms made it difficult, if not impossible, for the members with depression to enact their respective roles and caused difficulties in all areas of family functioning, including communication, problem solving, and marital satisfaction. Other family members, usually the spouse, assumed the role tasks of the ill member. The family atmosphere was described as tense or conflicted, and family members experienced guilt, anger, frustration, and pain. Spouses complained about the lack of emotional or material support from the members with depression and their frustrations with poor parenting:

What about me? When will he be well enough to give anything back again? . . . when will he be supportive back? (Ida)

He's been a good provider and we've been married for [many] years. He's been out of a job since last August, and he seems to be unable to hunt for one in a very productive manner. I feel some resentment because the fact that that was always his role. He was always the dependable breadwinner and now he isn't. (Cathy)

It's frustrating to me to see him and to see his kids. Yeah, when he gets home and there seems to be not much there. And time is going by, . . . and they're still young enough to be excited to see him. And there is going to be a time when all they're going to remember is, he was never around, or he was always tired, or he . . . (Ginger)

The parents of children with depression expressed similar feelings and sentiments: "my stomach would literally churn 'til she got out of bed" (Amy). Although frustrated with the child's behavior, separating from the child was not an option exercised by the parents, unlike spouses who considered separation.

A consistent theme for all family members was the simultaneous metamorphosis of others within the family and the increased physical and mental health problems of family members:

I never had any experience with depression growing up . . . everyone I knew including me was ok, so I didn't have any experience to draw on. . . . One counselor I went to said I had situational depression . . . I get all emotional but I'm working on it. . . . I think my trust is shot, and that [there are] all the other feelings of rejection and abandonment [crying—unable to continue] . . . I'm sort of a basket case. (Fran)

Several family members had been treated for depression, and others were sufficiently distressed to require counseling. Approximately one third of the family members reported that their children were affected by living with a parent with depression to the degree that they were beginning to display behaviors similar to the depressed parent. Family members were concerned about their children's genetic vulnerability to developing depression as well as the effect of the current social environment:

> My fear right now though is that my daughter has, is depressed. I don't know enough about this yet, but she is so much like her Dad. And the older she is getting, the more I see it . . . if this is hereditary . . . if children can have it, then I want to do something that will help her. . . . I don't know if I should be removing the children from it or not. Because I think they are sheltered from it because he is [either working or sleeping], but I'll probably find out in 10 years, they'll come back . . . and go " 'you know, Mom . . .' " (Ginger)

Children within the family expressed the loss of parental love and attention. One loss was due to the illness, and the other to the well parent's caring for the ill member. One daughter expressed their sentiments: "Although I didn't want to be sick like Dad, but in a way if I was, I would get all the attention" (Ida). Parental family members expressed that these comments supported leaving the marriage to avoid exposing the children to the parental depression.

Finding socially acceptable explanations was used to explain the metamorphosis and to protect against potential stigma. Reasons that would be considered rational explanations to the average person were used to explain the changes: relationship losses, job stresses, marital difficulties, other illnesses, or personal behaviors of other family members. Explanations, particularly those perceived as having little stigma attached to them, were usually suggested:

> Her mother died. . . . And [the change] was very, very dramatic. And understandable, . . . I shared in her grief, . . . I fully expected, as a normal person would, . . . to deal with the grief, and recover. . . . These were my expectations and that didn't occur. She did change, but she was not the same socially, sexually, or intellectually. (Ben)

> And at first we attributed it to his back pain and not that it was depression, but that his change and attitude change and personality change and response toward the children was all because of his pain and not really related to any depression. To this day even though he will admit he is severely depressed, it is seen as a tremendous sign of weakness. (Ida)

Almost all family members at one time questioned their responsibility in causing the behavior. Family members attributed particularly the irritability and anger to be caused by their own behavior:

> I would say in the last year that I even realized that that is what the problem was. . . . For a long time I thought it was me. If I did something, if I did it

> differently, if I reacted differently, . . . I thought, well, he's an alcoholic, and
> that's the problem . . . he's a workaholic and that's the problem or . . . (Ginger)

Unfortunately, finding socially acceptable explanations could prolong suffering because it interfered with or prevented the accurate recognition and treatment of depression.

Living two lives was used to maintain the illusion to the outside world that all was well within the family. This strategy also defended against potential embarrassment or stigma:

> In the beginning, I told no one. I guess I felt embarrassed and didn't want to
> admit that my son had problems, that he had [attempted suicide]. That was so
> hard, to come to work and act like all was well, with my friends too. (Hazel)

> I was living two lives, trying to live the life in the house, trying to survive in the
> house and raise two children, and then trying to maintain a job, and save face
> here, and never letting anyone know what was going on. That was real hard.
> (Diane)

> Now with his friends, it's been horrible, because I have to lie to them, I have to
> be evasive . . . [they ask] what is going on? . . . I [say] everything's fine, we've
> just been really busy with . . . (Karen)

Family members told no one about the problem, isolated themselves from others, and exhibited stoicism by suppressing painful feelings or selectively sharing them within the family home. While they were living two lives, family members expressed profound feelings of aloneness and additional stress from dealing with the members of the extended family. One family member stated, "my mother doesn't want to know when [she] is not doing well, it gets her too upset . . . so I just say, 'oh, [she's] all right' [when asked]" (Amy).

The member with depression was also living two lives. The ill member may have been able to maintain predepression behavior for limited amounts of time, often having just enough energy to function at work or for short periods outside the family home:

> I see him some days and wonder, How can you go to work and maintain? How
> can you make it? He says, "I smile a lot and I hide in my office a lot" . . . I don't
> know how he can do it . . . so I guess there is some strength there. (Fran)

Thus some family members believed the depressive symptoms and behavior could be controlled. This perception caused family members to express anger and hurt about what was perceived as unwillingness by the member with depression to control the behavior:

> He was irritable and unhappy, he would get angry, break things, stayed in his
> room and listened to [music]. . . . He became terrible at home. . . . The minute
> he left the house he could turn it off and click, he was fine. He would be all

smiles and talkative as if nothing was wrong. . . . He could be yelling and angry and get on the phone to his friends and be fine. Same old [person]. (Hazel)

Until reaching a crisis, finding socially acceptable explanations and living two lives were used sometimes for years. For some, a suicide attempt moved family members quickly into a crisis and toward seeking help for their ill member. Prior to the attempt, these family members were similar to other family members in using the strategies of finding socially acceptable explanations and living two lives. Others described this point as "spinning out of control" (Amy) or "being in a downward spiral with no end in sight" (Jenny). At the point when the family could no longer continue functioning, the family began searching for reasons and solutions to explain the metamorphosis.

Searching for reasons and solutions involved gathering information from both professional and lay literature, and requesting assistance from health care professionals (HCPs), usually the primary care physician. For some family members, their search was often serendipitous. They read about depression in popular magazines or heard about it on television. Interviews with famous people with depression were cited as important resources. One found information at her physician's office:

> We were in a doctor's office one time, . . . and there was a pamphlet on depression and he read it while I was in with the doctor. And when I came out it was like this light bulb went on. After I had been talking to him about this for probably 9 months . . . but he was reading it for himself and for some reason something connected . . . [he] wanted to look into it. And so we saw [the doctor] and asked about clinical depression. And he said, "Oh yeah, that's the real thing." (Ginger)

Unfortunately, many HCPs also used the strategy of finding socially acceptable explanations, resulting in misdiagnosis, ineffective treatment, or both:

> And this first [HCP] said that "you're not depressed, you are sad, there's something else other than depression that's wrong with you," and sent him on his merry way. So you know, obviously nothing happened, he wasn't getting any better. So then he decided to [find someone else]. (Fran)

> We got her into a couple of different kinds of therapies. I got her into [alcohol treatment] 'cause we thought alcohol was the problem . . . and when that didn't work we got her into extended care . . . and when that didn't work she saw a private psychiatrist. (Amy)

Family members expressed their frustrations with the health care and insurance systems during this stage. They described seeking help outside their current health care and insurance systems because they were so desperate for help for their ill family member:

> I couldn't tell you how many agencies I tried to get help from. We would go and have one visit and they'd say they couldn't see us anymore. I think if somebody would have sat down and told me what to do, that's really what I wanted. I

wanted somebody to say, "This is what's wrong with her, this is what you need to do," and I would have done it. (Amy)

Throughout this first stage and by searching for reasons and solutions, family members experienced hoping for what was. Hoping contained feelings of grief about what was lost and hope for what might be again. As one family member stated, "We had a fairly good relationship . . . so I'm dangling the carrot out here, saying remember how it was" (Ben). Another stated, "we had a wonderful life and I would love to just grasp hold just for a little bit of that" (Karen). Optimism about possible solutions increased the sense that the member with depression and the entire family would return to normal.

Stage 2: Fighting the Battle

Fighting the battle was described as the family members' daily efforts to deal with the interactional patterns within the family developed during the first stage that were perceived as different from predepression interactional patterns. These patterns were perceived as destructive to all aspects of family functioning such as communication or problem solving:

> We won't discuss it, we won't fight about it, we won't communicate in any way, shape or form about it. . . . So, not that I want to fight about it, I want to communicate about it and see my way through it. And I feel I don't want to just abandon her, because I know she's there, somewhere, this wonderful person, . . . but I don't know how to get in touch with her. (Ben)

> Probably for our family unit this has been tremendously destructive. . . . I feel it's kinda like living in hell . . . there has been no consistency in our lives. (Ida)

Family members alternated between the strategy of *holding our ground—protective* and the strategy of *moving forward—coercive* to deal with the fragile or vulnerable family member. Choices of strategies were determined by the family members' beliefs about which strategy would be most effective to counteract or control the metamorphosis and return the family to normal. Fighting the battle also involved *working the system* to obtain help for their ill family member.

The protective strategies were designed to prevent the situation from worsening and to protect the vulnerable individual from potential psychological and physical harm. The five protective strategies were *affirming affection, suggesting alternatives, reducing conflict, seeking social support,* and *maintaining vigilance.* Affirming affection was designed to assure the members with depression that they were loved and wanted. For example, some family members used frequent words of endearment to remind the members they were valued members of the family. Others reassured their ill family members that family members' feelings had not changed about them despite their illness. Affirming affection was also used to counter negative self-statements about the member's worth: "I've been able to reiterate how much I feel for her, how much worth she has. I've communicated how special I think she is" (Ben).

A second strategy—suggesting alternatives—involved providing the member with depression with ideas about how to increase pleasurable activities and to decrease depression. These included encouraging the member with depression to engage in hobbies, spend time with family and friends, exercise, return to school, and decrease work time. Family members expended considerable energy in suggesting alternatives. Most family members reported feeling frustrated and angry after using this strategy for any length of time. As family members became increasingly frustrated by their lack of success, they began to decrease communication with the ill family member:

> So I mentioned to him, "Why don't you do something you'll enjoy? Why don't you start trading in [art]?" And he says, "Oh, I couldn't do that." He's, he's just, every positive suggestion that flows from me seems to be met with a negative from him. And because of that, I get tired of even talking to him. (Cathy)

All family members reported using reducing-conflict strategies. These were designed to decrease the potential for conflict or tension within the family. Most often, reducing-conflict strategies were targeted at the negative affectively laden interactional patterns. Strategies included telling the members with depression what the family members believed they wanted to hear, withholding any actually or potentially upsetting news, and refraining from expressing emotion or criticizing the member with depression about expected role behaviors. For example, one woman assumed the task of family finances to avoid any potentially upsetting news or arguments about money. Another stated she no longer asked her husband to do any task because "It's a big deal . . . it's as if he can't cope really with anything" (Ida).

An integral part of reducing conflict was not expressing emotion. This was particularly used when the member with depression initiated conflict by name-calling or using verbal threats. One woman described leaving the house when her husband initiated conflict, but this strategy became increasingly ineffective over time:

> There was a time period that I was leaving the house so much that it was affecting what I was getting done in my own life. I didn't have any clean clothes to wear because I had to leave the house constantly. (Jenny)

Reducing conflict was difficult for other family members, especially children, who perceived that the member with depression was being difficult, angry, or unpleasant without the usual consequences. The most extreme method of reducing conflict was leaving the relationship.

A fourth strategy—seeking social support—was described as family members' attempt to mobilize the social network to maintain their health and well-being. Family members told only those within their social circle who they perceived would be supportive and understanding or who would be nondiscriminatory. All family members reported lacking energy for the typical reciprocity needed to sustain social relationships. They needed friends who could tolerate their lack of reciprocity and who would focus on subjects other than the ill member: "I live it, I don't need to talk about it." (Jenny)

Maintaining vigilance, the final protective strategy, was designed to protect the member with depression from potential self-harm and relapse. It contained elements of uncertainty about whether the vulnerable member would recover. Vigilance behaviors included changing family members' schedules to spend more time with the member with depression, checking on the member's physical and psychological safety, and monitoring progress in taking medication and other treatments. For most family members, maintaining vigilance was an effective method of protecting the vulnerable member during the acute episodes. Maintaining vigilance became counterproductive at remission, causing increased conflict. One woman stated that after her husband expressed suicidal ideation, she changed her work schedule to come home at frequent intervals to monitor him and to constantly check on his medication and other treatments. She continued these vigilance behaviors after her husband was better because of fears of relapse, causing increased conflict in the relationship.

The coercive strategies were also used in fighting the battle. These strategies were designed to force progress and recovery and involved more physical and verbal aggression than protective strategies. They also were described using controlling, tension-inducing, and rejecting terms. These strategies increased when family members became tired or frustrated by the ill member's lack of improvement; when the member with depression had dropped in and out of treatment; when protective strategies had failed to change the behavior; or when family members were unfamiliar with protective strategies.

The coercive strategies were *avoiding interaction, demanding change, expressing emotion, threatening the relationship,* and *managing treatment.* The first strategy—avoiding interaction—was described by family members as eliminating or avoiding communication or contact with the member with depression. Family members who used this strategy were frustrated that protective strategies had not worked. The following is one example of the avoiding-interaction strategy: "we lived separate in the house for [many] years" (Diane). Members with depression were excluded from scripted family routines (*e.g.,* mealtimes) or from particular areas within the house-hold (*e.g.,* spousal bedroom). Family members believed ill members would recognize the exclusion, understand the implications, and modify their behavior accordingly.

The strategy of demanding change was designed to force the members with depression to stop exhibiting depressive symptoms, to engage in treatment, or to resume their roles. Demanding change involved verbal and physical aggression. For example, family members used shaming to demand the person behave as the family members believed was proper. Family members might tell the person to "buck up, pull it together and you'll pull out of it" (Ida) or "act like a man." Shaming generally "made it, I think, even worse" (Ida). Other family members used physical aggression as a method to get the person to enact their roles. For example, one parent physically removed her adolescent from bed so the adolescent would get ready for school, and another family member moved all her husband's belongings into the living room to force him to deal with his withdrawal behaviors. Neither was successful in counteracting the metamorphosis.

Closely related to demanding change was the third strategy—expressing emotions. This strategy involved family members freely expressing their anger or frustration using either verbal or physical methods, and it usually caused escalation in an already-conflicted family situation. Family members used name-calling or profanity, and several reported abusing inanimate objects, such as slamming doors, to express their emotions.

Threatening the relationship was used by most family members unless the member with depression demonstrated signs of improvement and active involvement in treatment. For some parents, a modification of the strategy of threatening was asking the child to move outside the family home. The majority of family members questioned their abilities to continue in the marital relationships. For some, actually leaving was seen as a method to force the members with depression to care for themselves and to engage in treatment: "Because it seems to me that as long as I'm there to blame and to be angry at that he may not make any progress. . . . And so in a way, I feel like I'll be doing him a favor" (Cathy).

Managing treatment involved balancing issues of control and responsibility. For some family members, managing treatment was fueled by family members' fears of relapse because they perceived the member with depression as unwilling to engage in or unable to take responsibility for treatment. Others whose members had experienced relapses used this strategy more than other coercive strategies. As family members attempted to manage treatment, issues about control and responsibility surfaced that may or may not have been previous sources of conflict within the relationship:

> [He] was being really noncompliant with his appointments, and as far as medication refills, he hadn't really gotten them. And so then I was really more insistent on trying to make sure he went for help because once I realized that that was truly what it was, then I knew he really needed help. . . . I was driving myself crazy trying to make sure he did go somewheres and get some kind of help and I had to balance that with him not thinking I was being too controlling. (Ida)

Family members alternately engaged in protective and coercive strategies to deal with the interactional patterns between themselves and their ill members. As the ill member engaged in treatment and as depressive symptoms decreased, family members who remained in Stage 2 continued to alternate between these strategies, often regardless of strategy success.

Family members engaged in working the system to obtain help for their ill members. Working the system involved two strategies: *advocating with HCPs* and *mobilizing resources*. Family members advocated to obtain proper diagnosis and appropriate treatment:

> I've had to fight every inch of the way. And it's been a battle, not just with [my husband], but with the people that I would have thought would have been there to support me as far as the care that he needed . . . and I truly believe that if, and I've said this over and over again to [him], if it was a terminal illness, if it was cancer, MS [multiple sclerosis], anything else, the treatment would have been better. It would have been much better, more caring, more concern. And family members would have been more involved and more included. (Ida)

They also assisted their ill members with access, quality, and cost issues related to treatment. Family members mobilized resources. Often, they went outside their current health care and insurance systems and paid for care out-of-pocket. Although described as an economic hardship, all described this as necessary to obtain effective help for their ill members:

> And then even our insurance we found out they won't cover it. I don't know what the counseling or medication is going to cost . . . or whether we're going to be able to afford it. You know, which I really resent that and it makes no sense . . . if the [medication] will help him function normally and make some decent money so he can pay your bill, then you would think they'd want to help him out. (Ginger)

Family members expressed frustration and anger about the care received by the member with depression, the stigma associated with having a mental illness, and their exclusion in treatment.

By the end of Stage 2, family members reported they were physically and emotionally exhausted from fighting the battle. Family members described accepting the realities and limits of their involvement and shifting the focus of responsibility away from the members with depression to others within the family. This was a critical juncture that allowed family members to move into Stage 3:

> At a certain point where I found myself, the shift for me was, a shift of withdrawing emotionally. I started detaching a great deal from the relationship and I lived with him for quite a long time that I wasn't there. I just lost ways of trying to cope with it and I consider myself a very resourceful individual. (Jenny)

> It's really a horrible feeling to know that there is absolutely nothing you can do. If I'm up and happy, it is not going to bring him out of it. (Fran)

> We were talking about it and she told me, very angrily, that it was my fault that she lost her job. And if I hadn't tried to get her outa here, tried to push her to work, she probably would have gone on her own. And something just sorta snapped inside, . . . but it sort of freed me from her. It made me realize that I couldn't fix it. (Amy)

Stage 3: Gaining a New Perspective

Gaining a new perspective, the third and final stage, was described as shifting the focus away from the ill member to themselves and others within the family and as changing interactional patterns between family members and the member with depression. As family members moved into Stage 3, they expressed feelings of self-loss and a loss of the person who was. Gaining a new perspective involved *preserving oneself, refocusing on others, redesigning the relationship,* and *becoming hopeful.*

Preserving-oneself strategies were used to regain a sense of self lost while fighting the battle. Other aspects of life such as work, social life, and health practices were changed or put on hold as family members focused on the needs of the ill member. Family members used counseling, setting limits, setting priorities for their own lives, engaging in pleasurable activities, avoiding being around people with depression, and resuming their relationships with others to regain a sense of self:

> When I went back to school I discovered art. And I discovered that I had a love for it, uh, maybe a talent for it and that it was what I wanted to do. It felt right. And I began to feel like I was living my life, that I was really being me. And I became a happy person. I feel like at that point, somewhere along there, I learned how to live and how to live happily. (Cathy)

> I have to know what I want in a relationship, in life. I think that's important . . . good self-knowledge. The best advice I can give [other family members], if they have the capacity to step back and be patient, that's probably the best thing they can do . . . don't allow their lives to start [being] controlled by the other person [with depression]. . . . I don't want to become a victim of her depression. (Ben)

Family members realized that to care for others, they must care for themselves:

> I have to take care of me. I'm important for myself and my family, too. I couldn't live my own life because I was too preoccupied with theirs. I told them, and I said, "I cried a tub full of tears and it never changed a thing." I still care. I care about them, but I cannot live like this, I mean live my life for them completely. That's too much you know. (Diane)

For other family members, self-preservation required separating from or divorcing the member with depression. Those who chose this option expressed tremendous pain associated with the decision but discussed it as a critical step for self-survival and for maintaining their own sanity:

> Yea, that is the sadness part. Because to have that separation due to one person being depressed is a whole different kind of breakup than having a divorce because one partner has gone off and found another partner or whatever. For me, it's not over yet. It's a very definite sensation that I have a legal divorce, but there has not been an emotional divorce, no emotional divorce has occurred. . . . It just finally came down to self-survival. (Jenny)

Within families, refocusing on others involved reestablishing or repairing previous relationships with extended family members and friends. For some family members, it was only at this stage that the extended family was told the truth about the member with depression. For many, it was the first time the metamorphosis was attributed to depression rather than some socially acceptable explanation. Family members described increasing time with their children to counteract the negative effects of living with a parent with depression:

> My daughter has really been flown around in all this too. She doesn't know if we're leaving or staying from one day to the next . . . her life certainly isn't stable right now and that certainly adds to my pain. I try to reassure her that no matter what happens, . . . she'll never stopped being loved no matter where we may live. But I really try to make an effort and to leave her out of the day-to-day kind of stuff that I'm going through. (Fran)

Family members described redesigning the relationship between the member with depression and other family members as a necessary step to positively reconnecting with the person with depression. Family members learned to show love, care, and concern for the member with depression while maintaining emotional distance and limiting responsibility. Further, many learned to enjoy engaging in activities with them or resume living with the members with depression.

Family members accepted that the old patterns of relating were no longer productive and may have maintained the depression. Interactional patterns such as communication or problem solving were examined, and new interactional strategies were developed:

> Just a lot of family dynamics are going to have to change. What specifically I'm not sure, but I just think that things will have to be different . . . whether it's mental illness or anything two people go through that's this overwhelming that you can go back to things being the way they were . . . there's no way possible. (Ida)

> Once in awhile she will step back into a negative thing, but rather than ignore it like before, I tell her. And she'll see it and she'll stop. (Eddie)

> I still realize how it affects us when I talk to him . . . he tries to remind me that sometimes he is going to be down, but that doesn't mean he won't be all right. I just worry . . . and it has also affected my relationships with my daughters as well. (Hazel)

For a few family members, redesigning the relationship occurred through counseling and family sessions focused on the interactional patterns within the family. These family members reported more successful outcomes than family members who did not have such counseling. For some who were unable to redesign the relationship, they separated or divorced.

As part of this third stage, family members described becoming hopeful. One spouse described her mood following initiation of treatment as follows: "now I feel like there's hope" (Ida). Another family member stated, "medication helps. . . . I do believe that she's gonna be ok, whatever happens. So I am optimistic" (Amy). As part of their new perspective, family members accepted the new realities and limits. Their feelings of hope were mixed with caution, particularly for those ill members who had relapsed.

DISCUSSION

The social psychological process found in this study describes how all family members are transformed when living with members with depression. The grounded theory described the movement of the family members through stages of acknowledging the strangers within, fighting the battle, and gaining a new perspective. The negative symptoms (*e.g.,* hopelessness, irritability) were the most disturbing aspects of the ill member's metamorphosis for many family members, and the metamorphosis of all family members resulted in difficulties in family functioning and health that were sometimes unresolved at remission. These findings support those from previous studies of family functioning and depression (Coyne et al., 1987; Keitner et al., 1990). Some strategies (*e.g.,* avoiding, threatening) used in fighting the battle were also consistent with previous findings with couples that included one member with depression (Beach et al., 1990).

Aspects of the first stage described in this study were similar to stages experienced by caregivers of Alzheimer's patients and of other chronic illnesses (Hinrichsen et al., 1992; Skaff & Pearlin, 1992; Strauss et al., 1984; Wilson, 1989). For example, there were similarities found for observing the changes in the ill member and others, finding socially acceptable explanations, and hoping for what was. Regardless of the type of illness, family members used rational nonstigmatizing explanations to explain behavioral changes and hoped the person's behavior would return to normal. The stigma associated with depression according to most family members was greater than for other illnesses that have clearer biological bases, such as Alzheimer's. Despite educational efforts to the contrary, mental illness is still associated with moral weakness or failure. The stigma associated with depression often interfered with seeking or continuing in treatment. Family members described sharing the stigma with their member with depression. This phenomenon seems similar to stigma contagion usually associated with deviance research (Kirby & Corzine, 1981). The phenomenon of stigma contagion may explain why family members are often excluded from treatment by members of the health care community. Further, current public policies have made it difficult for families to obtain quality help at reasonable costs for themselves and their ill members.

The sense of self-loss described by family members is similar to that described for Alzheimer's caregivers (Skaff & Pearlin, 1992) and for heart transplantation partners (Mishel & Murdaugh, 1987), among others. As family members focus on the ill member in the initial stages, they assume role tasks previously enacted by the ill member, and they limit social, work, or other roles. Although family members initially believed their lives would eventually return to normal, the reality was that their lives had changed. A critical step for family members to move to the final stage in this and in other studies with other illnesses was accepting the new realities and limiting responsibility for the ill member.

There are some major differences between the illness of depression and other chronic or terminal illnesses. The majority of those with depression will respond favorably to treatment and resume much of their previous functioning. Unlike the typical course of Alzheimer's or AIDS, with progressive decline and eventual death from the illness, most symptoms of depression such as fatigue or poor concentration subside rather quickly following treatment with little or no long-term effects. Although there is a risk of self-inflicted death with depression, the majority of people with depression recover following treatment to live long, productive lives. Death is not the inevitable outcome. The favorable prognosis for depression was a double-edged sword for family members who alternated between hope and frustration while fighting the battle.

This study provides perspectives of family members not normally included in recent depression studies (Coyne, 1990). In contrast to women being the identified patient, most family members in this study were middle-aged women who were the wives and mothers of the members with depression. These perspectives provide a needed dimension for understanding the process of living with members with depression. Process-oriented research expands knowledge about interpersonal and social contexts of depression. Theories addressing the process of living with depression provide an important foundation for understanding and treating depression in families.

Terry A. Badger, Ph.D., R.N., Associate Professor, College of Nursing, University of Arizona, Tucson.

▧ NOTES

1. The funding for this study was provided by Sigma Theta Tau International, Beta Mu Chapter, Tucson, AZ. The author thanks Drs. Linda Phillips, Alice Longman, and Joan Haase for their consultation throughout this process and comments on earlier drafts of this article. Special thanks to the family members who gave so generously of themselves. An earlier version of this article was presented at the Western Society for Nursing Research Conference in San Diego, CA, in May 1995. Address correspondence to Terry A. Badger, Ph.D., R.N., College of Nursing, University of Arizona, P.O. Box 21023, Tucson, AZ 85721-0203. Electronic mail may be sent to TBadger@RN1.nursing.Arizona.edu.
2. This article will use the more accurate and more cumbersome phrase members with depression instead of depressed members to avoid reducing people to illness labels and to be consistent with the guidelines in the Diagnostic and Statistical Manual of Mental Disorders (American Psychiatric Association, 1994).

3. Examples have been slightly edited for clarity and to protect confidentiality. Alterations are noted within the brackets, and authorship using a pseudonym is cited within the parentheses.

References

American Psychiatric Association. (1994). *Diagnostic and statistical manual of mental disorders* (4th ed.). Washington, DC: Author.

Beach, S. R. H., Sandeen, E. E., & O'Leary, K. D. (1990). *Depression in marriage: A model for etiology and treatment.* New York: Guildford.

Biglan, A., Hops, H., Sherman, L., Freidman, L. S., Arthur, J., & Osteen, V. (1985). Problem-solving interactions of depressed women and their spouses. *Behavior Therapy, 16,* 431–451.

Billings, A. G., & Moos, R. H. (1985). Psychosocial processes in unipolar depression: Comparing depressed patients with matched community controls. *Journal of Consulting & Clinical Psychology, 53,* 314–325.

Blazer, D. G., Kessler, R. C., McGonagle, K. A., & Swartz, M. S. (1994). The prevalence and distribution of major depression in a national community sample: The National Co-Morbidity Survey. *American Journal of Psychiatry, 151,* 979–986.

Brink, P. J. (1991). Issues of reliability and validity. In J. M. Morse (Ed.), *Qualitative nursing research: A contemporary dialogue* (rev. ed., pp. 164–186). Newbury Park, CA: Sage.

Buckwalter, K. C., Kerfoot, K. M., & Stolley, J. M. (1988). Children of affectively ill parents. *Journal of Psychosocial Nursing and Mental Health Services, 26,* 8–14.

Chenitz, W. C., & Swanson, J. M. (1986). *From practice to grounded theory: Qualitative research in nursing.* Menlo Park, CA: Addison-Wesley.

Coyne, J. C. (1990). The interpersonal processes of depression. In G. I. Keitner (Ed.), *Depression and families: Impact and treatment* (pp. 31–54). Washington, DC: American Psychiatric Press.

Coyne, J. C., Kessler, R. C., Tal, M., Turnbull, J., Wortman, C. B., & Greden, J. (1987). Living with a depressed person. *Journal of Consulting and Clinical Psychology, 55,* 347–352.

Depression Guideline Panel. (1993). *Depression in primary care* (Vols. 1-2, Clinical Practice Guideline No. 5 [AHCPR Publication No. 93-0551]). Washington, DC: U.S. Government Printing Office.

Fadden, G., Bebbington, P., & Kuipers, L. (1987). Caring and its burdens: A study of spouses of depressed patients. *British Journal of Psychiatry, 151,* 660–667.

Glaser, B. G. (1978). *Theoretical sensitivity: Advances in the methodology of grounded theory.* Mill Valley, CA: Sociology Press.

Glaser, B. G., & Strauss, A. L. (1967). *The discovery of grounded theory: Strategies for qualitative research.* New York: Aldine.

Hinrichsen, G. A., Hernandez, N. A., & Pollack, S. (1992). Difficulties and rewards in family care of depressed older adults. *The Gerontologist, 32,* 486–492.

Hooley, J. M., Orley, J., & Teasdale, J. D. (1986). Levels of expressed emotion and relapse in depressed patients. *British Journal of Psychiatry, 126,* 164–176.

Hutchinson, S. (1986). Grounded theory: The method. In P. L. Munhall & C. J. Oiler (Eds.), *Nursing research: A qualitative perspective* (pp. 116–117). New York: Appleton-Century-Crofts.

Keitner, G. I., Miller, I. W., Epstein, N. B., & Bishop, D. S. (1990). In G. I. Keitner (Ed.), *Depression and families: Impact and treatment* (pp. 3–29). Washington, DC: American Psychiatric Press.

Keitner, G. I., Miller, I. W., Epstein, N. B., Bishop, D. S., & Fruzzetti, A. E. (1987). Family functioning and the course of major depression. *Comprehensive Psychiatry, 1,* 54–64.

Keitner, G. I., Miller, I. W., & Ryan, C. E. (1993). The role of the family in major depressive illness. *Psychiatric Annals, 23,* 500–507.

Kirby, R., & Corzine, J. (1981). The contagion of stigma. *Qualitative Sociology, 4,* 3–20.

Lincoln, Y. S., & Guba, E. G. (1985). *Naturalistic inquiry.* Beverly Hills, CA: Sage.

Merikangas, K. R., Weissman, M. M., & Prusoff, B. A. (1990). Psychopathology in offspring of parents with affective disorders. In G. I. Keitner (Ed.), *Depression and families: Impact and treatment* (pp. 3–29). Washington, DC: American Psychiatric Press.

Miller, I. W., Keitner, G. I., Whisman, M. A., Ryan, C. E., Epstein, N. B., & Bishop, D. S. (1992). Depressed patients with dysfunctional families: Description and course of illness. *Journal of Abnormal Psychology, 101,* 637–646.

Mishel, M. M., & Murdaugh, C. L. (1987). Family adjustment to heart transplantation: Redesigning the dream. *Nursing Research, 36,* 332–338.

Pruchno, R. A., Kleban, M. H., Michaels, J. E., & Dempsey, N. P. (1990). Mental and physical health of caregiving spouses: Development of a causal model. *Journal of Gerontology, 45,* 192–199.

Schwab, J. J., Stephenson, J. J., & Ice, J. F. (1993). Family research. In *Evaluating family mental health: History, epidemiology, and treatment issues* (pp. 157–226). New York: Plenum.

Skaff, M. M., & Pearlin, L. I. (1992). Caregiving: Role engulfment and the loss of self. *The Gerontologist, 32,* 656–664.

Strauss, A. L., Corbin, J., Fagerhaugh, S., Glaser, B. G., Maines, D., Suczek, B., & Weiner, C. L. (1984). *Chronic illness and the quality of life* (2nd ed.). St. Louis, MO: C. V. Mosby.

Wells, K. B., Stewart, A., Hays, R. D., Burnam, M. A., Rogers, W., Daniels, M., Berry, S., Greenfield, S., & Ware, J. (1989). The functioning and well-being of depressed patients: Results from the Medical Outcomes Study. *Journal of the American Medical Association, 262,* 914–919.

Wilson, H. S. (1989). Family caregivers: The experience of Alzheimer's disease. *Applied Nursing Research, 2,* 40–45.

Name Index

Index

Page numbers in bold type indicate glossary entries.